TEXTBOOK OF

Couples and Family Therapy in Clinical Practice

Sixth Edition

TEXTBOOK OF

Couples and Family Therapy in Clinical Practice

Sixth Edition

Ira D. Glick, MD
Professor Emeritus of Psychiatry and Behavioral Sciences
Stanford University School of Medicine
Stanford, CA, USA

Alison M. Heru, MD
Previously Professor of Psychiatry
University of Colorado
Denver School of Medicine
Denver, CO, USA

Danielle Kamis, MD
Assistant Clinical Professor of Psychiatry and Behavioral Sciences
Stanford University School of Medicine
Stanford, CA, USA

Wolters Kluwer

Philadelphia • Baltimore • New York • London
Buenos Aires • Hong Kong • Sydney • Tokyo

Acquisitions Editor: Chris Teja
Development Editor: Ariel S. Winter
Editorial Coordinator: Arvind Siddharth J.
Editorial Assistant: Kristen Kardoley
Marketing Manager: Kirsten Watrud
Production Project Manager: Frances M. Gunning
Manager, Graphic Arts & Design: Stephen Druding
Manufacturing Coordinator: Lisa Bowling
Prepress Vendor: Aptara, Inc.

Sixth edition

9 8 7 6 5 4 3 2 1

Printed in Mexico

978-19752-3936-7

Library of Congress Cataloging-in-Publication data available upon request

shop.lww.com

QUADM1024

DEDICATION

To our families—
past and present,
personal and
professional

FOREWORD

by Ellen M. Berman, MD

Edition Six focusing on the field of couples and family therapy continues our long-standing efforts to make family inclusion and family therapy part of the everyday life of psychiatrists and other therapists. The goal is to make this book a basic text for those working with families in psychiatric settings, medical settings, and couple and family clinics.

A new edition of a standard text needs to demonstrate growth and changes in the field and the culture. There have been remarkable changes in our country around the issues of culture and gender, from the complex and politicized issues of immigration and color to the rapid changes in the roles of both women and men. As marriage and childbearing come later and later in life, as life expectancy grows exponentially, as expectations around gender become more fluid and men struggle to understand their role in the world, all of our family systems change to meet these challenges. The sixth edition of this book pays particular attention to major changes in our understanding of culture, increasing variations in family forms and new research in the neurobiology of attachment and stress. Our understanding of the biological co-regulation of attached persons, and how that affects mental and physical health has broadened greatly. This has led to more focus on intimacy and connection, and emotional regulation, in addition to the traditional focus on communications and behavioral training. Understanding that culture, gender, and ethnicity can be fluid rather than binary has led to a more nuanced understanding of how biology, psychology, family, and culture interact. This edition explores these fascinating changes in addition to providing basic knowledge in the field.

Family therapy has a high success rate with children's issues, with couples in crisis, with three-generation families struggling with transitions, and with families with a mentally ill member. For some couples and families, including those dealing with marital stress, family transitions, affairs or a life crisis, a systems approach is the main form of treatment. Couple and family work is also a crucial adjunctive treatment for those with psychiatric disorders including depression, addiction, and anxiety. Studies dating back to the 1960s, supplemented by much recent research (see Chapter 24), provide evidence that families are important in recovery from illness, and that family psychoeducation can decrease relapse and rehospitalization in very ill psychiatric patients by up to 50%. The increasing number of family psychoeducation studies in those suffering from severe mental illness provides a deep evidence base for incorporating those treatments into the complete treatment model.

Family inclusion and psychoeducation are highly efficient tools for extending the scope of today's brief psychiatric visits. Teaching the family to support the patient, increasing hope, calm and good communication, and decreasing anxiety in family members, improves everyone's functioning. This would suggest strongly that family intervention and psychoeducation be part of every provider's armamentarium.

Nevertheless, psychosocial interventions, and particularly the use of family interventions, have, if anything, decreased in recent years as a biomedical focus has become more common. Training in family systems has yet to become an integral part of most psychiatrically based training programs. We believe that the treatment model is expanding and that we need to move in the direction of increasing the options for therapy and psychoeducation. The family therapy community, much of which in the past was strongly against individual treatment, is slowly finding rapprochement with the mental health system and incorporating medication and individual sessions into treatment. Dr. Glick and myself have worked at the boundaries of these field for our careers and are proud to have contributed to their growing integration.

For a field to grow, it is imperative that younger members become involved. We hope that this book will encourage young therapists and psychiatrists to join us in supporting families and family therapy research. I am happy to be a colleague of the two new authors, Dr. Alison M. Heru, a midcareer psychiatrist whose books on families and health and families and inpatients are widely read, and Dr. Danielle Kamis, an early career psychiatrist. I am so pleased to pass the baton to Dr. Heru and Dr. Kamis and hope that their example encourages many of you to join them in becoming family-oriented psychiatrists. We encourage the readers of this book to also join organizations which support growth in the field—Association of Family Psychiatrists (familypsychiatrists.org) and the American Family Therapy Academy (afta.org).

This book is designed for family therapists from many disciplines, especially psychiatrists, who wish to understand the basics of family work and begin to apply it to the patients they are seeing now. Therapists new to the field experience several challenges in beginning work. The most critical is a shift in vision from an individual and linear model to a systemic one, in which the person in interaction with others is the key. If an individual presents for treatment, it requires that the person in front of them be seen in context and that the person be understood as an actor interacting with other actors. How does the person's family affect their lives, and how does the person affect their family? How can we see the person-in-context? For example, an adult with attention-deficit disorder (ADD) may struggle in a marriage because some aspects of ADD (procrastination, forget-fulness) may provide aversive stimuli to family members, and therefore be met with disapproval and hostility, which increases their anxiety and ADD symptoms. In this case, the reverberating issues are the problems that must be addressed by the systems therapist. Without including the partner, the couple difficulties may persist even if the ADD is addressed by medication. If a couple or family presents to treatment with all family members, a systems approach requires that the family be seen as the unit of treatment rather than identifying one member as the patient.

The second challenge is learning a series of new techniques, including the ability to manage a session with multiple family members each with their own agendas. As authors of family therapy research and practice tend to publish mostly in their own journals, psychiatrists are less likely to be familiar "thinking family," or reading about clinical skills necessary.

A third challenge is a shift from a problem-focused model to one that incorporates strengths, and an awareness of the many varieties of normative behavior—variant family forms, differing life cycle trajectories, and fluid sexuality. It must include a deep understanding of how power and gender shape individuals and relationships. This may produce therapist anxiety when the family's life or value system is outside their own experience. In addition, beginning therapists must pay close attention to how culture/ethnicity/setting affects the family's life. Understanding a culture also includes familiarity with community resources for family support. All of these issues are well covered in the new edition and ground the new therapist in clinical realities. The current text should go a long way toward helping therapists integrate family work into their current models and supporting people who wish to learn family therapy.

It is with great pleasure that I introduce this edition to my colleagues, my students, and now to you.

Ellen M. Berman, MD
Clinical Professor of Psychiatry,
Perelman College of Medicine University of Pennsylvania
Past President Association of Family Psychiatrists

REFERENCE

Miklowitz D, Otto M, Frank E, et al. Intensive psychosocial intervention enhances functioning in patients with bipolar depression: results from a 9-month randomized controlled trial. *Am J Psychiatry.* 2007;164(9):1340–1347.

by Lloyd I. Sederer, MD

Marriages and families have changed, evolved, in ways that our grandparents could never have imagined! As have the methods by which we can serve them during times of both emotional upheaval and in sustaining their vital bonds over the course of what can be a troubled lifetime.

We have needed a rapprochement between family theory (and therapy) and contemporary psychiatric and mental health services. The latter has been mightily drawn to medication and case management, especially for severe mental disorders as well as to highly stylized therapies, like CBT, DBT, ACT, and analytic psychotherapy. But those now ubiquitous changes have considerably parted ways with the conceptual and therapeutic world of families and the range of ways we can attend to their needs.

Families are, in the great predominance of instances, the greatest resources and most enduring sources of support for a person suffering from any serious and chronic illness, including mental and addictive disorders. Not recognizing the power of the family, for good or ill, and swiftly handing them off to a case worker misses the forest for the trees, as does singularly relying on invaluable volunteer organizations like The National Alliance on Mental Illness (NAMI). Highly trained and capable clinicians have so much to offer families, especially those where a serious mental disorder has entered their lives.

Yet few mental health clinicians continue to be professionally trained to assess, engage and work with families. Graduate and residency training programs often want for a core text and training curriculum in families and couples, which you will find it in this text. For experienced clinicians wanting to learn or refresh skills essential to working with families, you have what you need right here.

"You can observe a lot by just watching." All good clinical work starts with knowing what and how to observe, which, in turn, requires a clear perspective on how a person or family functions and how it can veer toward and enter dysfunction. *Textbook of Couples and Family Therapy in Clinical Practice* depicts the major schools of thought and proven practices for intervening and restoring the capacity of a family or couple to care for themselves and their loved ones throughout the demands of our lives, which do not seem to be getting simpler or easier.

Informed observation makes possible a formulation, the way we summarize a problem in a manner that lends itself to action and remediation. We learn from the accomplished authors of this text how to fashion a clinical formulation that, *ipso facto*, directs a treatment plan—the agreement, replete with possibilities, choices, and hope between therapist and family. The prospect of change predictably evokes a counter force, the demand to stay the same, in families, not just in physics. Readers of this text will better learn how to recognize needed yet resisted change, and to work with families so their strengths can prevail.

Practical matters of family therapy are given, throughout the text, the attention they deserve: Who should participate in the treatment (including children)? How may we best work with colleagues caring for our patients, as well as with co-therapists? How can medications and other forms of therapy amplify family therapy, and vice versa? What are the particulars of initiating family therapy, including setting, scheduling, fees, and session times? What do we know about the intensity and duration of treatment? What can help us endure the bane of medical record keeping? Common and destabilizing events like marital separation and divorce are given their due as is the sexual life of couples. This book has its head in theory and practice and its feet on the ground.

Dr. Glick and his coauthors are mindful and teach us the advances in working with families who have a member with a serious and persistent mental illness, like schizophrenia, and bipolar disorders, and borderline personality conditions. They hew to evidence-based practices of therapy and family psychoeducation. They attend, as well, to how to help families where a member has an acute or chronic physical illness, noting, here too, the need to establish roles and responsibilities, ongoing problem solving, and ready avenues of communication.

Paraphrasing Tolstoy and his enduring claim about unhappy families, we learn from this text that we must consider and relate to every family as unique—shaped by its natural roots in race, ethnicity, and religion; the effects of immigration and trauma; of being born into a particular social class and respective social milieu; and when families are turned asunder by illness and misfortune.

In *Textbook of Couples and Family Therapy in Clinical Practice*, we are delivered a wonderfully comprehensive view of contemporary (Western) family life: married and unmarried yet committed partners, with or without children; serial relationships; divorces (now in half of marriages); hetero, LTBQ, and trans people and their pairings; as well as single-parent and blended families. We follow the natural stages of family life that parallel the "stages of man." The new norm is that we have entered the territory of no norms. Modern means varied and diverse, with all its textures, vitality, nuances, and demands. Yet if there is one constant, it is that we humans are devoted to coupling, creating families, and producing the next generation of our progeny.

Does marital and family therapy work? You will find out in the chapter on results. Because the authors are rigorous academics, we are provided with informed and experienced clinical evidence for what works, for whom and when, as well as the limitations and potential negative effects of family treatments. Our patients and we clinicians deserve more than testimonials about family therapy; we are owed an inventory of proven and feasible therapies, which are thoughtfully and clearly provided by the authors of this text.

As a young psychiatrist but a few years out of residency, I trained in family therapy at the Cambridge Family Institute in Massachusetts. What I discovered then has forever enriched my work, not only as a psychiatrist but also as a public health doctor and clinical administrator. Now, perhaps as a village elder, I see more than ever the need to value and work with families, too often the unsung heroes and advocates that people with mental and addictive disorders deeply need to find help, to sustain hope, and to build the life of dignity and contribution that we all want.

My hat is off to the authors of *Textbook of Couples and Family Therapy in Clinical Practice*, now in its sixth edition. Their writings continue to teach and guide us about families—often overlooked, underused, and critical in clinical practice—in ways that are fresh, accessible, and useful.

Lloyd I. Sederer, MD
Adjunct Professor, Columbia/Mailman School of Public Health
Former Mental Health Commissioner of NYC and Chief Medical Officer of the NYS Office of Mental Health
www.askdrlloyd.com

BACKGROUND

The five previous editions of this textbook of family therapy reflect the history and development of the family field, which has evolved rapidly since the 1960s. The first edition was an outline about a field that was just beginning to grow and gain momentum. The second edition was a statement that the family field, which began in the minds of creative individuals in diverse settings (and often unknown to one another), was blossoming with great enthusiasm. The field had arrived with full gusto, and many clinicians were doing family work and clamoring for theoretical clarity and more training in this form of intervention. The third edition heralded a field that had come of age. It had expanded in scope and was being commonly used in clinical practice.

In 2000, the fourth edition made a statement, like its predecessors, about the current state of the art of family intervention. As we saw it, the field had gone beyond its heyday of enthusiasm and advocacy of family intervention for every clinical condition, to a more sophisticated time of differentiation. This differentiation was taking place on many levels. Examples include differentiating when family therapy is indicated, when the symptoms are under systems control, and when they are more strongly determined by other factors such as biology and genetics; how one evaluates in order to make both individual diagnoses and a family diagnosis; when the whole family is the patient and when the family is best seen as part of the treatment team in order to help the individual with symptoms; and when behavioral or educational strategies of family intervention are particularly helpful. New developments in theory and technique, and a widened lens in terms of specific problem areas, have enriched the field.

Over the past two decades, the most critical changes in family theory are the incorporation of new attitudes and information about ethnicity, gender, sexual orientation, and social class into our theory building. The rules that govern all aspects of family life and the experience of persons in families may be vastly different for men and women. Families may operate by systems principles, but men and women bring to the system different ways of thinking and different types of influence. Norms of closeness and distance, emotional expression, basic aspects of viewing and disciplining children also vary greatly across ethnic group, social class, and age cohort. The integration of this knowledge into the broad principles of family therapy, enabling therapists to work with a wide variety of families, is one of our key goals. Theory building in this area is still in a period of rapid growth and will probably be altered again by the next edition.

More integrative ways of working have replaced narrowly based schools of family therapy, and brief therapy models such as solution-focused and narrative therapy have been added to our armamentarium. New information about previously ignored or inadequately researched issues—such as gay and lesbian and non-traditional families, the sequelae of abuse, the complexities of AIDS, and family response to reproductive events—have enriched our understanding of family life. Family systems medicine has become a new subspecialty in recent years. We hope that this sixth edition adequately reflects this growing sophistication of the field.

Since the publication of the first edition of this book, we have consistently been gratified by the response of both readers and many reviewers, as well as by its adoption by some teachers as the standard introductory text. Since the publication of the second edition, it has been translated into Japanese and Spanish, and parts into Chinese; it has been adopted widely in Italy, England, and other European countries. Because of the growth and changes in the field, as well as suggestions received, we have decided that this is an opportune time to expand and rewrite the text. Most important, we are convinced that the field has matured. Presently there are many established schools of thought that continue to evolve. At the same time, just as in the adjacent field of individual psychotherapy, there is growing interest in adopting a more integrative (rather than parochial) perspective that highlights some of the factors shared by these different models. **In this text, we offer our version of an integration of different models of family theory, that is, a framework for trainees and practitioners in the family therapy field and those persons in various fields that need an introduction to family therapy.**

SIXTH EDITION CHANGES

For this sixth edition, the primary aim was to update couples and family function from a variety of points of view of both females and males. The second aim was to include newer research on outcome. It is now DSM-5-TR updated.

The fifth edition brought the reader into the 21st century with a flowering of psychotherapies, especially couples and family intervention. As such, couples and family intervention have become important components of an integrated prescription for the treatment of most mental disorders. The key message is that there is new evidence-based data suggesting that combining family intervention with medication is better than either modality alone.

Our aim/hope is that the material in the text will be used as a core curriculum for both psychiatric residency programs and family therapy institutes. Family interventions have positive implications for the family system as well as the patient who can feel ambivalent about adhering to individual therapy and medications on their own without a family aboard as "a treatment team member."

As we mentioned, we have not provided detailed information on the details of specific approaches of couple and family psychotherapy. This is not to say other models do not have important virtues or clinical utility. Rather, we have tried to include in our integrated model, the best of their techniques, as such, we have provided some of the crucial elements of the classic models.

We have described some of the classic models, for example "systems, structural, behavioral" in Chapter 1. We mention a few of the newer models in Chapter 9 as they relate to our integrated theory of couples and family therapy. In Chapter 18, we discuss family interventions and certain models used to treat specific mental disorders such as psychoeducation in schizophrenia. We also borrowed heavily from the McMaster Model detailed in the Keitner, Heru, and Glick text entitled *Clinical Manual of Couples and Family Therapy* (2009).

Although the newer body of knowledge has required extensive rewriting, the basic organization of the book is largely unchanged. The history of the field precedes general concepts of how families function, which are followed by evaluation, treatment, indications, and finally, results.

For this edition, we have highlighted the essentials and have thoroughly updated our chapter on family life in its historical and sociological context, and throughout we have paid special attention to both classic and newer family forms. Our sections on function and dysfunction have been expanded and rewritten to present the latest information on how families globally cope with rapid changes in our society. Given the publication of DSM-5-TR, we have made a thorough review of understanding and treatment of dysfunctional families both for major psychiatric illnesses and for other problems of living together. In our treatment section we have added a special section on treating serious psychiatric disorders by combining medication with family therapy. We have thoroughly rewritten the chapter on treatment as modified by cultural, ethnic, racial, gender, and class considerations.

Telemedicine via Zoom or Facetime, for example, has made it possible to do sessions virtually. That is, rather than in person, as well, doing an in-person session and

including a family member, who was constrained from attending by work or travel time or even was unwilling to attend in person, but would be willing to attend virtually. We urge family therapists to use this innovation to improve treatment outcome.

Our section on marital/couples disorders has been revised thoroughly, including a focus on blended families. In addition we have rewritten the material on LGBTQ (an initialism that stands for lesbian, gay, bisexual, transgender, or queer) families. We have added a section on couples and reproductive health. We have expanded in a major way the section on relational disorders including both Axis I disorders and other problems. The chapter on incest, violence, suicide, and the family responses to these problems is also revised.

Based on new outcome data, we have updated the section on guidelines and results (i.e., efficacy). Throughout the text we have made suggestions (where possible) to practitioners regarding how to practice the art of family therapy based on implications of research studies.

The section on family systems medicine has been rewritten thoroughly, adding a general overview of the field from the point of view of the physician (taking care of the medical problems of the patients) as well as from the family systems perspective. We close the book with guidelines and an overview of ethical, financial, and professional issues facing the field, including issues involved with training (Rait et al., 2019).

CONCLUSION

Past readers have been very helpful and generous with their comments for revisions.

Partly because of their suggestions, we have been able to add new chapters, revise chapters from the previous editions, and update the book. For this edition, we have been fortunate to add two new authors, both clinicians and teachers in the field (Alison M. Heru, MD and Danielle Kamis, MD). David Kessler, MD, was a coauthor on earlier editions, and Ellen Berman, MD, and John Clarkin, PhD, were coauthors of the fourth edition. Doug Rait, PhD and Michael Ascher, MD were coauthors for the fifth edition. Much of their wisdom still can be found in this revision.

In the last edition, we had many colleagues who contributed to specific topics. In this edition, we have reviewed and updated their sections like "Treatment of a suicidal patient and family" and checked for consistency on such a topic with a related topic (e.g., family treatments of patients with depression). For many of these topics for the interested reader, we have given an overview of the topic and for some provided a detailed reference in "Suggested Reading" at the end of some chapters. Classic references still remain as relevant today as they did yesterday. We made every effort to include recent applicable research in this edition.

In the third edition, we invited readers to write with their suggestions. In the fourth edition, the response was not only astounding but also helpful in improving the text. We were fortunate to have a number of contributors who lent their specific expertise to the fourth edition. We listed many of these scholars in the acknowledgments section, while reviewing and updating their topics for this sixth edition. We offer the same invitation now in 2023, so that we can continue to make this book as helpful and practical as possible. **We want the text to be by your side, used and not sitting on a shelf.**

Ira D. Glick, MD
Alison M. Heru, MD
Danielle Kamis, MD

REFERENCE

Rait D, Heru A, Glick ID. *Whatever happened to Couples and Family Therapy in Psychiatry. Am J Psychotherapy.* 2019;35: 85–87.

ACKNOWLEDGMENTS

We wish to thank the many individuals and families who have helped to make this book possible. First, our own families of origin, who in addition to steadfastly attempting to socialize us, provided us with our first major models of family structure and function. Second, our teachers, who by their concern and enthusiasm, first helped to stir our interest in family study and treatment and provided us with a family model of understanding human functioning. Third, our colleagues in family therapy, who by their stimulating and provocative comments, tried their best to keep us honest. Fourth, our trainees, with whom we have been privileged to work on the teaching–learning process in family therapy. They have had the courage to ask the critical questions about the field, and it was for them that much of the didactic material in this book was formulated and used in courses we have taught. Finally, to our spouses who supported us as we spent long hours preparing the book.

Most of all, we are indebted to the couples and families whom we have treated. They shared our journey, lived with our successes (and errors), and have taught us at least as much as we have taught them.

A GUIDE FOR USING THE TEXT

There are three important changes in the title of this text. In the previous edition, we substitute the word "Couple/Couples" for "Marital," as the former includes both marital and non-married couples. For grammatical reasons, the field is moving toward encompassing the word "couple" rather than "couples." In this edition, the first change to the title is to add in the phrase "Integrated in Clinical Practice." In that context, we strongly believe that working with the family should be mandatory in almost all cases when the identified patient is being treated with medication. This is why we use the term "integrated in the title of the text. Readers of the previous edition wrote us to say what they found most useful was (i) essentials of this treatment and (ii) guidance on integrating this modality into their clinical practice in a wide variety of settings. Perhaps most important, the second is to add the word "Textbook" as we believe this word fully conveys the definition—"a book used in the study of a subject, such as one containing a presentation of the principles of a subject." (Merriam-Webster Dictionary) change the word "therapy" to "psychiatry." The third is to change the word "therapy" to "psychiatry."

The book is organized into six overarching sections, starting with the history of the field followed by general concepts of family function and dysfunction, evaluation, treatment, indications, and results. It is our hope that the reader will gain a broad understanding of the underlying principles and hypotheses behind family models of treatment. Readers will also become familiar with techniques that can be utilized in the therapeutic space to foster change and growth in both patients and their families. The text will address the need for the modern-day clinician to have a solid foundation in cultural competency and to be able to work with patients who come from myriad of cultural, ethnic, sexual, and socioeconomic backgrounds. Furthermore, the book will address ethical quandaries, professionalism, and training issues.

Because this book is intended to serve as a basic but comprehensive textbook for individuals at different training levels and orientations, complex clinical situations and their sequential management regimens have been simplified and compressed. We realize this may be a disadvantage for the more advanced therapist and so have included both current and classical references. The book probably will be most helpful when used with ongoing supervision or with an ongoing course, because most of the case examples and interventions are written in bare-bones detail in order to make one or two teaching points at a time. For the sake of clarity, some chapters reiterate concepts presented earlier in a different context. For example, goals are mentioned in the (a) discussions of evaluation, (b) the process of setting goals before starting treatment, and (c) the course of treatment.

Likewise, a number of sections and short chapters are (in our view) much too brief to be of value to the experienced family clinician. Here, too, we opted to take the route of maximum breadth of topics, providing appropriate references to flesh out the materials. References have been updated, but we retained classics and those that refer to a particular research project mentioned in the text.

We believe that the alternative path (i.e., to limit the subjects covered and to go into greater depth) would make this introductory text too narrow and less useful given the many situations in which the family model is now being used. We recommend that the beginner read the text sequentially, although obviously the more experienced clinician initially may prefer to read particular sections or chapters only. The book is written for use as you see your patients and families, not as a reference. Some chapters may be read out of order, like the chapters on results (Chapter 24) or the family in historical context (Chapter 2), because they are more specialized and should be read as needed, as appropriate, or as the reader's interest dictates.

In part, how this book is used depends on one's training goals. Accordingly, a reader may want to refer to the training section, where we discuss context, formats, and goals. That is, the material can guide the reader's priorities. The reason, of course, is that the learning needs of someone trying to master the family model at a family institute are quite different from a psychiatric resident who is learning family therapy as one model among other competing models.

A note on the teaching objectives—there are two reasons for their inclusion.

First, many fields in medicine, psychiatry, and psychology are attempting to define the core knowledge and skill competencies required for a practitioner in that field. We do so in that spirit. However, a second and in many ways more essential reason, is that the ground we cover is so broad and can be so confusing to the beginner. By using the enabling objectives for each chapter as a road map, the reader can use them to understand the logic, direction, and end point for each topic. Our overall objectives include but are not limited to:

- A general understanding of the underlying theoretical principles and hypotheses behind the family model.
- An acquaintance with the techniques of family intervention, including an understanding of the advantages and limitations of such techniques.
- Development of an appreciation, through experience, of one's abilities and difficulties in using such techniques.
- An understanding of how ethnicity, gender, sexual orientation, and social class affect the therapist and family as they work.
- An appreciation of the ethical issues involved in all areas of the practice of family intervention.
- **Having you, the practitioner, feel comfortable in making family intervention a core part of your clinical practice.**

CONTENTS

Forewords vii–x
Ellen M. Berman, MD
Lloyd I. Sederer, MD

Preface xi

Acknowledgments xv

A Guide for Using the Text xvii

List of Tables xxxv

List of Figures xxxvii

Section I Family Therapy in Context 3

1 The Field of Couples and Family Therapy: Development and Definition 5

Objectives for the Reader 5
Introduction 5
Development of the Family Therapy Field 6
Definition of Couples and Family Therapy 9
Core Concepts 10
General Systems Theory 10
Family Systems Theory and Homeostasis Over Time 15
An Integrative Interpersonal Model 16
Differentiation of Family Therapy From Other Psychotherapies 16
Clinical Practice Implications 18
Suggested Readings 19
References 19

2 Family Life in Historical and Sociological Perspective 20

Objectives for the Reader 20
Introduction 20
The Family in Early Civilizations 21
Structure and Function of the American Family 21
Immigration 22
Ethnicity 22
Examples of Ethnicity versus Race 23
Internalized and Structural Racism 23
Secular View of Marriage 24
Structures of Marriage 25
Divorce 25
The Functional Single-Parent Family 26

Stepfamilies 26
Lgbtq (Lesbian, Gay, Bisexual, Transgender, Queer) Couples 27
Polyamory 29
Parenting in Postmodern Relationships 29
Family Types 30
Culture and Race 30
Social Class 31
Aging of the Population 31
The Changing Family Life Cycle 32
Clinical Practice Implications 32
Suggested Reading 33
References 33

Section II Functional and Dysfunctional Families 37

3 Understanding the Functional Family 39
Objectives for the Reader 39
Introduction 39
The Family as a System 40
The Couples/Marital and Family Life Cycle 42
The Individual Life Cycle 42
The Couples/Marital Life Cycle 44
Phase of Relationship and Tasks 45
Marital Coalition 46
Sex, Intimacy, and Companionship 47
The Family Life Cycle 47
Family Tasks 50
Provision of Basic Needs 51
Rearing and Socialization of Children 51
Family Belief Systems 53
Family Resilience 53
Clinical Practice Implications 53
Suggested Readings 54
References 54

4 Understanding the Functional Family in a Variety of Family Forms 55
Objectives for the Reader 55
Introduction 55
Impact of an Extended Individual Life Cycle 56
Marriage 56
Divorce 57
Marital Separation 57

Divorce 58
Children and Divorce 58
Binuclear Families 59
Impact of Divorce Based on the Age of the Child 59
The Functional Single-Parent Family 60
Mother-Headed Single-Parent Families 61
Father-Headed Single-Parent Families 61
Remarriage and Blended Families 61
Remarried Couple 62
Stepfamilies (Blended Families) 62
Grandparent-Headed Families 63
Lesbian, Gay, and Transgender Families 63
Parents with a Gender Nonconforming Child 65
Multiple-Partner Fertility Families 65
Adoption and Families 65
Interracial Families 65
Trends in Parenting 66
Clinical Practice Implications 66
Suggested Readings 67
References 67

5 Problems and Dysfunction from an Integrated Family Systems Perspective 68
Objectives for the Reader 68
Introduction: The Dysfunctional Family System 68
A Systems Approach to Problems and Dysfunction 69
Historical Perspectives 69
Current Perspectives 70
Family Resilience Key Processes 71
Structural and Organizational Problems 71
The Solution as the Problem 72
Family Beliefs and Myths 73
The Larger Social System and Dysfunction 75
Implications for Treatment—the Development of Symptoms in a Particular Person 75
Life Cycle Problems and Dysfunction 77
Unresolved Grief 78
Toxic Secrets 78
Task Performance in the Dysfunctional Family 78
Providing for the Family's Basic Needs 78
Maintaining a Functional Marriage: Issues of Sex, Intimacy, and Commitment 79
Rearing and Socializing of Children 79
Clinical Practice Implications 79
Suggested Reading 80
References 80

Section III Family Evaluation 83

6 The Process of Evaluation 85

Objectives for the Reader 85

Introduction 85

Who to Include in the Family Evaluation 86

Progression of the Family Evaluation Interview 87

Dimensions of Couple and Family Assessment 87

Joining with the Couple or Family 88

Seeing Systemic Patterns 88

Recognizing Family Developmental Stage, History, and Culture 88

Identifying Family Structure 90

Working with a Systemic Model of Change 90

Role of Historical Material 91

Role of Individual and Family Diagnoses 92

Clinical Practice Implications 93

References 93

7 The Content of Evaluation 94

Objectives for the Reader 94

Introduction 94

Dimensions of Family Function 95

Family Evaluation Outline 95

Gathering Identifying Data and Establishing Current Phase of Family Life Cycle 95

Gathering Explicit Interview Data 96

What Is the Background of the Family Problem? 97

What Is the History of Past Treatment Attempts? 98

What Are the Family's Goals and Expectations of the Treatment? 100

The Family Genogram 101

Clinical Practice Implications 101

References 101

8 Formulating an Understanding of the Family Problem Areas 102

Objectives for the Reader 102

Introduction 102

Rating Important Dimensions of Family Functioning 103

Communication 103

Problem-Solving 103

Roles and Coalitions 103

Affective Responsiveness and Involvement 104

Operative Family Beliefs and Stories 105

Recent Family Events and Stresses 105

Family Classification and Diagnosis 105
Planning the Therapeutic Approach and Establishing the Treatment Contract 108
Case Example Illustrating Evaluation and Case Formulation 109
Suggested Reading 116
References 116

Section IV Family Treatment 119

9 Major Family Therapy Schools and Their Treatment Strategies 121
Objectives for the Reader 121
Introduction 121
Insight-Awareness Model 123
Family of Origin Model 123
Systemic-Strategic Model 124
Structural Model 124
Cognitive–Behavioral Model 125
Experiential Model 126
Narrative Model 126
Psychoeducational Model 126
Clinical Practice Implications 127
Suggested Readings 127
References 127

10 Goals 128
Objectives for the Reader 128
Introduction 128
Mediating and Final Goals as They Relate to Schools 129
The Most Common Mediating Goals 129
The Most Common Final Goals 130
Individualizing Goals with the Family 130
Goals and Their Relation to Process and Content Issues 132
Mediating Goals and Their Related Strategies 133
Goals and Related Strategies 133
Common to All Family Therapy Schools 133
Clinical Practice Implications 134
Reference 135

11 Family Treatment: Integrated Strategies and Techniques 136
Objectives for the Reader 136
Introduction 136
General Elements of Psychotherapy and Their Relationship to Family Therapy 137

Basic Strategies of Family Intervention 137

Techniques for Supporting Adaptive Mechanisms and Strengths: The Psychoeducational Approach 138

Techniques for Expanding Emotional Experience 139

Techniques for Developing Interpersonal Skills 140

Techniques for Reorganizing the Family Structure 143

Techniques for Increasing Insight and Conflict Resolution 147

Techniques for a More Effective Construction of Family Reality 149

Treatment Packages 149

Indications For Differential Use of the Basic Strategies 149

Clinical Practice Implications 150

References 150

12 The Course of Family Treatment 151

Objectives for the Reader 151

Introduction 151

Early Phase 152

Identifying Objectives of the Early Phase 152

Choosing Strategies to Get Started 152

Distributing the Available Time 153

Gathering History and Simultaneously Building a Treatment Alliance with the Family 153

Distinguishing Evaluation from Treatment 154

Middle Phase 155

Termination Phase 156

Conducting Brief Family Therapy: Treatment as It Is Influenced By Time Constraints 157

Indications for Brief Family or Couples Intervention 157

Course of Brief Therapy 158

Techniques 158

Setting Limited Goals and a Definite End Point 158

Active Focus: Reinforcement of Family Strengths, Reconceptualization 159

Active Exploration of Alternatives: Behavioral and Emotional Rehearsal 160

Homework and Family Tasks 160

The Problem-Oriented School of Brief Therapy 161

Crisis Intervention 161

Clinical Practice Implications 161

Suggested Readings 162

References 162

13 Promoting Change in Family Treatment: Issues of Alliance and Resistance 163

Objectives for the Reader 163

Introduction 163

The Therapeutic Alliance 164

Models for Dealing with Families That Have Trouble Forming an Alliance 165
Medical Model 165
Coaching Model 166
Conflict Model 166
Strategic Systems Model 166
Problems in Creating Change: Resistance and Disconnection 167
Problems in Creating Change: Emanating from the Family 167
Problems in Creating Change: Emanating from the Therapist 168
Problems in Creating Change: From the Therapist–Family System 168
Problems in Creating Change: Stages of Treatment: At Evaluation and Early in Treatment 169
Problems in Creating Change: In Ongoing Treatment 171
Problems in Creating Change: At the Termination Phase of Therapy 172
Problems in Creating Change: Family Secrets 172
Techniques to Deal with Resistances or Stalled Therapy 173
Assume Nothing 173
Collaboration 173
Emphasizing Family Responsibility 174
Focus on the Present 174
Clinical Practice Implications 174
Suggested Readings 174
References 174

14 Family Therapy: General Considerations 175
Objectives for the Reader 175
Introduction 175
Family Participants 176
Extended Family and Significant Others 177
Caregivers 178
Including Children and Adolescents in Family Therapy 178
Diagnostic Family Evaluation 179
Treatment 180
Therapist Combinations 181
Co-Therapy 181
Working as a Team 181
Setting 182
Time, Scheduling, and Fees 182
Keeping a Record of Treatment 183
Family Therapy in Combination with Other Psychosocial Therapies 184
Practical Guidelines 185
Effective Family Intervention 186
Comparison of Therapy Formats and Strategies 186
Clinical Practice Implications 186
References 187

Section V Couples Therapy 191

15 Dysfunctional Couples and Couples Therapy 193
Objectives for the Reader 193
Introduction 193
Marriage in Its Historical Context 194
Couples Difficulties, Problems, and Dysfunction 194
From a Dynamic Point of View 195
From a Behavioral Point of View 196
From a Systems Point of View 196
From a Psychiatric Illness Point of View 196
Couples' Development Dysfunction 197
Couples Therapy 197
The Issue of Commitment—The Problem of Affairs 197
Evaluation of Partners 198
Goals 199
Strategies and Techniques of Intervention 199
A Model for Intervention Based on Patterns of Interaction 199
Individual Models 200
Strategies and Techniques 201
Clinical Practice Implications 203
References 203

16 Sex, Couples, and Sex Therapy 204
Objectives for the Reader 204
Introduction 204
Diagnosis—Systems Issues 205
Some Parameters of Sexual Function 205
Assessment of Sexual Disorder 206
Treatment 209
Lack of Desire 209
Erectile Disorder 209
Premature (Early) Ejaculation 210
Painful Intercourse/Female Orgasmic Disorder 210
Sex Addiction and Pornography 211
Other Issues Related to Sexuality and Couples 212
The Spectrum of Sexuality 212
Sexual Functioning After Rape or Sexual Abuse 212
Sexual Problems After Medical Illness 213
Sexual Problems in the Elderly 213
Clinical Practice Implications 214
Suggested Readings 214
References 214

17 Couples and Families Breaking Apart: Separation and Divorce 215

Objectives for the Reader 215
Introduction 215
Separation 215
Separation Leading to Divorce 217
Communicating the Issue of Divorce to Children 218
Immediate Issues 218
Therapy for Families Facing Divorce 219
Divorce and Postdivorce Treatment 220
Single-Parent and Binuclear Families 221
Blended Families (Stepfamilies) 222
Goals 222
Evaluation and Treatment 223
Cohabiting Couples 225
Serial Relationships 226
Clinical Practice Implications 226
Suggested Readings 226
References 226

Section VI Family Treatment When One Member Has a Psychiatric Disorder or Other Special Problem 229

18 Family Treatment in the Context of Individual Psychiatric Disorders 231

Objectives for the Reader 231
Introduction 231
The Family Model and Individual Diagnosis 233
Schizophrenia 233
Rationale 233
Treatment Considerations 235
Patients with Schizophrenia Living with or Supported by Families of Origin 237
Patients with Schizophrenia Who Are Married, with or without Children 238
Mood Disorders: Bipolar Disorder 239
Rationale 239
Treatment Considerations 241
Mood Disorders: Persistent Depressive Disorder and Major Depressive Disorder 243
Rationale 243
Treatment Considerations 245
Borderline Personality Disorder 246
Rationale 246
Treatment Considerations 247

Anxiety Disorders 248
Rationale 248
Panic Disorder and Agoraphobia 249
Treatment 249
Obsessive-Compulsive Disorder 250
Rationale 250
Treatment 250
Posttraumatic Stress Disorder 250
Rationale 250
Treatment 251
Dementia, Amnesia, and Other Cognitive Disorders 251
Rationale 251
Treatment Considerations 252
Eating Disorders 253
Rationale 253
Treatment Considerations 253
Substance-Related Disorders 254
Rationale 254
Assessment and Treatment Guidelines 255
Children of Alcoholic Parents 256
Psychiatric Disorders of Childhood 256
Intellectual Disability 256
Treatment 256
Autism Spectrum Disorder 256
Attention-Deficit/Hyperactivity Disorder 257
Oppositional Defiant Disorder and Conduct Disorder 259
Anxiety Disorders 259
Mood Disorders 259
Childhood Obesity 260
Clinical Practice Implications 260
Suggested Readings 260
References 260

19 Family Treatment in the Context of Other Special Problems—Violence to Self and Others 264
Objectives for the Reader 264
Introduction 264
The Family Model and Violence 265
Description of the Problem 265
How Violent Acts Occur: The Cycle of Violence 269
Assessment of Individual and Family Systems Issues 269
Physical and Psychological Consequences of Violence 271
Treatment 271
Clinical Issues for Therapists 274

Intrafamilial Child Sexual Abuse 275
Individual Issues 276
Family Issues 276
Larger System Issues 276
Assessment 277
Treatment 277
The Family Model and Child Abuse 278
Incestuous Trauma 279
The Suicidal Patient and the Family 279
Acute Management 280
Evaluating the Family 280
Involving the Family 281
Treating the Family 281
Discharging the Hospitalized Patient 282
Clinical Practice Implications 282
Suggested Reading 282
References 282

20 The Family and Treatment of Acute and Chronic Psychiatric Illness 284
Objectives for the Reader 284
Introduction 284
Background 285
Acute Treatment 286
The Function of the Acute Team for the Family 286
Family Responses to Mental Illness of a Family Member 287
The Family Burden in Psychotic Illness 287
Rationale for Acute Treatment of Families 288
Process of Family Treatment in Acute Care 289
Common Goals of Acute Family Intervention 290
Particular Decisions in Acute Care and Family Intervention 292
Family Techniques 293
A Working Model of Acute Family Intervention 294
Guidelines for Recommending Family Intervention in an Acute Care Setting 294
Empirical Studies 295
Families of the Chronically Ill 296
Expressed Emotion 296
Community-Based Support Groups 298
Controversies in the Treatment of Acute and Chronic Psychiatric Illness 298
Clinical Practice Implications 299
References 300

21 Working with Families in the Medical Setting 302

Objectives for the Reader 302

Introduction 302

How Family Functioning Impacts Illness 303

Gender Matters 303

Family Health Beliefs 304

Family Adherence 304

How Illness Impacts Family Functioning 304

Family Coping and Adaptation to Illness 304

Learning to Cope and Adapt 306

Providing a Therapeutic Space 306

Caregiving 306

A Family Systems Interview For Families with Medical Illness 307

Problem Solving 307

Communication 308

Roles 308

Affective Responsiveness 309

Affective Involvement 309

Behavior Control 309

Family Interventions 310

Family Support 310

Family Psychoeducation 310

Family Systemic Interventions 310

Multifamily Groups 311

Clinical Practice Implications 311

Suggested Readings 312

References 312

Section VII Results of and Guidelines for Recommending Family Therapy 317

22 Indications for and the Sequence of Family Therapy Evaluation and Treatment 319

Objectives for the Reader 319

Introduction 319

Sequence of Evaluation and Treatment Planning 320

Step 1: Is Family Evaluation Indicated? 320

Step 2: Is Family Treatment Indicated? 322

Family Therapy Versus Individual Therapy 322

Managed Care 324

Individual, Couples, or Sex Therapy for Sexual Problems 325

Family Crisis Therapy Versus Hospitalization 325

Step 3: What Shall Be the Duration and Intensity of Family Therapy? 325

Family Crisis Therapy 326

Brief Family Therapy 326

Long-Term Family Therapy 326

Step 4: What Model of Family Intervention Is Indicated? 327

Clinical Practice Implications 327

References 328

23 Controversies and Relative Contraindications 329

Objectives for the Reader 329

Introduction 329

Couples Therapy 330

Couples Conflict and Dissatisfaction 330

Sexual Issues 331

Families in the Process of Divorce 331

Unmarried Couples 332

The Child as the Identified Patient 332

The Adolescent as the Identified Patient 333

Family of Origin Issues 333

Situations In Which Family Therapy Is Difficult and Perhaps Contraindicated 334

When Psychopathology in One Family Member Makes Family Therapy Ineffective 334

When the Family or Therapist Thinks the Risks of Therapy Outweigh the Advantages 334

When the Family as a Whole Denies Having Family Problems 335

When Cultural or Religious Prejudices Are Present 335

Skills and Attributes of the Therapist as They Affect Family Work 335

Clinical Practice Implications 336

References 336

24 Results: The Outcomes of Couples and Family Therapy 337

Objectives for the Reader 337

Introduction 337

Overview of Psychotherapy Outcome Research 338

1. Specificity 338

2. The Difference between Efficacy and Effectiveness 339

3. The Difference between Qualitative and Quantitative, or Exploratory and Confirmatory, Research 339

4. The Difference between Process and Outcome Research 339

What The Studies Show? 340

Couples Treatments for Adult Disorders 341

Insight-Oriented Marital Therapy for Marital Distress 341

Integrative Behavioral Couple Therapy for Marital Distress 341

Emotionally Focused Couples Therapy for Marital Distress 341

Behavioral Marital Therapy for Depression 342
Behavioral Couples Therapy for Alcoholism 342
Couples Therapy for Posttraumatic Stress Disorder 342
Family Treatments for Adult Disorders 343
Schizophrenia and Major Mental Illness 343
Focused Family Therapy for Bipolar Disorder 343
Family Treatments for Child and Adolescent Disorders 344
Brief Strategic Family Therapy for Children and Adolescents with Externalizing Disorders 344
Functional Family Therapy for Delinquent Adolescents 344
Multidimensional Family Therapy for Adolescent Substance Abuse 344
Multisystemic Therapy for Youth at Risk 345
Functional Family Therapy for Adolescents with Bipolar Disorder 345
Family-Based Treatment for Anorexia Nervosa 345
Family Interventions for Medical Illnesses 345
The Effectiveness of Combining Medication and Family Therapy 346
Limitations of Family Therapy 346
Negative Effects of Family Therapy 347
Inability to Engage and Premature Termination of Family Therapy 350
Clinical Implications of Data From Couples and Family Therapy Outcome Studies 351
Clinical Practice Implications 352
References 352

Section VIII Ethical, Professional, and Training Issues 357

25 Ethical and Professional Issues in Couples and Family Therapy 359
Objectives for the Reader 359
Introduction 359
Ethical Issues Inherent in Family Therapy 360
Conflicting Interests of Family Members 360
Understanding HIPAA 361
Secrets and Confidentiality 362
Issues Involving Gender, Gender Roles, and Sexuality 363
Ethics in a Managed Care World 364
Informed Consent 364
Financial Issues 365
Professional Issues 365
The Problem of Boundaries and Dual Relationships 365
Competencies 368
Training Issues 368
Clinical Experiences 370

Training Programs in Family Psychiatry 371
A Multidisciplinary Field 371
Family Therapy Fellowships 372
Training and Licensure 373
Clinical Practice Implications 373
Suggested Readings 373
References 374

Index 375

LIST OF TABLES

Table 1.1 Family therapy format compared with other psychosocial therapy formats 17

Table 3.1 Processes that characterize functional families 41

Table 3.2 The family life cycle and adult development 43

Table 3.3 The child-focused years of the family life cycle 43

Table 4.1 Keys to family resilience 66

Table 6.1 Family life cycle 89

Table 6.2 Thinking family and working systemically 91

Table 7.1 Family evaluation outline 95

Table 8.1 A comprehensive evaluation schema 107

Table 8.2 Setting goals after evaluation 108

Table 8.3 Proposed classification of relational disorders (CORD) 114

Table 9.1 Models of family treatment 122

Table 10.1 Determining strategies after goals are set 130

Table 10.2 Mediating goals of family therapy and their strategies 133

Table 14.1 Comparison of therapy formats and strategies 187

Table 15.1 Guidelines for interviewing couples—The process 202

Table 16.1 Assessment of sexual problems 208

Table 17.1 Differences between stepfamilies and nuclear families; therapeutic implications 223

Table 18.1 Alternative formats for psychoeducational family treatment 235

Table 18.2 Special issues in carrying out psychoeducational family programs with patients experiencing their first psychotic break 237

Table 18.3 Factors affected and not affected by a brief family education program 237

Table 21.1 Dyadic coping questions 305

Table 22.1 Relative selection criteria for treatment format: family versus individual 322

Table 22.2 Criteria for sex and couple therapy 325

Table 22.3 Criteria for family crisis therapy and hospitalization 326

Table 24.1 What constitutes a negative effect? 348

Table 25.1 Excerpt from AAMFT Code of Ethics 366

Table 25.2 Group for the advancement of psychiatry (GAP) proposal for specific family systems competencies 369

LIST OF FIGURES

Figure 1.1 Hierarchy of natural systems, showing levels of organization 11
Figure 1.2 Continuum of natural systems 12
Figure 1.3 Minuchin's description of the boundaries of the family system 13
Figure 1.4 Hoffman's time cable 15
Figure 3.1 The family life cycle 48
Figure 4.1 Poverty rates of various types of families 60
Figure 6.1 Genogram showing family with a symptomatic daughter 89
Figure 6.2 Structural map showing same family in therapy 90
Figure 7.1 The family genogram and symbols 98
Figure 7.2 Example of a genogram (Sigmund Freud's family) with demographic, functioning, and critical event information 99
Figure 8.1 Relational problems and abuse and neglect 106
Figure 11.1 Types of family coalitions 143
Figure 12.1 Schematic of the joining of therapist and family scenarios 155
Figure 18.1 A tentative, interactive vulnerability–stress model for the development of schizophrenic psychotic episodes 234
Figure 18.2 A quality treatment equation 235

For family therapists, context is everything. Family therapy is both a set of therapeutic techniques for treating family distress and a specific way of thinking about human behavior. The family is a critical context for understanding normal behavior and psychopathology. In Chapter 1, we speak of the following three issues: (1) How did family therapy develop? (2) How is it defined? and (3) What are the core concepts that every family therapist must know? Finally, we examine the elements that distinguish family therapy from other core psychotherapies. In this edition of the book, we pay particular attention to recent studies of how gender, ethnicity, race, class, and socioeconomic status can influence family therapy and to how DSM-5 and managed care affect this treatment approach.

We placed Chapter 2, which puts the family and family life in historical and sociologic perspective, early in the book to make the point that there is no way to understand family function and dysfunction as well as treat families without being aware of the changing, global landscape, and cultures within which the family is embedded.

To avoid unnecessary duplication, we often use the word *family* (as in family therapy, family system, and family unit) instead of the more cumbersome term *marital and family*. When we refer to marital issues specifically we use only the word *marital*. We use the term *couples* to refer to both married and unmarried couples. Throughout the text, we use a broad definition of family to include both blood and nonblood relatives who may not be under the same roof, including those who have been referred to as *significant others* or who are considered family members by the family itself. For historical purposes, we have chosen to leave in many of the original references from earlier additions of this book. Family "treatment" and family "interventions" are used interchangeably.

Section

I Family Therapy in Context

1 The Field of Couples and Family Therapy: Development and Definition 5

2 Family Life in Historical and Sociological Perspective 20

1 The Field of Couples and Family Therapy: Development and Definition

OBJECTIVES FOR THE READER

- To understand the historical development of family therapy as it influences present-day theory and practice
- To define family therapy and to begin to differentiate it from individual and group formats and strategies
- To recognize and be able to use basic family system concepts in evaluation and treatment

For easier reading, we emphasize that the descriptors "couples" or "marital" are used nearly interchangeably in this chapter.

INTRODUCTION

Family life has always been the main building block of human connections, but treating the family has only come into its own in the last 50 years. Families as basic human systems are different in several essential ways from other types of human groups and relationships. **Love of and bonding or attachment to family members are to some extent biologically built into the nervous system as survival devices, and our most intense emotions, both positive and negative, are reserved for family members.** Emerging research investigating the biology of attachment is growing. Scientists are looking at genetic factors and psychophysiological responses in infants that shape attachment. Hormones oxytocin and vasopressin, known as neuropeptides, are thought to play a role in forming attachments to others (Hanna S, 2014).

Marriages and families perform vital socialization tasks for children and for society at large. It has been a commonsense view that we are all shaped by what we experience in our *families of origin* (i.e., comprising our parents, siblings, and extended family). For most people what occurs in their current marital or family system is a significant element in their general sense of well-being and functioning. Furthermore, as we discuss in subsequent chapters, the family has important effects on the quality of life and on the course of psychiatric illness (e.g., a mood or psychotic disorder) and medical illness.

In the past four decades, mental health professionals have moved past a singular focus on individual dynamics to examine the enigmatic processes that lead to family distress. They have developed a set of theories grouped loosely under the name *systems theory*, which examines how people or aspects of a system affect one another. Using this theory, they have devised both a paradigm for explaining human behavior, one that looks past the individual, and a set of techniques for reducing distress and improving family functioning. As we discuss in this book, the mental health field is gradually incorporating these changes so that a comprehensive biopsychosocial model of behavior is becoming a reality.

DEVELOPMENT OF THE FAMILY THERAPY FIELD
DEFINITION OF COUPLES AND FAMILY THERAPY
CORE CONCEPTS
General Systems Theory
Organization
Control Over and Adaptation to the Environment
Energy
Family Systems Theory and Homeostasis Over Time
AN INTEGRATIVE INTERPERSONAL MODEL
DIFFERENTIATION OF FAMILY THERAPY FROM OTHER PSYCHOTHERAPIES
CLINICAL PRACTICE IMPLICATIONS

DEVELOPMENT OF THE FAMILY THERAPY FIELD

Although exciting and often efficacious, family therapy can be confusing for the beginner. Just as psychoanalysis has spawned a range of perspectives that include classical (Freudian), interpersonal, and relational, the family therapy field is differentiated by approaches that include (among others) family systems, structural, strategic, psychodynamic, experiential, cognitive–behavioral, integrative behavioral, behavioral, family focused, emotionally focused, narrative, and psychoeducational. For some, it may be difficult to distinguish the thinking that lies behind the personal styles of charismatic family therapists. For others, it may seem difficult to synthesize a coherent family theory from the variety of existing orientations. Yet, as in any field of academic study or clinical practice, family therapy's present state can be understood partly by looking at its own evolution. How did this state of affairs come about, and how is it changing today?

In a broad sense, the significance attributed to the family's role in relation to the psychic and social distress of any of its members has waxed and waned over the centuries. The important role of the family in the development of individual problems was mentioned by Confucius in his writings and by the Greeks in their myths. The early Hawaiians would meet as a kin network (i.e., family) to discuss solutions to an individual's problem. For a long time in Western culture, however, what we now call mental illness and other forms of interpersonal distress were ascribed to magical, religious, physical, or exclusively individual factors.

It was not until the early 1900s that individual psychodynamics was delineated as a major determinant of human behavior. Although Freud stressed the major role of the family in normal and abnormal development, he believed that the most effective technique for dealing with such individual psychopathology was treatment on a one-to-one basis.

At about this same time, others working with the mentally ill began to suggest that families with a sick member should be seen together and not as individuals removed from family relationships. In particular, psychiatric social workers in child guidance clinics began to recognize the importance of dealing with the entire family unit around child-focused issues. However, the psychiatric community in general was dominated by Freudian thinking until the late 1960s.

In the psychiatric literature, psychoanalysts reported experiences in treating a marital pair as early as the 1930s. They began to see a series of marital partners in simultaneous, but separate, psychoanalyses in the following decade. This approach was quite unusual because psychoanalysts generally believed that this method of treatment would hinder the therapist in helping the patient, on the assumption that neither spouse would trust the same therapist and consequently would withhold important material. As a result, the other marital partner was usually referred to a colleague. The two earliest marriage counseling centers in the United States began to treat couples in the early 1930s.

The early 1950s, which might be considered the heyday of American social psychiatry, witnessed the first consistent use of family therapy in modern psychotherapeutic practice. In New York, Ackerman began to use family interviews consistently in his analytic work with children and adolescents.

Not until the early 1960s did the modern field of family therapy begin to take shape. A backlash against psychoanalytic orthodoxy coupled with the social activism of the era propelled a handful of early theorists into leading roles in a social revolution within the fields of psychiatry, psychology, and social work. This group assumed that family, group, and community were the keys to effective intervention. Group therapy, family therapy, and milieu therapy in inpatient settings flourished during this period, as did community mental health. Various schools of theory and practice emerged, and leading journals (e.g., *Family Process*) were established. At the same time, teaching practices were marked by innovation, as the use of one-way mirrors and videotaped interviews moved the practice of therapy out into the open for study and discussion. As a result, many mental health professionals were drawn to learning about and practicing family therapy.

During the 1970s, the scope of family therapy was expanded to apply to a broad range of psychiatric problems with families differing widely in socioeconomic background. In particular, Minuchin's contributions to the development of briefer, crisis-oriented methods began to address the needs of families with multiple problems. This was a decade of ferment as well, as traditionalists proposing more psychodynamic or biologic models battled with family clinicians over territory, training funds, and the right to the "best" explanation for how psychopathology occurs, is maintained, and is remedied. During this period, researchers also began to look at process variables that contributed to treatment efficacy.[1,2] Finally, the number of available clinical models of marital and family therapy expanded exponentially. During meetings of the American Psychiatric Association, considerable prominence was given to family therapy topics. Interdisciplinary organizations such as the American Orthopsychiatric Association became a home for family therapy presentations. Except for relatively infrequent, small conferences, family therapists presented their major findings at meetings of these other professional organizations and were published frequently in other professional journals until the early 1970s. Later that decade, various clinical techniques in family therapy became more distinctively identified as schools, and family therapy began to become a distinct entity. As the American Family Therapy Association and the American Association of Marital and Family Therapists grew, training conferences nationwide evolved. For many mental health professionals, family therapy seemed to be the right treatment at the right time.

During the 1980s, the early polemics faded and clinicians and researchers continued to establish innovative practices and particular treatment packages for specific individual, marital, and family problems. For example, data had made clear the existence of an important biologic component in the etiology of schizophrenia and other mental disorders, and psychopharmacologic treatment became an accepted practice. Although most family therapists no longer viewed family therapy as the primary treatment for schizophrenia, they considered family psychoeducation—a particular form of family treatment—to be one important component of a multimodal intervention. In 1988, marriage and family therapy was added to the list of four core mental health professions eligible for mental health traineeships under the Public Health Service Act, Title III, Section 303(d). In addition, issues of gender and culture became more prominent in the field, and the differences and similarities in family function among ethnic groups were addressed clearly for the first time.

Throughout the 1990s, some family therapists expended much effort to establish marital and family therapy as a differentiated, autonomous profession. The marital and family therapy degree is now widely established, and marital and family therapy has become a separate and licensed profession. However, the downside of this is that family psychology, master's and doctorate degrees in family therapy, and family psychiatry seem to be moving further apart.

Psychology, social work, and counseling psychology have developed active subspecialties in couples and family therapy. At the same time the rapidly developing interest in the biologic treatment of psychiatric problems is to a degree overshadowing the development of new effective psychotherapeutic therapies. Couples and family work is more mainstream.

The aim of this book is to continue the tradition of integrating the best of theory and data from all disciplines into a coherent model of family theory applicable to trainees and practitioners in all of the mental health professions.

The health of the family therapy field has always resided in its diversity and its unwillingness to simply accept narrow, linear explanations for psychopathology or narrow, linear treatments. As members of a field originally composed of mavericks and rebels, family therapists were initially unwilling to accept the dominant psychodynamic and biologic ideas of American psychiatry. However, during the 1990s, the independence of family therapists receded somewhat as mental health professionals of every discipline and theoretical commitment were gradually recognizing that no one perspective owns the truth and that multimodal treatments are frequently necessary, even desirable. There is also a movement toward specificity of treatments, in the development of diagnostic classification systems for families (see Chapter 8) and in the development of selection criteria for the application, focus, duration, and intensity of family and marital interventions. In the 2000s, family therapists are integrating creative new theories like attachment with older models. These approaches are being studied and applied to work with an increasing number of cultural groups and emerging family forms that were previously thought of as "nontraditional."

The last two decades have witnessed the introduction of a new wave of couples and family treatments that include specific family-focused treatments for Axis I disorders such as eating disorders and bipolar disorder, as well as narrative and more integrative approaches (e.g., integrative behavioral couple therapy and emotionally focused couple therapy). Although treatment techniques have become more differentiated, so that one can speak of major orientations, such techniques must be integrated into a treatment package that is flexible and that meets the needs of individuals and families alike. The family therapy field is generating a body of treatment outcome research, primarily the fruits of systematic research by more behaviorally oriented marital researchers. These research efforts are growing in number and are becoming more sophisticated in design and execution. The findings that family therapy has demonstrated positive results with certain family problems, ranging from schizophrenia to childhood problems, are indeed encouraging (see Chapters 18 and 24 for a full discussion of these issues).

At the same time, an additional clinical and financial issue facing family therapists has been the effect of managed care and the need for treatment selection and provision to be increasingly based on outcome data that demonstrate evidence for efficacy. In many instances, the outpatient family therapist must provide care that is focused and feasible within the limits set by the managed care provider.

Likewise, managed care has had major effects on inpatient family therapy by decreasing the allowed length of stay (and accordingly the number of family sessions). It has also decreased the possibility of family outreach and long-term family support in publicly funded settings. To make matters even more complicated, families are expected to provide more illness monitoring and in-home care to loved ones discharged from the hospital prematurely due to managed care restrictions on length of stay.

The passage of the Affordable Care Act (ACA) will lead to profound changes in the way health care services are accessed and delivered. At the time of this publication, many of the specific details regarding implementation of the ACA as it relates to family oriented interventions are unknown. The ACA calls for the expansion of Medicaid and the unveiling of new exchange subsidies for those who have existing coverage. Mental health conditions must be covered the same way physical health services are covered. Many clinicians fear that while managed care insurers will attempt to provide mental health care coverage to more Americans, the type of interventions covered will be limited and clinicians will not be compensated appropriately.

More closely aligned with the strength-based and systemic thinking of family therapists, the recovery movement is gaining traction in America and is expected to have a transformational effect on professional practice. According to the National Consensus Statement on Mental Health Recovery,[3] recovery is defined as "a journey of healing and transformation enabling a person with a mental health problem to live a meaningful life in a community of his or her choice while striving to achieve his or her full potential." An essential aspect of recovery-oriented health care is family-driven care. Family participation is encouraged in all aspects and phases of care.

Rait and Glick[4] pointed out that consistent with the burgeoning evidence for the value of family interventions, the President's New Freedom Commission on Mental Health,[5] which established new priorities in the delivery of mental health services, emphasizes family-centered care. Current standards of treatment for the seriously mentally ill recognize the importance of family members' roles in the promotion of long-term recovery. In response to the Commission's findings, the Veterans Health Administration health care system, the largest health care system in the United States, developed an action agenda titled "VA's Achieving the Promise: Transforming Mental Health Care in the VA." One of the report's strongest recommendations was to implement consumer- and family-centered care programs in all Veterans Affairs medical centers.[6]

The most important subsequent developments over the past decade was the VA Health Care System's decision in 2010 following Public Law 110–387 to "include marriage and family counseling in the list of services that be provided... for the effective treatment and rehabilitation of a Veteran, as part of a Veteran's hospital care." VA medical centers must now offer services to couples and families, and the potential impact on the rest of the American health care system may be significant as evidence-based treatments for couples and families facing relationship issues, physical and psychiatric illness, and parenting challenges have been rolled out at VA medical centers throughout the country.

Finally, the trend toward couples- and family-centered, collaborative, biopsychosocial models of health care for patients with physical illness provides further impetus for family training in psychiatry. Rolland and Walsh[7] noted that consumers have increasingly advocated for health care that attends to the physical and psychosocial challenges of major health conditions for *all* family members (not just the sickest person). Heru[8] suggests that, "improving the family environment has important health implications equivalent to the reduction of risk factors for chronic illness." As consultants in medical settings, psychiatrists serve an important function in recognizing that chronic illness, disability, terminal illness, and loss represent changes that invariably affect every family member.

DEFINITION OF COUPLES AND FAMILY THERAPY

Family therapy is distinguished from other psychotherapies by its conceptual focus on the family system as a whole. In this view, major emphasis is placed on understanding how the system as a whole remains functional and on understanding individual behavior patterns as arising from and inevitably feeding back into the complex interactions within the family system. **In other words, a person's thoughts, feelings, and behaviors are seen as multidetermined and partly a product of significant interpersonal relationships.** From the family systems perspective, alterations in the larger marital and family unit may have positive consequences for the individual members and for the larger systems.

The family system under consideration may be either two or three generational, depending on the problem and the model used. A major emphasis is generally placed on understanding and intervening in the family system's current patterns of interaction. In some cases, a secondary interest is placed on the origins and development of those patterns (depending on the model).

Couples and family treatment can be defined as a systematic effort to produce beneficial changes in a marital or family unit by introducing changes into the patterns of family interactions. Its aim is the establishment of more satisfying ways of living for the entire family and for individual family members.

In many families, a member or members may be singled out as the *identified patient*. Occasionally a marital or family unit presents itself as being in trouble without singling out any one member. For example, a couple may realize that their marriage is in trouble and that the cause of their problems stems from interaction with each other and not from either partner individually.

Family therapy might broadly be thought of as any type of psychosocial intervention using a conceptual framework that gives primary emphasis to the family system and that, in its therapeutic strategies, aims to affect the entire family structure. Thus any psychotherapeutic approach that attempts to understand or to intervene in a family system might fittingly be called family therapy. This is a very broad definition and allows many differing points of view, in theory and in therapy, to be placed under one heading.

Family therapy might be thought of as any type of psychosocial intervention using a conceptual framework that gives primary emphasis to the family system and aims to affect the entire family structure.

A continuum exists between the individual's intrapsychic processes, the interactional or family system, and the larger social/cultural system. Different conceptual frameworks are used when dealing with these different levels. A therapist may choose to emphasize any of the points on this continuum, but the family therapist is especially sensitive to and trained in those aspects relating specifically to the family system—to both its individual characteristics and the larger social matrix.

Although many clinicians agree that problematic interactions may occur in families in which one family member has a gross disturbance, it is not always clear whether the faulty interactions are the cause or the effect of the behavior of the disturbed individual. Some practitioners continue to perceive and treat the disequilibrium in the individual's psyche as the central issue, viewing the family and larger social system as context, which adds an important dimension to the conceptualization and treatment. Others see and treat as the central issue the disequilibrium in the family, viewing the individual symptoms as the result of, or the attempted solution to, a family problem. There is reason to believe that both views are important. Clinicians should evaluate each clinical situation carefully, attempting to understand the phenomena and select intervention strategies designed to achieve the desired ends.

CORE CONCEPTS

General Systems Theory

Like other developing fields of knowledge, the family therapy field has needed to generate its own terminology. Although individual behavior and individual psychodynamics have had a long history and a wealth of sophisticated terminology attached to them, the language available to describe specific interactions among people is already substantial. Family therapy is based on a set of theories that combine a general systems view of interactions, a cybernetic epistemology, traces of interpersonal psychiatry, and the most recent contributions of social constructivism. Thus there is a need to begin by delineating the basic concepts underlying the developments in understanding family process and family intervention. These concepts are not numerous, but their paucity belies the profound shift in focus that occurs when progressing from concepts about the individual to describing a system and its functioning.

The biologist Von Bertalanffy is credited as the first to introduce the principles of *general systems theory*, which provide an organismic approach to understanding biologic beings.[9] Von Bertalanffy felt that the reductionistic, mechanistic tradition in science was insufficient to explain the behavior of living organisms, because this approach depended on a linear series of stepwise cause-and-effect equations. He developed general principles to explain biologic processes that include considerable complexity and levels of organization. General systems theory was described as a "new approach to the unity of science problem which sees organization rather than reduction as the unifying principle, and which therefore searches for general structural isomorphisms in systems"[10] (p. 7).

Thus a systems approach places an emphasis on the relationship between the parts of a complex whole, and the context in which these events occur, rather than on an isolation of events from their context.[11]

A system is a group of interacting parts. In nature, each system is nested within a larger one (see Fig. 1.1). In the most general terms, a living system is organized, exerts control over and adapts to its environment, and possesses and uses energy. Let's see how these notions apply to families.

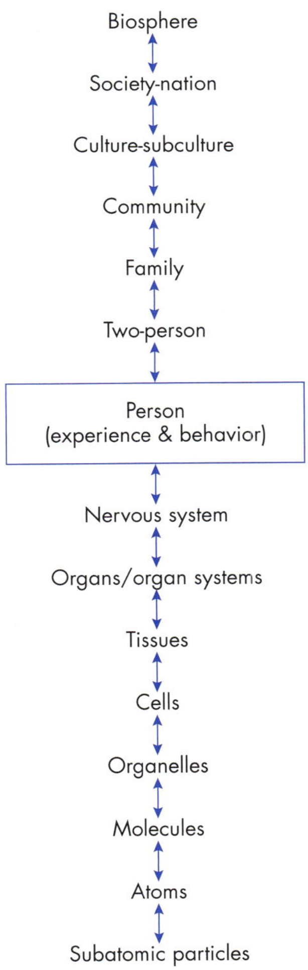

Figure 1.1 Hierarchy of natural systems, showing levels of organization. (Reprinted with permission from Engel GL. The clinical application of the biopsychosocial model. *Am J Psychiatry.* 1980;137(5):535–544. Figure 1. Copyright © 1980 American Psychiatric Association. All Rights Reserved.)

Organization

The first key concept relevant to living systems is that such systems have a high degree of organization; that is, there is a consistent relationship between the elements or parts of the organism. The systems view implies that the organism or entity is greater than the sum of the separate parts. No single element in the system can be thought of as acting completely independently. One might think of this as the difference between physiology and anatomy. According to Engel,[12] each hierarchy represents an organized dynamic whole, a system of sufficient persistence and identification to justify being named. Its name reflects its distinctive properties and characteristics. Each system implies qualities and relationships distinctive for that level of organization and each requires criteria for study and explanation unique for that level.

In order to regulate its exchange with systems outside itself, the living system must have boundaries (Figs. 1.1 and 1.2). The membrane around a cell defines the boundary or outer limit of that functional unit. While creating a boundary between the cell and the outside, the cell membrane also provides through its permeability an interactional relationship between the inside and outside of the cell, by selectively allowing the transfer of chemicals across itself.

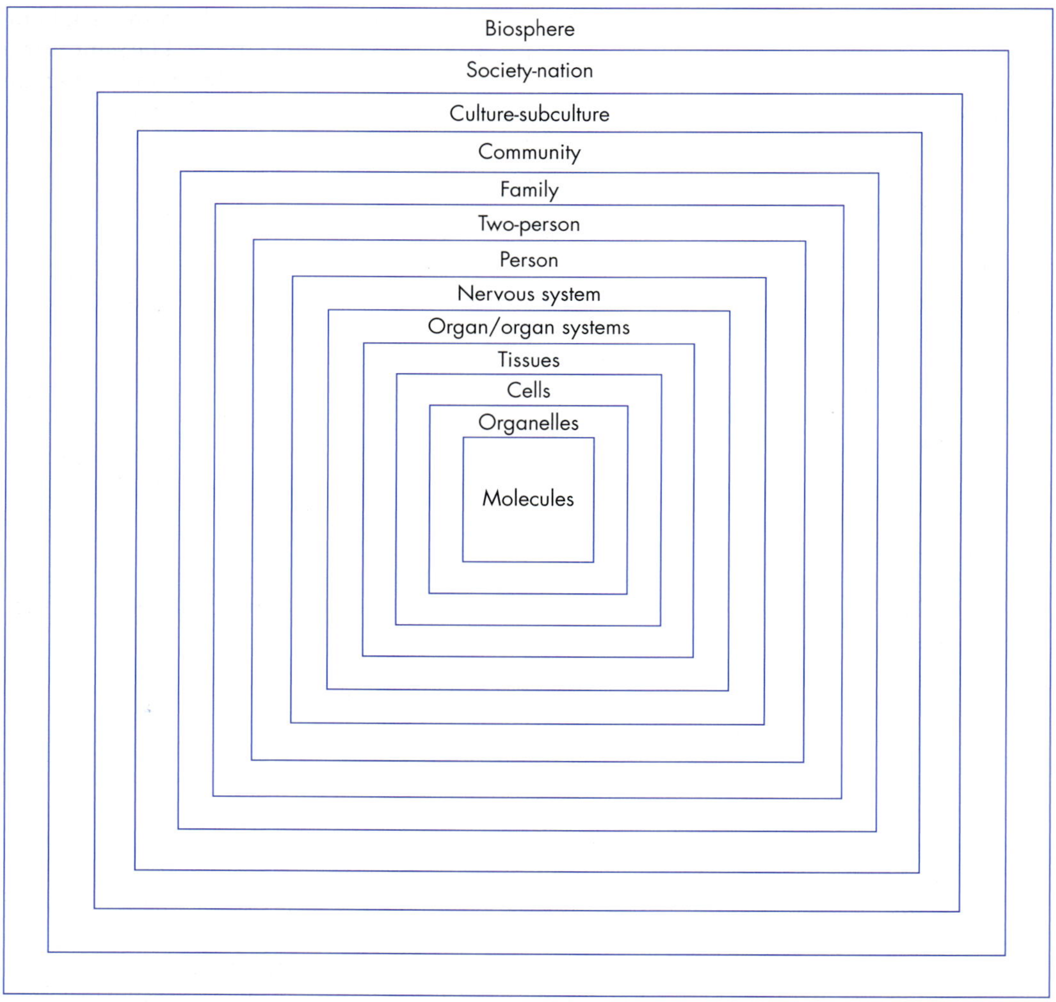

Figure 1.2 Continuum of natural systems. (Reprinted with permission from Engel GL. The clinical application of the biopsychosocial model. *Am J Psychiatry.* 1980;137(5):535–544. Figure 2. Copyright © 1980 American Psychiatric Association. All Rights Reserved.)

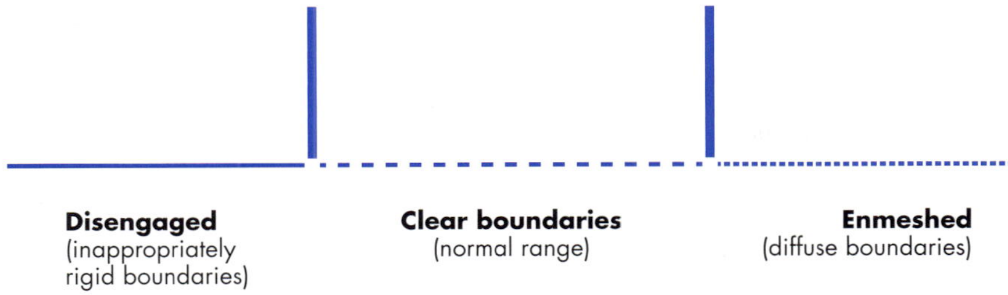

Figure 1.3 Minuchin's description of the boundaries of the family system. (From Minuchin S. *Families and Family Therapy.* Harvard University Press; 1974. Copyright © 1974 by the President and Fellows of Harvard College. Used by permission. All rights reserved.)

Analogously, the organized family system has a membrane, or boundary, between itself and the surrounding neighborhood and community.

This boundary is the set of implicit and explicit rules by which the family keeps information and activities to itself or allows outside information and contact with people in the neighborhood and the community. A family must have clear boundaries to be functional. The same is true for subsystems within the family. For example, in order for the marital subsystem to function, it must have a boundary that separates it from other subsystems such as the sibling subsystem.

A family's boundary comprises the set of rules by which the family keeps information and activities to itself or allows outside information and contact with people in the neighborhood and the community.

Minuchin[13] described families as being on a continuum from disengaged (i.e., having inappropriately rigid boundaries) to enmeshed (i.e., having overly permeable, diffuse boundaries). Families in the middle of this continuum (i.e., having clear boundaries) are considered to be the most functional (Fig. 1.3). Although no one-to-one correlation exists between extremes of boundary functioning and symptomatology, extremes are seen as more likely to lead to pathologic behavior in one or more members of the family system. Because normative boundaries may vary considerably from one ethnic group to another and still allow development and growth of the child, families need to be considered using the norms of their cultural group as a reference point. For example, it is normal for some groups, such as upper-class English families, to send their children to boarding school by age 9 or 10 years, whereas in other groups children live at home until they are in their 20s or are married.

Recognition of the existence of subsystems within the family system relates to the notion of a hierarchical organization. The system itself is organized on one or many hierarchical levels entailing systems or subsystems (see Figs. 1.1 and 1.2).

Control Over and Adaptation to the Environment

A second key concept relevant to living systems is that a functional living system must have some means of controlled adaptation to its environment. In 1948, Wiener introduced the notion of *cybernetics* as a branch of science dealing with control mechanisms and the transmission of information. He pointed out the similarities between the mechanisms of internal control and communication in an animal and in machines. A key concept in cybernetics is that of *feedback* and the feedback loop. In such a circular sequence of events, element A influences element B, which influences element C, which in turn influences element A.

For example, if the temperature in a room becomes too low, the thermostat initiates a mechanism, which turns on the furnace, which raises the temperature in the room, which registers on the thermostat, which then signals the furnace to shut off. Such mechanisms serve to control the state of the organism or environment.[14] Control concepts such as homeostasis and feedback have been used by family theorists to understand and change family systems.[15,16]

Corrective feedback (or negative feedback in the language of cybernetic theory) results in a sequence of events that returns a person to a previous, more balanced state.[17] Consider the following case example:

Mr. A, a young father who had bipolar disorder, noted that as his mood became more elevated at home, his wife would become anxious. She would then say things like, "Why don't you slow down? I'll help you with the chores."

This intervention appeared to help Mr. A to regain control of his activity level and his wife to become more comfortable. A system always has feedback, but the result of a particular behavior is determined partly by each person's internal processing. Consider this case example:

Mr. B, a 40-year-old patient with schizophrenia, responded to his wife's request to slow down by becoming angry because he believed she was chastising him. She became more insistent, and he became more angry and upset. She finally started crying, and he calmed down. After a while, whenever he became upset she began crying, which kept her calm, but then she developed depressive symptoms of low mood, anhedonia, and functional impairment.

In this instance, an attempted solution became a problem.

Energy

A third and final key concept relevant to living systems is that of energy and information. Living systems are open systems in which energy can be transported in and out of the system. Instead of a tendency toward entropy and degradation of energy, which happens in nonliving systems, living systems have a tendency toward increased patterning, complexity, and organization.

In human open systems such as the family, information (meaning knowledge from outside of the family) acts as a type of energy that informs the system and can lead to more complex interaction. For example, in families open to it, the women's movement brought many changes in how the spouses reacted to each other. In some families, however, these changes led to confusion and distress, whereas in others they led to improvement in function.

To summarize, a theoretical framework commonly used by family therapists is the family systems approach. The understanding of families is ecologic, in that the capabilities of the family are viewed as greater than an arithmetic sum of its parts. Each person is viewed in interactive relations with the other family members, all functioning to maintain the family system coherently but also striving for their own unique goals. The family system is maintained by its members so as to preserve its essential traditions, myths, patterns, identities, and values.

A key concept here is that although to an outside observer some of a family's behavior may appear crazy or self-defeating, the behavior is assumed to be the family's best solution to its problems. For example, in Mr. B's family (see the case example mentioned earlier in this chapter), the wife's depression seemed to decrease her husband's symptoms.

The boundaries of the system are determined by the family and sometimes by the therapist. Most family therapists think of a family system as comprising at least three generations; however, a particular subsystem of couple or parents and children can also be seen as a system. In remarried families the system boundaries are more complex and permeable, and the total number of people involved tends to be much larger. Family organization shifts over time.

Often the family returns to an apparent steady state, but it must always deal with the inevitable changes that time and biologic development bring. Sometimes it responds to stress with creative solutions but at other times with stagnation. The notion of the evolution of families as life events occur (e.g., when a child goes away to college) differentiates this view of coherence from that of a fixed homeostasis.

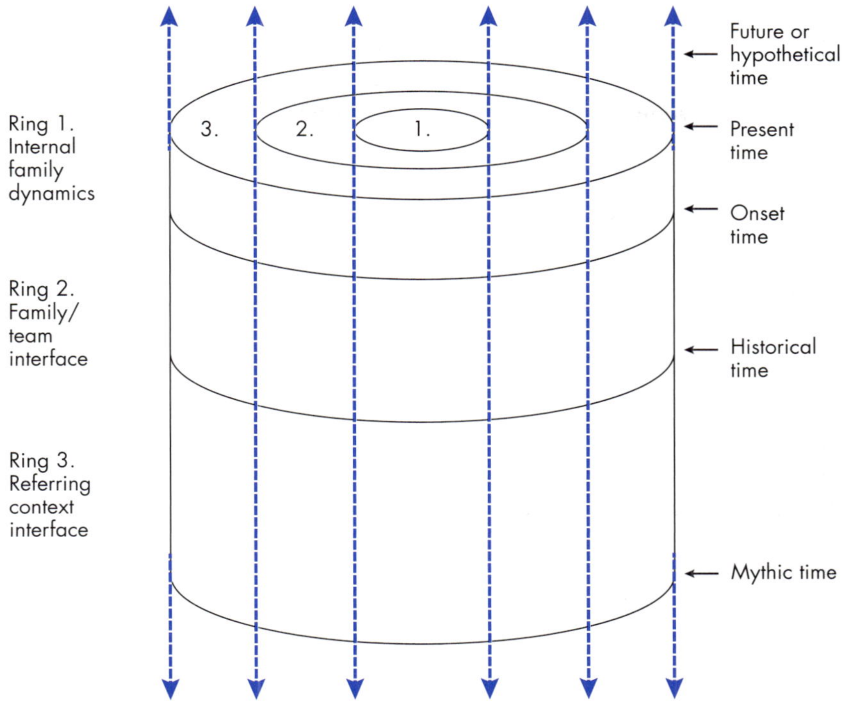

Figure 1.4 Hoffman's time cable. (From Hoffman L. A co-evolutionary framework for systemic family therapy. *Aust N Z J Fam Ther.* 1983;4(1):9–21. Copyright © 1983 Australian Association of Family Therapy. Reprinted by permission of John Wiley & Sons, Inc.)

Family Systems Theory and Homeostasis Over Time

It can be said that the critical issue for families is which homeostasis to evolve toward, that is, what to preserve of the past (in order to manage the present competently) and what to look forward to in the future. Hoffman[18] has developed a useful diagram (Fig. 1.4), which she calls a time cable, to illustrate the concepts of (1) how the family (and treating team) interface with the community and with its internal dynamics and (2) how each family has a long history (so-called mythic time) and is evolving constantly.

Hoffman[18] (p. 42) describes the time cable as follows:

The figure presents a diagram of this construct, sometimes still referred to by me as my Cosmic Sausage, because so much depends on where you cut it. In this case, we will assume that the cable's outer skin ends at the boundary of that imaginary entity called the family. The cuts in the cross-section correspond to different dimensions of time: present time, onset time, historical time, mythic time, and future or hypothetical time. At each position depicted by the Time Cable, "different" questions work to clarify family alignments in relation to the problem, by revealing five aspects:

1. *Family alignments as they relate to the problem in the present*
2. *Family alignments as they relate to onset of the problem*
3. *Family alignments as they furnish a historical matrix for the problem*
4. *The effect on family alignments if the problem were to change*
5. *Family alignments related to paradigmatic values that the problem metaphorically represents*

Information thus gathered can be used both to build a hypothesis and to suggest a positive connotation of the problem in whatever temporal context seems most relevant.

The cable also contains subcylinders: Rings 1, 2, and 3, indicated within the cross-section, in the present. The idea of the rings is to show that there are several systems interfaces one might have to consider in targeting an intervention, and there seemed to be an order of priority, too. Interface dynamics within the family took second place to team/family system and professionals from the referring context. As I said before, the interface that seems most important in any interview can be called the "presenting edge."

To summarize, classical family therapy examines interpersonal relationships—rather than biologic, intrapsychic, or societal processes—when attempting to understand human distress. That is not to say that family therapy ignores the intrapsychic or the biologic, but its primary vision and interventions are focused on interpersonal relationships. For example, both chemistry and physics use versions of relativity theory and quantum theory. They are not separate disciplines because they embrace unique scientific approaches; rather, they are distinct because each uses its overlapping theories to concentrate on different natural phenomena.

AN INTEGRATIVE INTERPERSONAL MODEL

An integrative model connects the systems concepts above with Lewis's work on interpersonal relationships and individual outcome. Our model is based on the notion that there is an ongoing and consistent interplay between psychopathology (related to biologic and developmental factors) and the individual relationships with significant others. As Lewis[19] noted,

At its center this perspective holds that relational structures—the more or less enduring patterns of interaction—either facilitate or impede the continued maturation of the participants. It is important to note that the relationship between an individual and their relational system is not linear; rather, individual characteristics influence system properties, and these properties shape individual characteristics.

We discuss Lewis's ideas about relationships in later chapters (see Chapters 14 and 15).

DIFFERENTIATION OF FAMILY THERAPY FROM OTHER PSYCHOTHERAPIES

Family therapy as a format of treatment can be distinguished from other psychotherapies by its fundamental paradigm shift, which assumes that people are best understood as operating in systems and that treatment must include, either in person or in theoretical understanding, conceptualization of all relevant parts of the system. From this assumption comes different goals, foci, participants, and so on (Table 1.1). The term *family therapy* connotes a format of intervention that attempts to include the relevant system members—this means at least the nuclear family but most often the three generation family and perhaps significant others such as lovers, friends, or important adoptive kin (persons without ties of blood or marriage whom the family has designated as members of itself). The presence of family members is considered crucial to addressing the goal of family treatment, which is the improved functioning of the family as an interlocking system and network of individuals. This context allows a focus on the family system as a whole in order to understand current individual behavior as rising from, and inevitably feeding back into, the complicated matrix of the general family system.

The goal of family treatment is the improved functioning of the family as an interlocking system and network of individuals.

The final and the intermediate goals of the family format are different from those in the individual and group formats. The final goal of the family model is improved family functioning and improved individual functioning of its members. This goal is reached, for example, by

Table 1.1 Family therapy format compared with other psychosocial therapy formats

Therapy format	Intermediate goals	Final goals	Focus	Participants	Length or frequency of sessions	Mean overall duration of treatment
Family	Improve family communication; decrease family conflict	Improved family functioning	Family intervention: family coalitions and roles	Nuclear family unit; extended family; 1–2 therapists	Most 1–2 hours per week	2 mo–2 y
Individual	Insight into intrapsychic conflicts; insight into interaction (transference)	Individual personality/ symptom change	Unconscious conflicts: individual's thoughts, wishes, and behaviors	1 patient; 1 therapist	1 h, 1–5 times per week	2 mo–5 y
Group	Sharing with group; improved relating skills in group	Improved individual social functioning	Group participants and feedback	6–8 patients; 1–2 therapists	1½ h, 1 time per week	6 mo–2 y

intermediate goals of improving family communication and decreasing family conflict. Thus the focus of the family model is on the current family interactions with the various coalitions, boundary difficulties, and other features of systemic dysfunction.

This model assumes that because a large part of a person's problem is connected to malfunction in the family system, mobilizing and reorganizing the system may be an effective way to solve the problem. In contrast, the final goal of the individual model is personality, symptom, or behavior change in one particular individual. In order to reach such a final goal, the focus of the individual format is often on the individual's behaviors, unconscious conflicts, or cognitive schema. With this final goal and focus, the intermediate goals of individual intervention (depending on the particular therapeutic strategies) include insight into intrapsychic conflicts or interpersonal interactions with others, or knowledge of one's individual cognitions/behaviors, and a progressive change therein. The group format has as its final goal improved individual social functioning. The focus (somewhat similar to family treatment) is on current group interaction and intermediate goals but would include the individual sharing with the group and manifesting an improved relating skill with other group members. The following case example illustrates how three different approaches could be applied to the same situation:

> *Ms. C, a young woman with depressive illness, is living at home and not dating. An individual therapist might determine that Ms. C's intrapsychic conflicts around dependence and autonomy and her early interactions with her father led her to be afraid of men. The therapist might choose an individual format to increase understanding or a group format to increase interpersonal interaction. A family therapist might see that Ms. C's grandmother just died, that her mother is grieving and hostile to her father, that she is the youngest child and last one home, and that she is staying at home because her mother desperately needs her as a companion. The family therapist would see the girl with her parents. A psychopharmacologist might see the phenomenology of classic depression and prescribe medication without individual or family treatment.*

The strategies and techniques of family therapy (see Chapters 9 and 11)—whether structural, strategic, behavioral, psychoeducational, experiential, supportive, or psychodynamic—overlap with these same techniques as they are used in individual and group formats, but they may take on added dimensions in a family session. For example, in individual insight-oriented psychotherapy, the therapist may interpret an individual's interaction with his wife as it relates to his earlier developmental interaction with his mother. A family therapist, with both spouses in the room, might also make a related interpretation about the wife's reaction to her husband's behavior and how it related to her behavior with him and perhaps to her earlier interactions with her father.

The individual patient, hearing the therapist's interpretation alone, may integrate it in such a way that his behavior toward his wife changes. The couple hearing the family therapist's interpretation together can use it to jointly understand and shift their interaction. A therapist using a family-of-origin approach might ask the husband and wife to bring in their parents for a family-of-origin session, so that they could deal with unresolved conflict directly with their families rather than playing it out with each other. In that way, the larger family system is used as a resource instead of a source of aggravation.

The model of psychopathology underlying family treatment is quite different from other forms of intervention. The family model is based on the assumption that personality development, symptom formation, and therapeutic change result, at least in part, from the family's function as an interdependent transactional unit. The individual psychopathology model is based on the view that these factors are determined largely by the dynamic, intrapsychic function of the individual. If one takes a psychodynamic point of view (or a biologic point of view), the individual has been the major focus of attention. In contrast, Schatzman[20] states in his critique of the individual model that although this model is helpful, it is ultimately inadequate for understanding how people affect one another:

> *Psychoanalytic theory cannot render intelligible someone's disturbed experience or behavior in terms of disturbing behavior by someone else on that person. In order to comprehend a relationship between two individuals—husband and wife, mother and child, or father and son—we must take into account that each individual experiences the world and originates behavior. Of course, psychoanalysts know that other persons' experiences act upon their patients and that certain persons who dealt with their patients as children influenced them greatly by their behavior. But insofar as psychoanalysts speak of object relations, their theory does not adequately account for this influence.*

Schatzman's formulation (although somewhat dated) can be related to other therapeutic models. Modern biopsychiatry is concerned with the biologic correlates of emotional disorders, whereas personality psychology and the psychotherapies are concerned with individual psychodynamics and their relation to mental disorders. Family therapy is concerned primarily with the relationships among persons and how these family relationships and disruptions are linked both to physical and mental disorders of individuals and to larger contexts in the community.

CLINICAL PRACTICE IMPLICATIONS

"Thinking family" can help clinicians become aware of the need to include "family" into the assessment and treatment room. For a patient, "family" might mean their case worker, their AA sponsor, their neighbor, or church leader. Including family deepens the formulation, and provides more opportunity for intervention and therefore a successful outcome. Little training is needed for simple family inclusion except to "think family."

For more extensive family involvement, family psychoeducation which includes the ability to support family emotional responses as well as education about the specific illness, is a more sophisticated intervention but can be taught in about 6 hours, according to McFarlane.[21] Multifamily psychoeducation is especially helpful for targeted illnesses.[22]

The most sophisticated family intervention is systemic family therapy which requires more intensive training with supervision over time. Nevertheless, it is highly effective treatment for many illnesses.[23]

SUGGESTED READINGS

Heru AM. *Working with Families in Medical Settings*. Routledge; 2013.

Heru AM. The context of our lives; 2022. Clinical Psychiatric News. https://www.mdedge.com/psychiatry/article/252824/neurology/context-our-lives

REFERENCES

1. Gurman AS, Kniskern DP. Research on marital and family therapy: progress, perspective and prospect. In: Garfield SL, Bergin AE, eds. *Handbook of Psychotherapy and Behavior Change: An Empirical Analysis*. 2nd ed. John Wiley & Sons; 1978.
2. Wells RA, Dezen AE. The results of family therapy revisited: the nonbehavioral methods. *Fam Process*. 1978;17:251–274.
3. Substance Abuse and Mental Health Services Administration. National Consensus Conference on Mental Health Recovery and Systems Transformation. Department of Health and Human Services; 2005.
4. Rait D, Glick I. Reintegrating family therapy training in psychiatric residency programs: making the case. *Acad Psychiatry*. 2008;32:76–80.
5. President's New Freedom Commission on Mental Health. *Achieving the Promise: Transforming Mental Health Care in the United States*. Department of Health and Human Services Publication No. SMA-03-3832; 2003.
6. Office of the Assistant Deputy Under Secretary for Health. *A Comprehensive VHA Strategic Plan for Mental Health Services*. Veterans Health Administration Mental Health Strategic Plan; 2004.
7. Rolland J, Walsh F. Systemic training for healthcare professionals: the Chicago center for family health approach. *Fam Process*. 2005;44:283–301.
8. Heru AM. Family psychiatry: from research to practice. *Am J Psychiatry*. 2006;163:962–968.
9. Von Bertalanffy L. *General Systems Theory*. George Braziller; 1968.
10. Gray W, Duhl FJ, Rizzo ND. *General Systems Theory and Psychiatry*. Little, Brown; 1969:7.
11. Anonymous. Towards the differentiation of a self in one's own family. In: Framo JL, ed. *Family Interaction: A Dialogue Between Family Researchers and Family Therapists*. Springer; 1972:111–166.
12. Engel G. The clinical application of the biopsychosocial model. *Am J Psychiatry*. 1980;137:535–544.
13. Minuchin S. *Families and Family Therapy*. Harvard University Press; 1974.
14. Wiener N. *Cybernetics or Control and Communication in the Animal and the Machine*. MIT Press; 1948.
15. Jackson DD. The question of family homeostasis. *Psychiatr Q Suppl*. 1957;31:79–90.
16. Minuchin S, Baker L, Rosman B, Liebman R, Milman L, Todd TC. A conceptual model of psychosomatic illness in children. *Arch Gen Psychiatry*. 1975;32:1031–1038.
17. Strauss JS, Hafez H, Lieberman P, Harding CM. The course of psychiatric disorder, III: longitudinal principles. *Am J Psychiatry*. 1985;142:289–296.
18. Hoffman L. A co-evolutionary framework for systemic family therapy. In: Hansen JC, Keeney BP, eds. *Diagnosis and Assessment in Family Therapy, The Family Therapy Collections*. Aspen; 1983:42.
19. Lewis JM. For better or worse: interpersonal relationships and individual outcome. *Am J Psychiatry*. 1998;155:582–589.
20. Schatzman M. The Schreber case. *Fam Process*. 1975;14:594–598.
21. McFarlane WR. *Multifamily Groups in the Treatment of Severe Psychiatric Disorders*. Guilford Press; 2002.
22. Libbon R, Rothberg B, Baker S, Heru A. Multifamily group psychotherapy for patients with nonepileptic seizures and their families. *Am J Psychother*. 2023;76(2):62–68.
23. von Sydow K, Beher S, Schweitzer J, Retzlaff R. The efficacy of systemic therapy with adult patients: a meta-content analysis of 38 randomized controlled trials. *Fam Process*. 2010;49(4):457–485.

2 Family Life in Historical and Sociological Perspective

OBJECTIVES FOR THE READER

- To understand how family structure and family function evolve over time
- To recognize the importance of ethnicity and culture in families
- To appreciate how immigration affects families
- To understand the role of the family life cycle in family life

For easier reading, we emphasize that the descriptors "couples" or "marital" are used nearly interchangeably in this chapter.

INTRODUCTION

An understanding of evolving family structures is important for all mental health professionals. Understanding how ethnicity, culture, and social changes shape families and guide treatment. It is important to identify variations in cultures and societies. One often assumes that the family forms we grew up with are the "normal," or "correct," family forms, when instead they are simply a product of a specific time and place. Family and cultural differences have implications for treating families. This chapter includes the impact of immigration on families. Immediate, extended, and stepfamilies, kinship networks, and families of choice are included in the term "family." Families move through the family life cycle as parents age and children mature. Understanding where a family is in their family life cycle provides a frame for family therapy.

THE FAMILY IN EARLY CIVILIZATIONS
STRUCTURE AND FUNCTION OF THE AMERICAN FAMILY
IMMIGRATION
ETHNICITY
Examples of Ethnicity versus Race
Internalized and Structural Racism
SECULAR VIEW OF MARRIAGE
STRUCTURES OF MARRIAGE
DIVORCE
THE FUNCTIONAL SINGLE-PARENT FAMILY
STEPFAMILIES
LGBTQ (LESBIAN, GAY, BISEXUAL, TRANSGENDER, QUEER) COUPLES
POLYAMORY

PARENTING IN POSTMODERN RELATIONSHIPS
FAMILY TYPES
Culture and Race
SOCIAL CLASS
AGING OF THE POPULATION
THE CHANGING FAMILY LIFE CYCLE
CLINICAL PRACTICE IMPLICATIONS

THE FAMILY IN EARLY CIVILIZATIONS

In early civilizations, people found food through hunting and gathering while men went out in search of animals, women remained near the campsite to care for the children. Women also trained the children in the culture of the group.

When civilization developed, men gave up hunting and became farmers, but women continued some of the farming. Men were responsible for farming and for making metal products such as weapons. Women were responsible for managing the family and for making, in the home, items necessary for survival. Women also probably invented pottery and weaving.

Religion was important in the lives of early families. Early people believed in many gods and in the unseen forces in nature.

The families in early civilizations were large. In addition to mothers, fathers, and children, they consisted of grandparents, aunts and uncles and cousins. Medical knowledge was limited and most children died as infants. When people grew older, they expected to be taken care of by their children. People looked to their relatives for help in everyday affairs.

In most early civilizations, the father was considered the head of the family. But because women were responsible for managing the family, they also had great authority—however, this authority did not extend into other areas of social activity, such as politics or religion.[1]

STRUCTURE AND FUNCTION OF THE AMERICAN FAMILY

This continent was originally settled by Native Americans. Approximately 1.5% of the U.S. population identify as having some American Indian or Alaska Native ethnicity (www.census.gov/). The majority of American Indians and Alaska Natives live in western states and in non-reservation areas. There are 564 federally recognized tribes and 100 additional state-recognized tribes, and over 200 native languages. Native Americans have a lower educational level, are more likely to be unemployed or hold low-paying jobs, and are twice as likely to live in poverty compared with the general population. They have a lower life expectancy, a higher infant mortality rate, and higher rates of adoption and foster care placement than any other segment of the population. The attempt of early settlers to "civilize" the Native Americans resulted in their experiencing multiple traumas of social, economic, and political injustices. The intergenerational repercussions of these traumas still resonate.

Tribal elders provide guidance and direction to their community. Loyalty to the group is more important than the individuality of each member. Family members are expected to share and care for other family members. Grandparents are key decision-makers and may have a central role in parenting. Children are controlled by shaming and teasing. Developmentally disabled people are considered "special," and encounter little rejection and stigma. When children mature, they are not expected to separate from their family. Taking care of an elder is a continuation of the custom of lifelong care for family. Elders prefer to stay at home in their communities, despite the lack of appropriate services. In general, Native Americans do not differentiate psychological symptoms from physical symptoms. The most significant mental health concerns are depression, substance use, suicide, and anxiety including posttraumatic stress disorder (PTSD). Traditional healers are consulted at the same time as Western practitioners. A strong identification with culture, a sense of family, an enduring spirit, a connection with the past, and wisdom of the elders are recognized strengths of Native American communities.

IMMIGRATION

In the 1600s, European immigrants, who were predominantly of Catholic and Protestant religions, brought their beliefs about family life and structure to the New World. Their family life was based mostly on religious beliefs and practice and on the traditional "productive" view of marriage. Marriage was considered as a strategic alliance between families to strengthen family ties and acquire or keep land within the family. Today, immigrants bring with them their own, perhaps unfamiliar, family structures and practices. They bring assumptions, values, and behaviors about family life. Family members assimilate at different speeds. Many immigrant families experience conflict when Americanized children do not want to comply with the traditions of their parents who then feel that their culture and tradition are being disrespected. Immigrants may hold differing views on marriage, gender, parenting, and religious practices. For example, marriage may be arranged, take place across nations and continents, and be of mixed race or ethnicity. A social justice approach focuses on the racism and discrimination that is common in the life of immigrants. Therapy that acknowledges these complexities is helpful.

A postmodern term, "transnationalism," describes a new way of thinking about family relationships that extend across national boundaries and cultures.[2] Transnationalism describes the pattern of immigration that allows strong connection between family members in their country of origin and in the United States. In these families, children may be parented by parents, grandparents, or other extended family members and may move back and forth between countries. Money also travels across borders and American dollars frequently support poorer relatives back home. Family members use Skype, often daily, to connect with the matriarch or patriarch who urges the family members to remain true to the culture of their home country. We still need to improve our understanding of global family life, how relationships evolve over long distances, and how to develop systemic and transnational interventions for family separations and reunifications.

ETHNICITY

In the 2020 Census, new questions were created to more accurately assess the concept of race alone, race in combination, and race alone or in combination. The 2020 Census showed that nearly all population groups gained since 2010, with the exception of White alone, which decreased by 8.6% since 2010. The largest increase was in the Two or More Races population (the Multiracial population), by 276%.

The category noted as "Some Other Race alone or in combination group" increased to 49.9 million, surpassing the Black or African American population (46.9 million) as the second-largest race alone or in combination group. The next largest racial populations were the Asian alone or in combination group (24 million), the American Indian and Alaska Native alone or in combination group (9.7 million), and the Native Hawaiian and Other Pacific Islander alone or in combination group (1.6 million). The Hispanic or Latino population, which includes people of any race, increased to 62.1 million. Of note, the 2020 census changed the way information was gathered about people of Hispanic origin and race.

Race and ethnicity are two concepts related to human ancestry. Race is defined as "a category of humankind that shares certain distinctive physical traits." The term ethnicities is more broadly defined as "large groups of people classed according to common racial, national, tribal, religious, linguistic, or cultural origin or background." "Race" is usually associated with biology and linked with physical characteristics such as skin color or hair texture. "Ethnicity" is linked with cultural expression and identification. However, both are social constructs used to categorize and characterize seemingly distinct populations. Neither race nor ethnicity is detectable in the human genome.

According to the American Anthropological Association "the 'racial' worldview was invented to assign some groups to perpetual low status, while others were permitted access to privilege, power, and wealth. The tragedy in the United States has been that the policies and practices stemming from this worldview succeeded all too well in constructing unequal populations among Europeans, Native Americans, and peoples of African descent."

Scientific research demonstrates that racism, prejudice against someone because of their race and a belief in the inherent superiority and inferiority of different racial groups, affects biology, health, and well-being. Institutional and structural inequities (racism) that have emerged in tandem with such beliefs in European colonial contexts are among the most damaging elements in human societies.

Examples of Ethnicity versus Race

When Italian, Irish, and Eastern European immigrants began arriving in the United States, they weren't considered part of the White race and entered as "non-White" immigrants.

Two people might identify their ethnicity as American, yet one is a Black person and the other is White. A person born of Asian descent growing up in Britain might identify racially as Asian and ethnically as British. An Indian-American woman might display her ethnicity by wearing a sari, or she could conceal it by wearing Western garb.

Ethnicity is fluid and crosses racial lines: Born in Korea to Korean parents, but adopted by an Italian family in Italy. Ethnically, she feels Italian, speaks Italian, knows Italian history and culture, and knows nothing about Korean history and culture. When in the United States, classified racially as "Asian."

Internalized and Structural Racism

The American Association of Biological Anthropologists Statement on Race and Racism published in the *American Journal of Physical Anthropology* (2019;169(3):400–402) includes the following comments: While human racial groups are not biologic categories, "race" as a social reality—as a way of structuring societies and experiencing the world—is very real. The racial groups we recognize in the West have been socially, politically, and legally constructed over the last five centuries. They developed in tandem with European colonial expansion and the emergence of American and European societies with well-documented histories of being shaped and structured by racial hierarchies, power inequities, economic exploitation, dispossession, displacement, genocide, and institutional racism. These practices are rooted in assumptions of innate, natural differences between Europeans and other peoples, and systems of racial classification are intimately tied to histories of European settler colonialism, empire, and slavery. Classifying human beings into different races has never been wholly innocent, unbiased, or apolitical; racial classification has long served to justify exploitation, oppression, discrimination, and structural racism.

The Smithsonian Museum of African American History and Culture: Racial identity, however, is very real. And, in a racialized society like the United States, everyone is assigned a racial identity whether they are aware of it or not. Institutional racism is the policies and practices within institutions that benefit White people to the disadvantage of people of color. An example of institutional racism is how children of color are treated within the U.S. education system. On average, children of color are disciplined more harshly than their White peers. They are also less likely to be identified as gifted and have less access to quality teachers.

The Smithsonian National Museum of the American Indian: American Indians devised and have always lived under a variety of complex systems of government. Tribal governments faced rapid and devastating change as a result of European colonization and the development of the United States. Tribes today still govern their own affairs and maintain a government-to-government relationship with the United States and other governments. Today, tribal governments operate under self-chosen traditional or constitution-based governmental structures. Based on treaties, laws, and court decisions, they operate as sovereign nations within the United States, enacting and enforcing laws and managing judicial systems, social well-being, natural resources, and economic, educational, and other programs for their members. Tribal governments are also responsible for interactions with American federal, state, and municipal governments.

Long before European colonization, American Indians had developed a variety of complex systems of government that embodied important principles for effective rule. American Indian governments and leaders interacted, recognized each other's sovereignty, practiced diplomacy, built strategic alliances, waged wars, and negotiated peace accords.

After 1492, American Indians suffered diseases and genocidal events that resulted in death on a catastrophic scale and the rapid decimation of Native populations. These episodes greatly compromised the continuity of existing tribal government structures. A variety of political, economic, legal, military, and social policies were used by Europeans and Americans to remove and relocate American Indians and to destroy their cultures. U.S. policies regarding American Indians were the result of major national debate. Many of these policies had a devastating effect on established American Indian governing principles and systems. Other policies sought to strengthen and restore tribal self-government.

SECULAR VIEW OF MARRIAGE

Marriage can be described as religious or secular. A religious marriage is one sanctioned by a specific religion. In the Catholic Church, marriage is considered one of the seven sacraments. A secular or nonreligious view of the institution of marriage considers how marriage is shaped by social and economic forces. A traditional or "productive" marriage is based on a division of labor. Usually the male works outside the home and the female works in the home, caring for her husband and children and the running of the house. In the traditional or productive marriage, marriage is functional, and each partner is expected to fulfill role obligations which are associated with gender roles. Marital failure, in this model, is synonymous with role failure. In this model, a known set of role functions is expected if one accepts marriage; if a person does not want to perform these functions, then they may decide not to marry. If love occurs in a traditional marriage, it is frequently not the essential requirement in the decision to marry; rather, a potential partner is chosen based on their ability to perform role functions (e.g., will he be a good provider? or will she be a good mother?).

In contrast to traditional marriages, hedonic or companionate marriage occurs when people who marry are of similar age, educational background, and perhaps occupation. The hedonic marriage suits people who seek a companion, and thrives when time and resources are available to enjoy companionable life. Same-sex marriages make sense when considered in this broad frame. Supporting this conception is the fact that couples who have married in recent years are more likely to stay together than their parents' generation. The companionate style of marriage can be viewed from a process perspective; that is, how the marriage works. Communication and negotiation skills are vital in companionate marriage, and it is important that each partner knows what they want from the marriage. Roles in the companionate marriage are created by the partners so that role competency is more difficult to evaluate, and marital failure is synonymous with a poor relationship rather than role or gender incompetency. Within the companionate model, wide discrepancies in power and influence can occur but the key concepts are love and choice. The partners in companionate marriages have high expectations of each other and the relationship, and disappointment can occur when romance settles into routine and the relationship is no longer exciting. Marital enrichment workshops have evolved to help partners work on maintaining a fulfilling companionate marriage.

Romance is thought to be both essential and inessential to marriage; depending on the purpose of the marriage. Henry Grunebaum[3] states that we do not have control over our feelings of romantic/erotic love, that these feelings occur relatively infrequently during most people's lives, that being with a partner whom one loves, is valued and regarded as a good, that it sometimes conflicts with other values and goods, and that although love is regarded as one essential basis for marriage, other qualities and capacities are important in sustaining a long-term relationship such as a marriage. He states that, currently, the greatest demand we make is that marriage should combine passion and stability, romance and monogamy, transports of tenderness and excitement from the person who will also perform the many mundane tasks of daily living. In other words, meld everyday love with romantic/erotic love.

STRUCTURES OF MARRIAGE

In the first half of the 20th century, the typical family life cycle included a long courtship and a long-term marriage. In the second part of the 20th century in Western countries, women gained access to education and birth control, changing their expectations of marriage and family life. Prior to this, college-educated women were less likely to choose to marry and men did not consider educated independent women as suitable home makers. The high divorce rate among those who married in the 1970s reflects growing discontent with this model of marriage. After the 1960s, serial long-term relationships became more common, resulting in the creation of serial families.

Serial long-term relationships may mean marriage or cohabitation. Cohabitation has become normative in the United States, although in other parts of the world, cohabitation has been common for centuries. Couples cohabit for many reasons, ranging from convenience to a trial marriage to a permanently committed relationship for emotional or economic reasons. Although the basic tasks of couple coalition are present, by definition, cohabitation implies less agreement on beliefs about permanence. When relationships are less stable, separation is more common.

Separation in the early stages of a relationship occurs when infatuation dies. Separation is more likely when a relationship is based on shaky footing, such as unplanned pregnancy, to get away from the parental home, or in desperation about an inability to ever attract anyone else. Other reasons for separation include difficulty coping with chronic illness, personality disorder, substance misuse, violence, mistreatment, or incompatibility. Incompatibility can occur when there is skewed individual development or when the children leave home and there is little emotional or functional viability left in the marriage.

DIVORCE

Divorce is painful. Divorce is a process with its own developmental path.[4,5]

1. A predivorce phase of growing disillusionment and dissatisfaction.
2. Separation phase with emotional distress, confusion, and grief.
3. Reorganization phase (1 to 2 years) of life structure, parenting issues, financial and family, and legal issues. Negative life stresses are most marked during the first 2 years following divorce. Children are most likely to experience diminished parenting during this period because of the parents' preoccupation with divorce issues. Children are likely to respond with noncompliant, angry, demanding, or depressed behavior.
4. Reforming an identity as a single person. The sense of narcissistic injury may be profound for one or both partners. Later events may include fierce fighting over custody, money, or the story of what went wrong—this fighting may serve the purpose of punishment or revenge, or it may

be a way of staying connected to the spouse. For many spouses, attachment may last long after love or respect is gone, leading to confusing attempts to reconnect. The process of coming to grips with the self, recognizing one's own part in the marital dissolution, and beginning to date again often provokes a great deal of anxiety. Regardless of how bad the marriage was for both spouses, many divorced people find that the transition to living alone is very painful.

During the first 2 years, children of both sexes are apt to exhibit problem behavior; boys may exhibit problems for a longer period of time than girls. Adolescent girls may have problems with precocious sexual behavior. Situations likely to lead to more severe problems include postmarital fighting between all the adults over the children, persistent custody battles, disappearance of or irregular contact with the noncustodial parent, poverty due to a decrease in income in a single-parent family, and lack of parental supervision.

THE FUNCTIONAL SINGLE-PARENT FAMILY

Families with only one responsible adult may decrease the hierarchical structure common to two-parent families and give the children more power and responsibility. Some parents, particularly fathers, may find themselves closer to their children than they were before because they are directly responsible for the daily care of their children for the first time. In other cases, particularly those of mothers with no financial or family support, the need to work full time may decrease the parent's time with and energy for the children. Single-parent households formed after a divorce or a death go through a transition period during which family structures have to be reformed. Evaluation of the effect of an absent spouse on the rest of the family unit must take into account the phase of family development during which the absence occurred, the length of the absence, the feelings of the remaining family members about the absent member, and the mechanisms the family has used in coping with its reconfiguration.

The effectiveness of parenting depends on the qualities of the specific parent. Being the only parent, or the only custodial/residential parent, creates family issues that may include the following:

- Social isolation and loneliness of the parent
- Difficulty dating with jealousy from the children
- Demands by small children for the continuous physical presence of the sole parent
- Children fending for themselves and carrying a greater share of the domestic responsibilities because the sole parent is working
- Less opportunity for a parent to discuss pros and cons of decisions and to get support and feedback when decisions are made
- Crises and shifts caused by the introduction of a potential new mate or companion

STEPFAMILIES

A stepfamily system is composed of many people: the remarried family plus former spouses, grandparents, aunts, uncles, and others who may have significant input into the remarried family system. The children are part of each of their biologic parents' household systems. The system has permeable (i.e., open) boundaries, and input from significant others can have a marked effect on the remarried family's viability and functioning.

Stepfamilies must manage the following:

- The impact of loss and change.
- Incongruent individual, marital, and family life cycles. For example, if a 55-year-old man with two grandchildren marries a 35-year-old woman with two young children, he may be a grandfather, a new husband, and a new father all at once.

- Children and adults all come to the stepfamily with a history of experiences and convictions from previous families, leading to differences of opinion that must be resolved so that new traditions can be established.
- Parent–child relationships predate the new couple relationship. A couple bond and new relationships with others in the stepfamily must be developed consciously.
- Cooperative parenting relationships between biologic parents.
- Children are often members of two households, and everyone must cope with shifting household composition and complicated relationships. Children are frequently caught in loyalty conflicts.
- There is little or no legal relationship between the stepparent and stepchildren, so that there is a perceived risk in forming new relationships with little legal and societal support.

Forming new relationships and finding solutions to stepfamily challenges take time. Teenagers take longer than younger children. In general, stepfamilies start from a position in which the adults expect everything to go smoothly—the so-called fantasy stage. The adults try to make the fantasy come true, but as a rule, there are tense times, and stepparents start to feel that something must be wrong with them and the way they are feeling and doing things. When things go wrong the family splits along biologic lines and pressures build. Getting past this stage is difficult and takes time and understanding. As things become clearer and the two adults begin to work together as a parenting team, changes take place in the household so that biologic divisions begin to blur. The stepparent becomes an "intimate outsider." A stepparent can develop multiple types of relationships with a stepchild: friend, "aunt" or "uncle," or parent. Mastering difficult interpersonal situations increases self-esteem for both children and adults. Everyone has a basic human need for belonging to an accepting group, receiving individual support from someone who really cares about them, and having some control over their life. Those families that work out ways of satisfying these needs will become integrated more quickly.

LGBTQ (LESBIAN, GAY, BISEXUAL, TRANSGENDER, QUEER) COUPLES

America's families are changing. Public discussion about American families often assumes the nation is largely made up of married heterosexual couples raising their biologic children. In fact, Census Bureau data show that less than a quarter of all U.S. households fall into this category. Today, just 69% of children live with married, heterosexual parents, down from 83% in 1970. Today's children may be raised by grandparents, single parents, stepparents, aunts, uncles, or foster parents. Their parents may be married or unmarried or belong to the LGBTQ (lesbian, gay, bisexual, transgender, and queer) community. Currently, between 2 million and 2.8 million children are being raised by LGBTQ parents, with 24% of female same-sex couples and 11% of male same-sex couples are raising children. A recent survey of transgender Americans finds that 38% identify as parents.

Overall, LGBTQ families are more racially and ethnically diverse than married, heterosexual couples raising children. Same-gender couples with children are more likely to include people of color in their families and 59% of same-sex couples with children identify as White compared to 73% of married heterosexual couples with children. Similarly, 55% of children raised by same-sex couples are White compared to 70% of children raised by married heterosexual couples. Reflecting trends in the broader population, same-sex couples of color raising children are more likely to be poor, than White same-sex couples raising children. Information about families headed by transgender parents is limited, but it is known that transgender people face economic challenges with rates of extreme poverty being four times that of the general population.

LGBTQ families are geographically dispersed, living in 93% of all U.S. counties. States like California and New York have high numbers of same-sex couples, yet same-sex couples are most likely to raise children in Mississippi, followed by Wyoming, Alaska, Arkansas, Texas, Louisiana, Oklahoma, Kansas, Alabama, Montana, South Dakota, and South Carolina. Historically LGBTQ families have existed outside of the legal framework as states only recently began to pass legislation recognizing same-sex couples. In 2015, the U.S. Supreme Court made its landmark Obergefell v. Hodges decision that the U.S. Constitution guarantees same-sex couples the right to marry. However, in 2023, state legislatures have introduced more than 400 antitransgender bills. About 100 failed in the legislature, but more than 60 have passed. There are also dozens of other anti-LGBTQ bills targeting gay and lesbian rights and bills attempting to limit any discussion of sexuality at school. Recent research has highlighted the impact of the sociopolitical context on LGBTQ parent families, citing events such as the Trump Presidency, the COVID-19 pandemic, and racial justice movement. Pervasive stigma and discrimination toward families headed by LGBTQ parents remains.

The LGBTQ community remains strong and reflects the fact that many LGBTQ individuals are ostracized from their family and friends, and has been actively creating support networks for decades. LGBTQ parents and their children fare better when they have adequate resources and when they live in supportive environments. LGBTQ parents and their children do not differ in well-being or in multiple developmental outcomes from parents and children in the general population. Despite the improvement in the legal climate in the United States for LGBTQ people and their families, significant legal and practical difficulties remain, including greater poverty.

LGBTQ people take many paths to parenthood. Some pursue parenthood using assisted reproductive technologies such as donor insemination or surrogacy. Donors and surrogates may be friends or relatives, or they may provide services through a clinic and remain unknown to the family. Other LGBTQ individuals become parents through adoption or serve as foster parents. Still others may conceive via sexual intercourse with a different-sex partner.

Research shows that despite the diversity of paths to parenthood, positive adjustment among the children is found, across varying ages and several domains of child development. Children of transgender parents have also been found to be well adjusted, and family processes have been found to be more important to individual and family outcomes than parents' gender identity or expression. Qualitative work has also revealed important strengths among members of transgender parent families, such as adaptive strategies for navigating parental disclosure of gender identities.

Among diverse LGBTQ-parent family forms, lesbian and gay stepfamily arrangements formed post heterosexual relationship dissolution represent the most common form. Early studies with mothers who came out as lesbians showed that they were just as likely to have good mental health and positive relationships with their children as were heterosexual mothers, and that their children were no more likely to show emotional and behavioral difficulties, poor performance at school, or atypical gender role behavior than were children with heterosexual parents. In the last two decades, some longitudinal studies have been conducted with adoptive lesbian- and gay-parent families confirming that the quality of family processes and the stigmatization occurring in the outside world are more relevant to child adjustment than family structure.

The negative experiences of children of lesbian and/or gay parents with regard to homophobic teasing or bullying from peers, can be countered when school curricula and policies are explicitly inclusive of them. Founded in 1973, PFLAG is the first and largest organization dedicated to supporting, educating, and advocating for LGBTQ+ people and their families. LGBTQ individuals and families may cause tension with members of members of their family of origin.

Lastly, it is important to acknowledge the destruction to the LGBTQ+ community by the AIDS epidemic from the 1970s until 1999. More than 267,500 men are estimated to have died, leaving behind families torn apart by symptoms of trauma, grief, and loss.

POLYAMORY

Due to our longer life span, it is more challenging to remain sexually exclusive with a single partner for an entire lifetime. Serial monogamy has become common, where people partner with one person for a period of time, break up, re-partner with someone else, break up, and re-partner again. Other arrangements include maintaining multiple concurrent partners.

Polyamory, or consensual nonmonogamy (CNM), is in a resurgence, CNM is in its third wave in the United States, having started with the anarchists of the 1880s and enjoyed a robust resurgence in the 1960s. Its current wave is the most socially significant and widespread, partly as the result of internet access. CNM is the practice of having multiple intimate relationships, whether sexual or just romantic, with the full knowledge and consent of all parties involved. Polyamory is not gender specific; anyone can have multiple partners of any gender. Some polyamorous people have a primary relationship and engage in casual hookups, but most begin secondary relationships with the consent of their primary partner, to whom they are generally married or committed. Introducing a secondary partner requires the primary couple to agree on a set of stipulations, such as date, times, and the type of intimacy allowed. Research has found that, despite the complications, polyamory offers benefits ranging from greater satisfaction and extra help with childcare to increased relationship commitment. The American Psychological Association's Division 44 has developed tow evidence-based resources on CNM (https://www.div44cnm.org/).

Polyamory is not to be confused with polygamy which is a marital arrangement in which one person has multiple spouses. This can be polygyny, where one man has various wives, or polyandry, where one woman has multiple husbands. Polygamous relationships have been practiced in different cultures around the world, though it is currently illegal in many countries, including the United States, due to concerns about power imbalances and potential abuse.

PARENTING IN POSTMODERN RELATIONSHIPS

Blended families are common with children from prior marriages and prior relationships either living full or part time in the home. Linda Burton highlights the role of "othermothers" in raising children in low-income families. Othermothering is a form of co-parenting, distinct from stepparenting. Othermothers take care of children that are their romantic partners' children from previous and concurrent relationships. Compared to stepfamilies, these multiple-partner fertility relationships are more prevalent among young couples with limited financial resources, contentious relationships, and relationships characterized by serial childbearing through serial repartnering. This style of co-parenting helps the biologic parents of relatives and friends who have limited social and psychological capital, with the goal of protecting and raising "good children."[6] It is important that we approach family arrangements and structures that we find "different" with an open mind, looking for the strengths that are often present but not recognized or given voice.

About 2% of children under 18 years of age are adopted. Many children are adopted from overseas, resulting in families of mixed ethnicities. Parents of transracially adopted children have to help their children confront racism openly and learn about the culture of their biologic parents. Transracial adoptees aren't necessarily motivated to learn about their birth cultures, but it is helpful for family therapists to support a continuous effort in parents. Although most adoptees are well adjusted, children placed after infancy, or who have experienced multiple changes in caregivers and/or who were abused or neglected prior to adoption placement, are more vulnerable. Compared to nonadopted peers, adopted children experience more emotional, behavioral, and academic problems.[7] Positive social and emotional adjustment in adopted children is facilitated by openness about adoption.

Sexual identities (including gender identity, gender-role behavior, and sexual orientation) develop in the same way in all children. The development, adjustment, and well-being of children with lesbian and gay parents are no different from that of children with heterosexual parents (http://www.apa.org/about/policy/parenting.aspx). Adoption and fostering children are more common in LGBT couples and childrearing among same-sex couples is most common in Southern, Mountain West, and Midwest (content/uploads/LGBT-Parenting.pdf). These families are also more likely to be poor.

In a society that sees gender as a binary concept, raising a child who has gender nonconformity can be a challenge. Most parents are supportive of their child, and consider their child psychologically healthy but having a social problem. Some parents react very negatively and gender nonconformity can become a significant source of conflict between parents and result in disconnection between parent and child. Whether accepting or struggling, parents need to nurture their child's sense of self as well as help with their adjustment to social realities. Parents can advocate for flexibility of gender norms in their families, schools, and community.

FAMILY TYPES

Culture and Race

It is important to develop a strong working alliance when ethnic or racial differences are present. Patients may hide their reactions from the psychiatrist out of culturally sanctioned beliefs such as fear of rejection if there is a disagreement or through deference to authority. Patients and families may also get angry if they feel slighted or misunderstood. Well-meaning therapists may hold egalitarian beliefs but may not be aware of subtle negative attitudes and stereotypes about people of color or may not have had sufficient contact with people different from themselves. Strategies to reduce bias and to promote a healthy and constructive therapeutic alliance include increasing awareness of possible negative attitudes, immersing oneself in other cultural experiences, working hard to stay attuned to patients, demonstrating cultural empathy, and being respectful and open to alternative worldviews.

Historical racism may interfere with an African American patient's seeking treatment. Ethnic minority populations underutilize psychotherapy services and have high rates of dropping out of treatment. Dovidio et al.[8] demonstrated in a series of studies that contemporary racism among Caucasians is subtle, often unintentional, and unconscious. White physicians may display negative body language (less eye contact, voice tone not as warm or natural) in response to those who are different from themselves. Caucasians who demonstrate these behaviors report not being aware of negative attitudes toward them in studies that examined these interactions. A genogram can be used to explore how the family understands culture difference and ethnicity and can also be used as a training tool for therapists.

It is always important to recognize that "cultural" issues can sometimes be best understood as family problems that need to be resolved. For example, Mrs. J, who is Catholic, and Mr. J, who is Jewish, fought about how to celebrate the December holidays. Exploration revealed that neither member of the couple had been very religious before marriage and had seldom celebrated holidays. However, when Mrs. J's father died and her mother became depressed, Mrs. J began to spend more time with her mother, a very religious woman, and was less available to her husband. Conflict over her return to her family of origin was being expressed by the couple through their inability to compromise over religious rituals.

Cultural competence means being aware of one's own attitudes, being knowledgeable about cultural issues, and having the clinical skills to understand the cultural context of the patient's concerns. Establishing rapport with a patient can be enhanced by listening to the patient's story. Demonstrating humility and concern can also be effective in this regard, although the former is not a common physician characteristic. Self-reflection regarding personal, institutional, internalized, and subtle forms of bias is an important part of cultural competence in general. Cultural competence training requires both general attitudinal approaches and specific advice based on cultural aspects of minority life. Some teachers, concerned about stereotyping, discourage the knowledge approach to cultural competence training and argue that cultural humility is superior to cultural competence. Cultural competence education should be tailored for the ethnic and racial minorities that are present in the community served by specific health care providers. However, when faced with an unfamiliar culture, the therapist can ask the family members to talk about their culture and what important information the therapist should know in order to be of help. This position of naivete helps engage the family and encourages a sense of competence in the family.

SOCIAL CLASS

Society recognizes four social classes; the ruling class, which comprises 90% of the nation's wealth, professional-managerial class, where people usually have a college education, working class, where children usually complete a high school education and lastly the underclass, which consists of the disenfranchised such as the chronically unemployed, those on disability and welfare, and undocumented workers.

As a society, we focus erroneously on individuals, without giving much attention to the social structures and social context that impact and shape us. Most people stay in the income group they start life in and the single biggest determinant of one's class identity as an adult is not one's education level or job, but a parent's occupation and income. Expectations about family life are likely to be more contingent on family of origin than actual income. Someone born into a U.S. family that is White, owns property, and has a higher education level competes in our economy with clear advantage over someone who is born outside the United States, is a person of color, and has less family wealth, property, and educational opportunity. The majority of poor people in the United States are White, but because class has been racialized in the United States, a greater percentage of people of color live in poverty. Poverty and unemployment rates for African-Americans, Latinos, and Native Americans are more than double that of White Americans (www.census.gov/).

Many families have experienced downward mobility due to the current changing economic times and have associated feelings of shame, worthlessness, and helplessness. A loss of job means loss of health insurance, house, and perhaps support from family and friends. A family without financial resources can quickly find itself in poverty and homeless. The impact of chronic medical or psychiatric illness is associated with a fight for disability status that can at least provide a basic income.

Social class determines expectations about financial support from parents, when independence from parents is expected, who is a suitable marital partner, and help with childcare. Marriage across classes can lead to family conflicts about expectations and aspirations that may need to be clearly articulated in therapy. (For a detailed discussion about social class and family life, read Kliman, 2011.[9])

AGING OF THE POPULATION

The population aged 65 and older is expected to reach 92.0 million in 2060, representing just over one in five U.S. residents. Those people who are 85 and older are projected to reach 18.2 million (www.census.gov). A greater life expectancy affects family life by increasing the number of multigenerational families and increasing the number of family caregivers. The majority of caregivers are middle-aged women, who are also caring for children. They are referred to as the "sandwich generation." There are also over 1.3 million children who are caregivers (www.caregiving.org/data/youngcaregivers.pdf), usually caring for a parent or grandparent. More than 50% of the child caregivers helped with bathing, dressing, and toileting and all children helped with shopping, household tasks, and meal preparation. Almost all of the children (96%) stated that they keep the care recipient company. About 75% stated that they have someone else helping them.

Companion animals are regarded as family members by 85% of pet owners and attachment to pets provides many important family functions such as unconditional acceptance and support.[10] Children, especially single children and those in single family homes, appreciate the companionship and security that pets provide. Pets can be very helpful for children recovering from illness and for the elderly living alone.

Many families in the United States have been impacted by recent wars. Children and families can struggle with changes resulting from an absent parent or spouse and returning service members may have PTSD that can affect their family members adversely. How children cope with deployment and with the effects of war is dependent on the mental health of the at-home parent. Resources are available both within and outside the Veterans Administration Medical Centers to help families, including books for children and teens.[11]

THE CHANGING FAMILY LIFE CYCLE

Understanding where a family is in their life cycle is an important key to determining what the appropriate concerns are for the family. Family life stages are birth, marriage or coupling, bringing up children, launching children, retirement, illness, and death. The tasks of a young family are establishing a work career and child rearing, whereas older couples focus on retirement, looking back over their lives, coming to terms with what they have and have not been able to accomplish.

When these normal stages occur out of sequence, the family is faced with additional difficulties or adjustments. For example, if the wage earner gets sick early in the family life cycle, then the financial security of the family is jeopardized. If the wage earner becomes ill in late life, while this is still stressful, it is somewhat expected, and the children will hopefully be independent and able to provide support and care. A child is not expected to become ill, and mourning the death of a child is one of the hardest tasks of a family. When a young person develops a chronic illness such as schizophrenia, then the parents may have anticipatory grieving.

The current societal climate has brought several changes to the traditional expectations of how life progresses in the family. Launching a child used to occur at about age 18, when the young adult would marry, obtain independent employment, and establish their own life. It is not uncommon to hear of children, sometimes with their own children, returning to the parental home. This re-entry is considered temporary and the adult child continues to strive to become independent. As life span lengthens, people are choosing to continue working through their 70s or start other careers.

CLINICAL PRACTICE IMPLICATIONS

The family has maintained itself as an institution throughout history and in all recognized cultures. Postmodernism provides family therapists with a new set of theories and a new language for describing the variety of families. The traditional belief about marriage is referred to as "heteronormativity"; the belief that a viable family consists of "a heterosexual mother and a father raising heterosexual children together." Rather than focus on the gender of a partner or the assumption of particular roles, the family therapist should focus on the quality of the family relationship.[12]

Many families consist of people of different ethnicities, cultures, religion, and class, leading to a clash of values and beliefs that need to be resolved, respected and hashed out for effective family functioning. Raising children in an environment where differences are respected and tolerated is important as they will internalize how to tolerate and respect the values and beliefs of others. A family therapist can invite the family to explain and describe how the cultural and ethnic differences play out in their family.

The take-home message from this chapter for family therapists is that couples and families of different ages, ethnicity, race, gender will have very differing attitudes about intimacy, gender equality, divorce, and child rearing. The family therapist must ascertain clearly the attitudes and beliefs of the couple or family and pay special attention to the structure of that family, its goals, resources, motivation, and potentialities. Only after understanding the specifics of a particular family can the therapist begin to think about treatment. No family therapist can be expected to understand and master all the variants of family that have been covered in this chapter. The use of culturally and ethnically sensitive questions and the inclusion of expanded kinship networks will yield the best results.

In this chapter, we have discussed the variations of family life with specific attention to context and background. In Chapters 3 and 4, we begin to look at how families function.

SUGGESTED READING

This paper presents an overview of marriage and explores the complexities of the institution from historical, anthropological, legal, and sociological perspectives. We think that it is important for clinicians to be sensitive to the many dimensions of marriage as it relates to their patients.

Carone N, Bos HMW, Shenkman G, Tasker F. LGBTQ parents and their children during the family life cycle. *Front Psychol*. 2021;12.

Cheah CSL, Leung CYY, Zhou N. Understanding "Tiger Parenting" through the perceptions of Chinese immigrant mothers: can Chinese and U.S. parenting coexist? *Asian Am J Psychol*. 2013;4(1):30–40.

Falicov CJ. From rigid borderlines to fertile borderlands: reconfiguring family therapy. *J Marital Fam Ther*. 1998;24(2):157–163.

Hoff CC, Beougher SC. Sexual agreements among gay male couples. *Arch Sex Behav*. 2010;39(3):774–787.

Karasu SR. The institution of marriage: terminable or interminable? *Am J Psychother*. 2007;61(1):1–16.

Martin JL, Dean L. Effects of AIDS-related bereavement and HIV-related illness on psychological distress among gay men: a 7-year longitudinal study, 1985–1991. *J Consult Clin Psychol*. 1993;61(1):94–103.

Patterson CJ, Farr RH, Goldberg AE. *LGBTQ+ Parents and Their Children*. NCFR Policy Brief; 2021.

Sheff E. *The Polyamorists Next Door: Inside Multiple-Partner Relationships and Families*. Rowman and Littlefield; 2014.

Shernoff M. Negotiated nonmonogamy and male couples. *Fam Process*. 2006;45(4):407–418.

Watson M. *Facing the Black Shadow*. 2013. www.drmarlenefwatson.com/

REFERENCES

1. Mazour A, Peoples JM, Rabb TK. *People and Nations: A World History 1987*. Harcort Brace, Jovanovich; 1987:12–13.
2. Falicov CJ. Working with transnational immigrants: expanding meanings of family, community, and culture. *Fam Process*. 2007;46(2):157–171.
3. Grunebaum H. Thinking about romantic/erotic love. *J Marital Fam Ther*. 1997;23(3):295–307.
4. Kessler S. *The American Way of Divorce: Prescription for Change*. Nelson-Hall; 1975.
5. Salts CJ. Divorce process: integration of theory. *Journal of Divorce*. 1979;2:233–240.
6. Burton LM, Hardaway CR. Low-income mothers as "othermothers" to their romantic partners' children: women's co-parenting in multiple partner fertility relationships. *Fam Process*. 2012;51(3):343–359.

7. Keyes MA, Sharma A, Elkins IJ. The mental health of US adolescents adopted in infancy. *Arch Pediatr Adolesc Med*. 2008;162(5):419–425.
8. Dovidio JF, Glick P, Hewstone M. *The Sage Handbook of Prejudice, Stereotyping and Discrimination*. Sage Publications Ltd; 2010.
9. Kliman J. Social class and the life cycle. In: McGoldrick M, Carter EA, Garcia-Preto N, eds. *The Expanded Family Life Cycle: Individual, Family, and Social Perspectives (75-88)*. Allyn & Bacon; 2011.
10. Walsh F. Human-animal bonds I: the relational significance of companion animals. *Fam Process*. 2009; 48(4):462–480.
11. Sherman MD, Sherman DM. 2005. www.seedsofhopebooks.com/
12. Hudak J, Giammettei SV. Doing family: decentering heteronormativity in 'marriage' and 'family' therapy. *AFTA Monograph Series: Expanding our Social Justice Practices: Advances in Theory and Training*; 2010:49–58.

In the opening sentence of the book *Anna Karenina*, Tolstoy (1960) declares, "Happy families are all alike; every unhappy family is unhappy in its own way." Although one hesitates to disagree with Tolstoy, this and the next two chapters describe the ways in which functional families are alike, yet diverse, as well as the ways in which dysfunctional families are alike and yet unique.

Our bias is that to treat families, the family therapist must understand not only how families function but also how dysfunction develops. In Chapters 3 and 4, we consider the family as an organized system, its life cycle, and the family's tasks and functional characteristics as they relate to traditional and to newer, alternative family forms. In Chapter 5, we describe how dysfunctional families, which often have symptomatic members or members with problem areas, operate in these three dimensions.

Multiple models are available for understanding how families operate, but much remains to be learned. In this section, we provide information on what is known, so that readers can formulate a working model for use in clinical situations. In Section 3, we discuss the assessment of families. In Section 4, we will move on to the treatment based on the material in this section.

Section

II Functional and Dysfunctional Families

3 Understanding the Functional Family 39

4 Understanding the Functional Family in a Variety of Family Forms 55

5 Problems and Dysfunction from an Integrated Family Systems Perspective 68

3 Understanding the Functional Family

OBJECTIVES FOR THE READER

- To understand the concept of the family as a functional system
- To be able to characterize the phases of the family life cycle
- To be able to describe family structure
- To understand basic family tasks
- To understand characteristics of the functional family

For easier reading, we emphasize that the descriptors "couples" or "marital" are used nearly interchangeably in this chapter.

INTRODUCTION

There is probably little need to stress the general importance of marriage and the family. These social institutions have existed throughout recorded history and, despite the talk in some quarters about the death of the family, marriage and the family are clearly very much with us. It is also true, however, that expectations regarding marriage and the family have changed, especially when we compare the traditional American family of the 1950s with multiple current alternatives. There are a variety of accepted patterns (including cohabitation, blended families, single-parent and two- and three-generation families, same-sex marriages) but for some people, marriage and the family remains a cause for uncertainty, instability, and distress. Nevertheless, this diversity offers richness of solutions that a more rigid, unchanging pattern could not offer. As we have learned over time, some dimensions of functional families are stable, regardless of family form. All families, for example, need some form of organization, stable and clear ways of communicating, and protection for young children. The specifics, however, can vary considerably. In this chapter we try to locate the universals of family life as well as its diversity.

The frame of reference we provide for understanding the family is intended as a model for understanding what a family therapist encounters. This model will be supplemented by individual and sociologic frames of reference. Exclusion is not meant to imply that other models are unimportant, only that they are not in keeping with the general tenor of this book—that of presenting ideas of particular interest or use to the family therapist. Undoubtedly our model will not completely describe or explain the richness, complexity, and variety of marriages and families, nor will all of the categories used in our model fit precisely into every specific family system. It is hoped, however, that this material will offer a useful structure for thinking about all families, including those members in distress, who present themselves to professionals for help.

In this chapter, we examine the concept of the family as a functional system by exploring the phases of the individual, marital, and family life cycles, from courtship and early marriage to older adulthood when children have moved on and started families of their own. We also discuss the basic family tasks, including providing for basic needs and socializing children, and the evolution of characteristic beliefs and patterns of behavior among family members.

Since this is both a long chapter and a key one, we provide here an outline to guide the reader:

THE FAMILY AS A SYSTEM
THE COUPLES/MARITAL AND FAMILY LIFE CYCLE
The Individual Life Cycle
Early Adulthood
Mid-Adulthood
Older Adulthood
The Couples/Marital Life Cycle
Phase of Relationship and Tasks
Courtship and Early Marriage
Marriage in Mid-Adulthood
Marriage in Older Adulthood
Marital Coalition
Sex, Intimacy, and Companionship
The Family Life Cycle
Children and Shifts in Function
Family Structure as It Relates to the Life Cycle
FAMILY TASKS
Provision of Basic Needs
Rearing and Socialization of Children
Use of Age-Appropriate Childrearing Techniques
Maintenance of the Parental Coalition and Generational Boundaries
Sexuality
Support of a Sibling Coalition
Enculturation of Offspring
FAMILY BELIEF SYSTEMS
FAMILY RESILIENCE
CLINICAL PRACTICE IMPLICATIONS

THE FAMILY AS A SYSTEM

Families and married or unmarried couples differ from other human groups in many ways, including duration, intensity, and function of relationships. For most people, the family constitutes their most important group in relation to individual psychological development, emotional interaction, and maintenance of self-esteem. The family is a group in which they experience their strongest loves and strongest hates, enjoy their deepest satisfaction, and experience their most painful disappointments. The characteristics of the family (or couple) as a unit are different from the mere sum of its components. Knowing the attributes of all the individuals in the family is not the same as understanding the family system as an entity. **The family has a history and function of its own, the specifics of which differ from those of its individual members.**

As we discussed in Chapter 1, couples and families need to be thought of as interactive contexts in which transactions between component parts are continually taking place. From this perspective, the action of one member will affect the entire family (and vice versa). A ripple set off anywhere, internally or externally, that impinges on the family will reverberate throughout the family system.

At the same time there is a basic, underlying stability in every family that maintains each member's position within the family. The family is a system in dynamic equilibrium, oscillating between periods of relative balance and periods of disequilibrium. Family members are usually bound together by social roles, mutual support and needs, expectations, and intense and long-lasting ties of experiences. Factors are at work constantly, more or less successfully, to keep the family system in equilibrium and to keep it from undergoing a too severe or rapid change.

As we pointed out in Chapter 1, *family homeostasis* refers most generally to the concept that the family is a system designed to maintain a relatively stable state so that when the whole system or any part of it is subjected to a disequilibrating force, feedback will restore the preexisting equilibrium. However, it is often necessary for the family to move to a new equilibrium. This happens at transition points in the family's life cycle, after a major life change (e.g., if the mother goes back to work), or after a major trauma (e.g., if a family member is injured in an auto accident and cannot continue their usual roles).

If one thinks of characteristic patterns of achieving equilibrium for the family, then families can be thought of as having personalities or styles analogous to those of individuals. These styles consist of patterns of problem solving and preferred patterns of thinking, feeling, and interacting (e.g., fun loving and somewhat chaotic, organized and cheerful, angry and confusing). Studies have characterized families by their cognitive and problem-solving styles, by types of pathology, and by boundary patterns and organizational structure. No model has taken into account all variables. **The key to defining a functional family is in whether the characteristic patterns allow for flexibility and movement in response to stress (Walsh, 1993).**

For the family system to be functional, it must have certain characteristics. Walsh (1993) identified 10 processes that characterize functional families (Table 3.1). Another model is based on only three dimensions—problem solving, organization, and emotional climate. These dimensions are considered central for a rapid overview evaluation. They represent the core of the Global Assessment of Relational Functioning Scale now used in many clinical settings.[1] We discuss this scale in detail in Chapter 8.

Table 3.1 Processes that characterize functional families

1. Connectedness and commitment of members as a caring, mutually supportive relationship unit
2. Respect for individual differences, autonomy, and separate needs, fostering the development and well-being of members of each generation, from youngest to eldest
3. For couples, a relationship characterized by mutual respect, support, and equitable sharing of power and responsibilities
4. For nurturance, protection, and socialization of children and caretaking of other vulnerable family members, effective parental or executive leadership and authority
5. Organizational stability, characterized by clarity, consistency, and predictability in patterns of interaction
6. Adaptability: flexibility to meet internal or external demands for change, to cope effectively with stress and problems that arise, and to master normative and nonnormative challenges and transitions across the life cycle
7. Open communication characterized by clarity of rules and expectations, pleasurable interaction, and a range of emotional expression and empathic responsiveness
8. Effective problem-solving and conflict-resolution processes
9. A shared belief system that enables mutual trust, problem mastery, connectedness with past and future generations, ethical values, and concern for the larger human community
10. Adequate resources for basic economic security and psychosocial support in extended kin and friendship networks and from community and larger social systems

All families have conflicts, and family members' feelings toward one another may be mixed, or their love may not always be constant. Furthermore, the completely well-functioning, growing, long-term marriage is a rarity (estimated by clinicians to represent about 5% of all marriages). Different cultures place differing emphasis on certain processes listed in Table 3.1.

For example, some cultures place far more importance on the child's role as a family member than on fostering autonomy; patriarchal cultures are more interested in maintaining a clear hierarchy than in equitable sharing of power.

Most of these processes are necessary for family function, regardless of form. Focusing on the couple (as a system), Lewis[2] suggested that **the most important decision (and process) each partner in a couple makes is selecting the person they are going to spend their life with, jointly constructing a relationship.** That decision does not occur in a vacuum and is aimed not just at autonomy but, more important, at connecting intimately with others. Marriage is commonly the most important relationship for individual growth of each spouse.

THE COUPLES/MARITAL AND FAMILY LIFE CYCLE

Because a central family function is to raise children to adulthood, the system needs to ensure that various psychosocial tasks are mastered at each phase of the family life cycle. The extent to which this mastery is accomplished will depend on the individual adaptation of family members and on the flexibility and functionality of the family as a whole. Stressors during any of these phases may interfere with the accomplishment of normal developmental tasks. Although the family's ability to pass successfully from one specific developmental phase to another may depend on how prior phases have been negotiated, families sometimes find themselves better suited to meet the challenges of one phase than another. For example, a couple may be at odds in the childrearing phase of a marriage but function quite well during the post-childrearing phase.

A couple's ability to communicate clearly, to solve problems, and to have a relationship reasonably free of projection and incompatible agendas is based on the intrapsychic needs of the individuals, the reflexive behaviors they bring from their families of origin, the evolving marital dynamics, and the state of marital development. In our version of these life cycles (Tables 3.2 and 3.3), certain normative patterns of stress are determined by the individual and family life cycles described in the next sections.

A central issue in marriage is the meshing of individual needs with relationship needs. The behaviors and beliefs of dysfunctional couples tend to be more rigid than those of well-adapted couples.

The Individual Life Cycle

Issues of marital and family life are affected strongly by the age of the adult participants. One's attitudes, prospects, and emotional availability for intimacy and family life vary to some extent with age. In addition, the age at which one has children has become widely variable. Many young women have children in their teens—producing a family consisting of the teen, her child, and her parent(s). The other biologic parent may or may not be involved. The mother may choose to marry later in life. At the other end of the spectrum, many men and women are taking much longer to explore job opportunities and are marrying much later, so that a substantial number of couples do not begin their families until their 30s or 40s. Second marriages between 30- to 40-year-old women and 50- to 70-year-old men have produced a phenomenon of many men in their later years who are both grandfathers and new parents.

Adult developmental phases can be divided roughly into early adulthood (age 20 to 40 years), mid-adulthood (age 40 to 60 years), and older adulthood (age 60 years and older).

Table 3.2 The family life cycle and adult development

Early adulthood (age 20–40 y)	Mid-adulthood (age 40–60 y)	Older adulthood (age 60+ y)
Age 20–30 y	**Age 40–50 y**	**Age 60+ y**
1. Establish an independent life structure—home, friends, etc. 2. Renegotiate relationships with parents 3. Make first set of decisions around occupational choice 4. Explore intimacy/sexuality 5. Possibly deal with parenthood	1. Deal with complexities of being command generation: may be responsible for children and/or aging parents 2. Midlife transition: reevaluate life goals, work, and relationships 3. Forgive self for sins of omission and commission	1. Conduct a life review 2. Give up being command generation 3. Find function and direction in a world that values youth 4. Deal with physical changes of aging
Age 30 transition	**Age 50–60 y**	**Age 75+ y**
Sometimes rethink early choices—"course correction"	1. Settle into life one chose in the 40s 2. Accept who one has become 3. Deal with grandparenthood 4. Deal with issues of aging and mortality	Focus on functioning despite physical aging
Age 30–40 y		
1. Settle into chosen life structure 2. Deepen commitment to work and intimate relationships 3. Experience self as fully adult		

Table 3.3 The child-focused years of the family life cycle[a]

Childbearing family	Family with preschool children	Family with school-aged children	Family with teenagers	Family with launching center
Adjust from dyad to triad and beyond	Maintain couple connection	Maintain couple connection	Support children's autonomy while maintaining connection	Renegotiate marital dyad Develop adult–adult relationship with children
Apportion household tasks	Find ways to balance home and work that support child's development	Realize increasing complexity of children		Include children's spouses and children in system
Renegotiate position in extended family	If additional children are born, restructure to make room for all			

[a]This period, lasting perhaps 20–25 years, most commonly occurs when individuals are age 25–55 years.

Early Adulthood

Developmental issues in early adulthood include launching from one's family of origin and developing a sense of identity and life structure, a job or career track, and an intimate and committed relationship.

The 20s tend to be a time of maximum energy and minimum life experience. By the 30s most people experience themselves as older and more settled. Particularly in the 20s, with a need to attend to all developmental tasks at once, both marital choice and couple development can be altered profoundly by one's relationship with parents and work. Early love relationships, in particular, can be in response to perceived parental demands, to wishes to prove oneself adult, or to a need for closure as a result of insecurity. In their 20s, men in particular, but many women also, may channel much time and emotional energy into work rather than relationships. However, the need to establish the security of emotional ties is high, and most people, no matter how hard they work, begin intense long-term relationships by their late 20s and want to establish a family soon after. For people who are pleased with their choices, their 30s can be a particularly stable and settled time.

Mid-Adulthood

Midlife issues are complex. The early 40s are not always a crisis period but are usually characterized by a sense of transition and a need to reevaluate one's life structure after 20 years of functioning adulthood. The sense of mortality and potential aging prompts many people to conduct a life review and to redirect some portion of their lives. In addition, people in midlife have often exchanged some measure of their enthusiasm for more patience and wisdom, which makes them less demanding and more accepting of themselves and others. Some people may be depressed and bitter. As spouses, people in midlife may be more willing to let go of an obsession with work and become more intimate or to let go of a focus on the family and become more world oriented. Some people become very dissatisfied with their marriages as part of their life review and seek affairs, separation, or divorce. Later midlife can be a source of satisfaction, in which people come to terms with who they have become. If a couple's marriage is good, it can be a particular source of comfort and strength at this time. Many separated and divorced individuals begin new relationships at midlife, starting new families with young children.

Older Adulthood

The tasks of older adulthood focus on developing a sense of purpose for the rest of life and conducting a life review. Because many older adults now can expect to live into their 80s or 90s, finding purpose and function in a society that values youth and denigrates age is difficult. Key questions include how much to rely on adult children and how to construct a meaningful life. For widows and widowers the question of whether to date is an important one. Because women live on average 7 years longer than men and tend to marry men older than themselves, the oldest population consists primarily of widowed and divorced women, who are subject to sexism, ageism, and poverty.

The Couples/Marital Life Cycle

The marital life cycle for most people in first marriages begins in their 20s, with both partners in the process of building a life structure. Generations of researchers have studied mate selection, with complex and confusing results. Some of the factors involved are propinquity, cultural similarity, and some complex matching of psychological needs. In addition, many researchers speculate that biologic preference factors such as odor are involved.

Phase of Relationship and Tasks

In this section we first discuss tasks involved in the beginning family and then examine those tasks concerning the adult life cycle as they relate to the family form.

Courtship and Early Marriage

For many people, the most important decision made in the course of a lifetime is their intimate partner. Couple formation is best done when both individuals have completed tasks of restructuring their relationships with their parents, learned enough about themselves to become aware of their characteristic problems, and had enough freedom and adventure that the demands of an intense relationship feels comforting rather than constricting. The new couple must establish an identity as a couple, develop effective ways of communicating and solving problems, and begin to establish a mutual pattern of relating to parents, friends, and work. Decisions regarding sexuality and some patterns of sexual relating commonly occur before marriage. Marriage is not simply about establishing a family, finding the right person, or being chosen by the right person. It is also about providing a setting for personal growth.

If the couple did not live together before marriage, they will deal with sexuality and mutuality in the early months of the marriage. Because ways of communicating and dividing tasks set up in the first months are often difficult to alter later on, it is critical to address these issues directly and early.

Marriage between people younger than 21 years can occur in religious families, for example, those who practice Orthodox Judaism. In some cases, early marriage represents a search for a substitute parent, a way of getting out of a troubled home or getting revenge on a parent, or a search for security. Some early marriages function well and allow the partners to grow in them, but some interfere with further individuation.

Marriages undertaken between the ages of 21 years and the mid-30s are embedded in the set of multiple, complex tasks of early adulthood. Competency in intimate life, work life, and parenting may need to be developed simultaneously. As more women have moved into the labor force before marriage and remain in it after marriage, marriage has become more egalitarian. Spouses born before 1950, however, usually began marriage with the woman having little sense of herself as a person in the world and seeing her identity as tied to her role in the marriage.

In general, marital satisfaction is greatest in the first year and begins to decline thereafter, reaching a low point with adolescent children. However, divorces are also highest in the first year as poorly matched couples dissolve. Common stress points in early adult marriages are childbearing, attempting an egalitarian marriage in a nonegalitarian culture, and enduring an age 30 transition if one or both of the partners go through a major reevaluation period. Dysfunctional courtship patterns often worsen during marriage. Couples married in their 20s or 30s often find a stable and well-functioning style in their 30s.

Marriage in Mid-Adulthood

Marriages between people in midlife differ depending on whether they are long-term first marriages or new marriages. Long-term marriages are often threatened by the stirrings of midlife transition, the launching of children, and the beginning of illness. They may be stronger and deeper or may be structural shells. New marriages are usually second marriages and may profit from the mistakes of the past. Both partners may be more mellow about themselves and their work and more available for family life. As a result, the children of second marriages may be easier to raise; however, stepfamily issues may greatly complicate second marriages.

Marriage in Older Adulthood

Marriages between older people may be relationships of habit and convenience, or they may involve a deep connection. Spouses have usually stopped trying to change each other and may be more accepting; however, the divorce rate has risen even in this age group in recent years. The husband's retirement (if he retires first) may put stress on the marriage, but illness and health, including changes in each member of a couples' needs for intimacy/sex, are the biggest determinants of the couple's functioning in later years.

Marital Coalition

The core of the family is the *marital coalition* (i.e., the spouses working together). This term implies that the spouses have been able to loosen their ties appropriately from their families of origin and develop a sense of their own individuality and self-worth in addition to a joint identity as a couple. Marriage is not merely a joining together of two individuals; it is also a distillation of their families of origin, each with its own experiences, history, lifestyle, and attitudes. **One marries not only an individual but also the individual's family of origin.** For example, if the parents are alive, they may be involved very clearly and specifically in the daily operations of the new couple. They may take sides, comment on childrearing practices, or live next door. Even when the extended family is not physically present, the patterns experienced by the spouses in their original families inevitably influence their current marital and family interactions.

The process of working out a satisfactory marital relationship involves tacit, shared agreements between the two people involved. These agreements may consist of explicit rules, implicit rules (rules that the couple adhere to without discussing), and rules that an observer would note but that the couple themselves probably would deny. Seen this way, conflicts in marriage arise when there are disagreements about the rules of living together, about who is to set those rules, and about who is to enforce those rules that are mutually incompatible. For example, there may be disagreements as to whether the husband or wife should wash the dishes, but there may be further disagreements as to who should make this decision. More complex still is the situation in which one spouse forces the other to agree "voluntarily" to wash the dishes.

The basic issues of interpersonal relationships are found in the following five dimensions, which determine the quality of a relationship[2]:

1. **Power**. Who is in charge? This is a complex area because there are many kinds of power, ranging from expertise to physical coercion to custom. Although no one is completely without power in a relationship, and power may be shared in many ways, there is general agreement in most couples about who is in charge if a joint decision is impossible, and whose needs come first in the family. How a couple resolves conflict makes this factor most important of all.
2. **Closeness-distance (emotional intensity) and amount of shared activities and values**. Partners negotiate what type of emotional distance feels close and intimate and what feels too distant. Also, because different kinds of behaviors may connote intimacy to one partner and not the other, there usually are agreed-on behaviors that represent a bid for closeness.
3. **Inclusion and exclusion**. Who else is considered to be part of the marital system? This question of boundaries applies not only to relatives and other persons but also to time allocated for career and recreational interests.
4. **Marital commitment**. Both partners need to feel that they and their spouse are committed to the relationship and are primary in each other's lives.
5. **Intimacy** *(i.e., the reciprocal sharing of vulnerabilities)*. Partners often vary in their need for verbal sharing, but for most couples, this is an important or essential part of bonding.

In married couples, the spouses do not start with equal access to power or with similar ways of looking at issues of closeness and inclusion. Gender differences, both intrapsychic and sociocultural, affect the ways in which these issues play out. Traditionally men have been seen as family leaders and wives as the support system (i.e., the helpmate). Women were supposed to use indirect methods of influence rather than direct requests or, worse yet, demands.

Although this tendency has changed, it has certainly not vanished. In addition, men's typically superior physical strength makes physically coercive behaviors by them more threatening, and their commonly superior earning power gives them other sources of power in the home, so that structural equality is difficult even when desired. In addition, men in general have been taught to have more ambivalent feelings about intimacy than women because intimacy is seen as unmanly or as linked to being controlled. Intimacy is also more difficult in situations of grossly disparate power.

Couples matched for variables of socioeconomic class; religious, ethnic, and racial backgrounds; political and social attitudes; and values tend to be more successful. However, dissimilarity or complementarity of personality styles may enhance a partnership, as might other subsidiary interests. The determining factor seems to be a match of roles to goals—that is, to achieve a specific goal, do you need to pick a partner the same as or different from yourself? **Temperament and personality factors are other key determinants.**

In our experience, marriages that seem most stable over time are those in which both partners are willing to be influenced by each other and share power. Predictors of divorce include overt anger, criticism, and contempt toward one's spouse; defensiveness; and an unwillingness to discuss issues.

Sex, Intimacy, and Companionship

Marriage presents an opportunity for the spouses to deal with their sexual needs. It may offer, in part, a relationship more like a friendship, in which there is mutual sharing of feelings, interests, activities, availability, and emotional support. Marriage offers a practical and acceptable way to conceive and raise children. It offers a sense of stability, continuity, and meaningful direction into the future. For some people, marriage is a response to a variety of social pressures that sanction and reinforce it as an institution. For any two individuals, marriage may afford the opportunity for the meshing of particular psychological traits and needs. It is key for the family therapist to evaluate this dimension as it changes over time in all couples.

The Family Life Cycle

Although stability and homeostasis are important elements of marital and family systems, inevitably other forces also are continually changing the family, pushing it in the direction of development and differentiation. Some of these forces constitute the growth pattern known as the *family life cycle*. The life cycle can be thought of as the expected life events that most families go through in a fairly predictable but varying sequence.

Other stresses can be thought of as unexpected in that they are extraordinary. They are not necessarily experienced by most families, or they occur outside of the usual sequence of the life cycle. Thus each family finds its own balance between those forces that tend to keep it stable and those that encourage change.

The longitudinal view (what we refer to as the traditional view) of the family's development is analogous to the individual's life cycle.[3] Figure 3.1 offers one model of the family life cycle. This model integrates both individual and family life cycle issues.

Various authors have studied the specific tasks for each phase in an individual's and in a family's life. As in individual development, the family evolves through expected phases. The traditional phases include (1) couple formation (love, cohabitation or engagement, marriage); (2) the childbearing family (birth of the first child, oldest child younger than 5 years); (3) the family with school-aged children; (4) the family with teenagers; (5) the family as a launching center

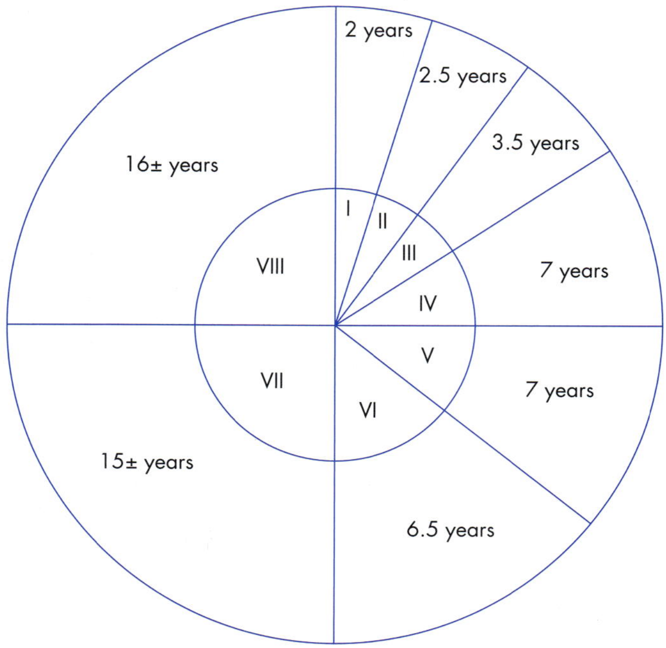

Phase	Family phase	Family description
I	Beginning family	Married couple without children
II	Childbearing family	Oldest child up to age 30 months
III	Family of preschool children	Oldest child age 30 months–6 years
IV	Family of schoolchildren	Oldest child age 6–13 years
V	Family with teenagers	Oldest child age 13–20 years
VI	Family as launching center	First child gone to last child leaving home
VII	Family in the middle years	Empty nest to retirement
VIII	Aging family	Retirement to death of both spouses

Figure 3.1 The family life cycle.

(the offspring begin their own adult life structure, usually but not always moving away from home); (6) the family in its middle years (which may include one or both spouses retiring and often includes grandparenthood); and (7) the couple as part of a three-generation family (and eventual death of a spouse). When one or both partners come to the marriage with a child, the couple may face the complex situation of having to deal with couple formation and child-related issues at the same time. In addition, families with many children, or with children spaced widely apart, may be dealing with issues of several phases at once.

Children and Shifts in Function

Family structure and organization change with each major developmental phase. For example, the marital couple's organization alters dramatically with the birth of the first child, the structure of this threesome will necessarily shift with the birth of a second child, and so on. Over time, it is to be hoped, the couple's ability to cope flexibly emerges.

In assessing the life cycle stage of the family, the therapist can anticipate the tasks and challenges that family members of different generations usually face.[4]

The family with young children is characterized by closeness, bonding, and intense inward focus on the children. The family can also expect that boundaries formed during the formation of the couple will be relaxed as relatives and friends move into and out of the expanded family, although in some families boundaries tend to be tightened around the nuclear family members.

In acquiring their role as parents, the married couple faces new responsibilities. Both parents cannot return to work full time without providing for the needs of the child, and parents must develop and revise strategies for meeting their own as well as their child's emerging requirements.[5] The couple must learn to operate in a triangular situation, to handle rapid decision making around the child's needs, and to negotiate around what are often very different ideas and styles of childrearing. Most often the mother is the one who does most of the child care and cuts back on her work, leaving the couple to find a way to negotiate roles in a system that pushes them back toward a traditional model.

Although adults may not think like children, children can be very observant and even insightful to what is going on among adults. The family with school-aged children is opened up to the larger world of the school, families of the children's friends, and new peers. As children interact with others outside the family, so too are parents freed up to pursue their own interests. This is also a time when children and parents can become good companions and is often a warm and easy time for the family. Even grandparents contribute to the opening up of the family system by introducing their grandchildren to experiences in different contexts. Issues of discipline, values, and amount of freedom for growing children may become major areas of argument. Religious or cultural differences between the parents must be negotiated around the children because this issue directly affects the family's rituals and functioning. As the children become adolescents, they press for greater autonomy. At the same time, parents also begin to struggle with contradictory desires for family closeness and safety on the one hand and freedom on the other. The years of adolescence are often difficult ones for many families. For the first time, the teenager appears to be half in and half out of the family. They are neither part of the parental subsystem nor comfortably identified with the child subsystem. To manage these developmental tasks, the family must be strong, flexible, and able to support growth. However, for the majority of families, adolescence is not a time of chaos and rebellion. Parents and children still connect and learn from one another in powerful ways. At the same time, parents also may contend with changes in their own parents' health, leaving many spouses feeling sandwiched between the needs of their children and their parents. Sometimes, parents face midlife issues of mourning lost youth or wishing to change themselves or their situation, all of which complicate matters.

The situation changes again with young adult children. The primary task of the family is to continue the letting-go process that began when the children were in adolescence, which involves restructuring the relationship while continuing to be related. American folk wisdom has placed autonomy as the only goal of this stage, whereas most people remain connected in different ways.

Young adults particularly are still in the process of launching and are deeply connected to their parents. For parents, the process of watching and participating in the life course as their children marry, have children, and become middle aged is a continuous process of relationship shift. Some families experience this later stage as a time of fruition and completion, whereas for others this stage prompts reevaluation of life and marital goals. Parents eventually encounter illness and loss as their own relatives and friends become ill or die. As their own health status changes, children again reenter the family to provide support and assistance.

Family Structure as It Relates to the Life Cycle

In healthy families, the basic roles and functions necessary for family adaptation are carried out by their subsystems (e.g., marital, spousal, sibling). These subsystems can be categorized according to the division of labor, or psychosocial tasks, within the family. For example, spouses generally offer each other social and emotional companionship and sexual intimacy, whereas parents provide nurturance, support, and guidance for children. In the sibling subsystem, children learn to share, trust, negotiate for resources, and develop social skills. Children provide parents with loyalty and a sense of purpose (or problems). The family's subsystems are arranged not only functionally but also hierarchically, with parents typically occupying positions of authority in relation to their offspring. From a developmental perspective, we would expect the family's structure to change over time. For example, the arrival of children signals the need for the marital partners to broaden their roles to include those of being parents. The task is to form an appropriate parental coalition with respect to childrearing practices. It is beneficial to have parental agreement and consistency in these areas, with a sharing of responsibility and mutual support.

Children may become confused if they do not know what is expected of them, or if they receive continually conflicting messages from each parent. Clearly, parents cannot agree on everything, and there may be danger in attempting to present a facade of agreement. **On basic, important matters, such as discipline, money, and central family values, however, it is preferable for parents to follow some sort of mutual, consistent childrearing guidelines.**

The maintenance of generational boundaries tends to lessen role conflicts that follow the blurring of roles and the ambiguity this fosters. A totally democratic family in which all members, regardless of age, responsibility, and experience, have an equal voice in all decisions seems wholly unrealistic. Far from being something to be decried, a generation gap between parents and children is a necessity, if we mean by the term a difference in responsibilities, roles, and maturity. Such a gap, however, should not consist of a deficiency in communication. Different relationships need to exist between parents and between parent and child. At the same time, the parents must give the child emotional room to learn, interact with peer groups, develop an identity, and begin to acquire responsibility and maturity themselves.

There must also be a reliable way for family members to relate to the larger society in which they live. The overall style of family involvement in relation to outsiders is also dictated by beliefs and behaviors (i.e., boundaries) that protect the family unit. In some families, the boundary is permeable, permitting free movement in and out of the system. In other families, the boundary is more rigid. A family with rigid boundaries may be isolated from social input, whereas a family with boundaries that are too diffuse may be unable to protect itself from external stresses. In either case, the family's structure or organization must be flexible enough for a variety of family aims and tasks.

These issues are complicated by the rapid shift since the 1970s from a traditional gender-differentiated marriage to a more egalitarian one. The traditional model specified separate domains of responsibility for men and women and set the man at the head of the hierarchy. It also specified fairly rigid emotional roles for men and women, with men being valued for strength and aggressiveness and women for intuition and emotionality (although intuition and emotionality tend to be undervalued in American society). **In the new model, roles are flexible, and both partners earn money, make decisions, have emotional sensitivity, and care for the children.** Most couples are the most traditional behaviorally, if not emotionally, when their children are young. In couples with widely differing expectations of male/female behavior, communication and problem solving become more complex and difficult.

FAMILY TASKS

Families can be viewed as laboratories for the social, psychological, and biologic development and maintenance of family members. In providing this function, couples and families must accomplish vital tasks, including the provision of basic physical and material needs (e.g., food, shelter, clothing), the development of a marital coalition (see section "Marital Coalition" earlier in this chapter), and the socialization of children. Therefore, not only do families have a given structure that expresses the family's underlying belief system, but families also serve to fulfill essential functions.

Provision of Basic Needs

Some of the essential life-maintaining tasks of the family group may be overlooked by therapists treating middle-class families. Therapists working with families from a lower socioeconomic class recognize immediately the fundamental requirement of addressing the family's basic needs. Depending on the extent to which these needs are not adequately met, the family's more complex functions will be affected in one way or another and become distorted or deficient. A therapist must pay attention to the family's safety, shelter, and nutrition, and, when indicated, the major or at least the initial effort may have to be to help the family deal more adequately with its basic needs. A family system already overwhelmed by gross deficiencies in basic needs will not usually be motivated to deal with more sophisticated or symbolic considerations.

Rearing and Socialization of Children

Although much of a child's essential temperament is inborn, the child's ultimate stance in relation to the world, their knowledge of cultural norms, and their attitudes toward men and women are developed within the family and the neighborhood and through traditional forms of media and now social media. Early neglect, trauma, or a chaotic upbringing can produce permanent damage in a child's brain structure and function.

Use of Age-Appropriate Childrearing Techniques

Parents need to understand or intuit their children's capacities at different ages in order to parent adequately. For example, expecting a 1-year-old to demonstrate patience and self-control, or trying to reason with a 3-year-old who is having a temper tantrum, will result in rage and confusion for both child and parent. In addition, some parents may have difficulty when their children are at a particular age because of what they experienced in their own family of origin. For example, a parent who was sexually promiscuous as an adolescent may become frightened when their child reaches the same age and may be untrusting and overly controlling as a result.

Maintenance of the Parental Coalition and Generational Boundaries

It is beneficial to both the parents and the children for the parents to be clear that they are functioning as a team to parent the children, and that grownup roles are different from child roles. Although parents cannot agree on everything, they should follow some sort of mutual, consistent childrearing guidelines. Even when parents disagree, their children should know that their parents will find a way to deal with the disagreement rather than leave the children in limbo. Problems arise when the parents are in so much conflict that one or both turn to the children for support, leaving the children either with a loyalty conflict (e.g., "If I side with Dad, Mom will not love me") or in a parentified, caretaking role.

Many single-parent families do extremely well by any standard of functioning. The most destructive for the children's development is fierce conflict between two parents (whether married or divorced) who are using their children as a weapon, or highly inconsistent, primarily neglectful behavior on the part of one parent, divorced or not.[6]

Sexuality

Parents do powerfully influence children's attitudes toward sexuality, their sense of whether it is good to be a boy or a girl, how one exhibits masculine and feminine behavior, and whether one can trust members of one's own or the opposite sex. Because much of this behavior is nonverbal (e.g., a man who is happy with his masculinity will appear masculine whether he is cooking or playing football), it is learned mostly outside awareness. Parents still need to teach their sons to be warm and empathic and their daughters to be strong and self-confident in a culture that still defines masculine in terms of aggression and control and that devalues women.

Support of a Sibling Coalition

The history of developmental theory has largely neglected the role of siblings in families. There has been greater emphasis on dysfunctional than functional relationships. For example, disproportionate attention has been paid to sibling rivalry.

A key issue is *microenvironments* for siblings (here meaning the world of the siblings as opposed to that of their parents). Research has found that siblings have a small degree of similarity in personality, but the commonalities in personality appear to result mostly from shared genes rather than from shared experience. Obviously, other factors influence how siblings turn out differently, for example, the so-called nonshared environment such as life events, each child's perceptions about the parents, different attitudes of the parents to each sibling, and the friends that each child develops.[7] The differences in family and environment are more obvious to the children themselves than to the parents. This research overlaps with Thomas and Chess's[8] work (discussed in Chapter 5), which has focused on the child–parent fit—the point being that some parents may make the same demands on two different children and get two different results (presumably because of the differences in the personality of each sibling).

Family theory has stressed the important role that siblings play in normal family functioning. Each sibling has a crucial role in the maintenance of homeostasis for that particular family system. Siblings often work together when their parents are continually at odds, when their parents have divorced, or when one or both parents have severe mental illness. That sibling bond is often the link that keeps a family functional when one or both parents cannot carry out parental roles.

Siblings can be both a source of stress and an enormous support to one another. Whether siblings support or befriend one another in childhood is to some extent a matter of temperament and age, but it is also a reflection of the parents' encouragement of kind behavior and their ability to keep the children out of parental conflict. In dysfunctional families, siblings often play stereotyped roles—the good kid, the bad kid, the clown, or the charmer—leaving little room for them to work out their own issues. How siblings connect in childhood does not always say much about how they will behave toward one another as adults.

Dysfunctional families often exhibit dysfunctional sibling relationships. For example, siblings may mimic the parental relationship by always bickering in the same way the parents bicker or by one being dominant. **The family therapist must see each sibling as a separate individual.** Family therapy should not presume that all siblings share the same experience.

Interventions focused on siblings may be included in family treatment models. Treatment can use older siblings as change agents or can focus on sibling conflict. When one parent has died, siblings are important in maintaining the family system while coping with the parental loss. When one sibling has a mental disorder, other siblings can be active supports. In addition, if one sibling has a serious mental illness, siblings need to know very specific information about the disorder, particularly the prognosis, and about how to deal with difficulties in communication and problem solving.[9]

Enculturation of Offspring

Parents teach the younger generation the basic adaptive techniques of their culture. They must transmit ways of thinking, feeling, and acting that are culturally appropriate. These include basic communication skills but also beliefs, values, and attitudes. For minority or oppressed groups, this is particularly problematic—for example, an African American family must teach both pride of heritage and ways of understanding and dealing with White privilege and racism. Social class attitudes are transmitted through the family, as are beliefs about the proper place of men and women. Parents who are themselves outside the mainstream culture (e.g., recent immigrants) must allow their children to find a way to learn mainstream culture. Families that wish their children to remain outside mainstream culture (e.g., Amish, Lubavitch) generally require a powerful and overarching community to provide boundaries.

FAMILY BELIEF SYSTEMS

Over the family's life course, characteristic beliefs and patterns of behavior evolve among family members. For example, in one family both parents may believe that neatness is very important. Everyone, including the children, learns to put things away and keep them clean. The family judges others by how organized they are and takes great pride as a family in its organization.

This may be a way of carrying on an extended family tradition of neatness and organization (e.g., certain cultural groups emphasize this behavior). Conversely, such behavior may be a way for the family to differentiate itself from a chaotic (and messy) extended family. In a different family, the mother may value neatness whereas the father may want a house that is emotionally warm and not focused on order. As the parents struggle, the children may take sides with one or the other, or they may shuttle between sides, playing peacemaker.

Key areas of belief revolve around what constitutes loyalty and proper behavior; however, all areas of family life include a system of beliefs. Family beliefs centered around fundamental issues determine what choices are considered normal or acceptable in times of change. A therapist who does not consider family beliefs in framing the problem or solution is likely to miss critical aspects of the situation.

FAMILY RESILIENCE

The concept of *family resilience* is the ability of the family to deal with crisis and adversity. Families that possess high levels of cohesion, connectedness, and mutual support and are able to communicate in clear and direct ways possess high levels of family resilience. These families are able to grow and recover from disruptive life challenges.

CLINICAL PRACTICE IMPLICATIONS

Each family should be approached as a unique cultural system that is influenced by ethnicity, race, religion, social class, and immediate social context. To develop a clinically meaningful picture of family functioning, the family therapist should evaluate the three dimensions of family functioning we have presented in this chapter: family structure, family life cycle, and the family's ability to accomplish tasks. The goal of a family systems assessment is to account for the salience of these factors and then to generate a kinetic understanding of the couple's or the family's general functioning. This assessment evolves through the generation of a series of systemic hypotheses or explanations and the systematic testing of each hypothesis with the family.

There are many paths to healthy family adjustment and effective functioning. In Chapter 4, we discuss alternatives to traditional two-parent families. Many, if not all, of the characteristics of healthy functioning that pertain to the families described in this chapter hold true for single-parent families, divorced and remarried families, and other family types.

SUGGESTED READINGS

Bigner JB, Wetchler JL. *Handbook of LGBT-Affirmative Couple and Family Therapy*. Routledge; 2012.

Falicov CJ. Working with transnational immigrants: expanding meanings of family, community and culture. *Fam Process*. 2007;46(2):157–171.

Gilmore KJ, Meersand P. *Emerging Adulthood: A Psychodynamic Approach to the New Developmental Phase of the 21st Century*. American Psychiatric Association Publishing; 2024.

McGoldrick M, Carter BA, Garcia-Preto NA. *The Expanded Family Life Cycle: Individual, Family, and Social Perspectives*. 4th ed. Pearson Allyn & Bacon; 2011.

Walsh F, ed. *Normal Family Processes: Growing Diversity and Complexity*. 4th ed. Guilford; 2012.

Walsh F. Family transitions: challenges and resilience. In: Dulcan M, ed. *Textbook of Child and Adolescent Psychiatry*. 3rd ed. American Psychiatric Association Press; 2022:637–652.

REFERENCES

1. Guttman HA, Beavers WR, Berman E, et al. A model for the classification and diagnosis of relational disorders. *Psychiatric Services*. 1995;46:926–932.
2. Lewis JM. For better or worse: interpersonal relationship and individual outcome. *Am J Psychiatry* 1998; 155:582–589.
3. Duvall E. *Family Development*. JB Lippincott; 1967:44–46.
4. Rapoport R. Normal crises, family structure and mental health. *Fam Process*. 1963;2:68–80.
5. Feldstein M, Rait D. Family assessment in an oncology setting. *Cancer Nurs*. 1990;15:161–172.
6. Hetherington EM, Law T, O'Connor T. Divorce: challenges, changes, and new chances. In: Walsh F, ed. *Normal Family Processes*. 2nd ed. Guilford; 1993:208–234.
7. Reiss D, Plomin R, Hetherington M. Genetics and psychiatry: an unheralded window on the environment. *Am J Psychiatry* 1991;148:283–291.
8. Thomas A, Chess S. *Temperament and Development*. Guilford; 1985.
9. Landeen J, Whelton C, Dermer S, et al. Needs of well siblings of persons with schizophrenia. *Hosp Community Psychiatry* 1992;43:266.

4 Understanding the Functional Family in a Variety of Family Forms

OBJECTIVES FOR THE READER

- To understand the functioning of the variety of family forms that include unmarried couples, same-sex couples and parents, single-parent families, blended families, constructed families, and transnational families
- To be able to delineate how families with differing structures and forms function well

For easier reading, we emphasize that the descriptors "couples" or "marital" are used nearly interchangeably in this chapter.

INTRODUCTION

There is a wide variety of family forms. Having a broad definition of family helps us understand the range of family forms. To this end, we define family as a group of people, related by biology or selected by choice, such as marriage, who are committed to each other's welfare. Family members may live together as a "traditional" family, or may live in a variety of homes. Children of divorced parents may live in two homes. Children of working parent(s) may spend most of their time in their grandparent's or neighbor's homes. In transnational families, family members live in two or more countries and may travel back and forth between the "new" and "old" homes. The impact of transnational living depends on factors such as legal or immigration status. If the migrated parent is sending money back home for the upkeep and education of children, then both grandparents and children benefit economically. However, if there is prolonged separation from parent(s), the children may suffer emotionally. With the introduction of social media and especially Skype, family members can keep in touch with each other and still have significant influence over each other's lives.

With such fluidity in the types and forms of relationships and families, it is important to remember the purpose of family. People form families to meet the human need for attachment, to gratify the need for a sense of belonging and often to raise children. This chapter examines the changes in family forms over the past decades, with the aim of providing a brief introduction. The family therapist can follow up for more specific details in the books and articles identified under further reading.

"The crucial scientific fact is that growing up in "loving homes" is the best predictor of good life outcomes. The presumed mechanism is that 'intimate touch,' turns on possible emotions which connect the neurons and brain fibers for life. Invasive, negative touch like sexual or physical abuse does the opposite, i.e. increases anxiety, depression and poor life outcome." —David Brooks

IMPACT OF AN EXTENDED INDIVIDUAL LIFE CYCLE
MARRIAGE
DIVORCE
Marital Separation
Divorce
Children and Divorce
BINUCLEAR FAMILIES
Impact of Divorce Based on the Age of the Child
The Functional Single-Parent Family
Mother-Headed Single-Parent Families
Father-Headed Single-Parent Families
REMARRIAGE AND BLENDED FAMILIES
Remarried Couple
Stepfamilies (Blended Families)
GRANDPARENT-HEADED FAMILIES
LESBIAN, GAY, AND TRANSGENDER FAMILIES
PARENTS WITH A GENDER NONCONFORMING CHILD
MULTIPLE-PARTNER FERTILITY FAMILIES
ADOPTION AND FAMILIES
INTERRACIAL FAMILIES
TRENDS IN PARENTING
CLINICAL PRACTICE IMPLICATIONS

IMPACT OF AN EXTENDED INDIVIDUAL LIFE CYCLE

We can now expect 60 to 75 years of functional adulthood. Life expectancy in the United States is currently 76.4 years (http://www.cdc.gov/nchs/fastats/life-expectancy.htm). This longer life cycle affects how we think about our individual lives and in turn, how we think about our relationships. Several common examples follow.

1. A couple may marry young and enjoy raising children together, but find they are not compatible when the children leave home. They may then decide to divorce and seek more compatible partners. Their "new" families will involve new roles and relationships with "new" family members.
2. In developed countries, women are increasingly choosing to establish a career in their twenties, and then seek a relationship/family in their thirties. Men are adapting to this change with an expectation that they will be more involved in the raising of their children and in the running of their home. These families tend to be wealthier and more educated, with the ensuing privileges.
3. A person may have a series of committed relationships, resulting in a series of distinct or overlapping "families." These "families" may consist of biologic and nonbiologic children, grandchildren, and other relatives. A child may have a more significant relationship with a relative, such as an aunt or grandparent, who was nurturing during their childhood rather than with a parent's newer partner and their family. It is important for the family therapist to consider the existence of hidden family loyalties.

MARRIAGE

Healthy marriages are good for couples' mental and physical health and for children; growing up in a happy home protects children from mental, physical, educational, and social problems.

In Western societies in recent decades, we have developed a more open attitude toward cohabitation, marriage, and child bearing. We have become more accepting of a wider variety of relationships. Marriage has traditionally been sequenced as "marriage with simultaneous cohabitation and subsequent childbearing." Common alternative sequences are "cohabitation, marriage, and subsequent childbearing," "cohabitation, childbearing, and subsequent marriage" or "cohabitation and subsequent childbearing without subsequent marriage."

The National Survey of Family Growth (NSFG [2017–2019]) gathers information on family life, marriage and divorce, etc. (http://www.cdc.gov/nchs/). They recently reported that 38.9% of men and 38.9% women were married, 12.0% of men and 13.9% of women were cohabiting, but they do not report on same-sex marriages, which are now legal in the majority of states, although some areas of the country still oppose same-sex unions. The family therapist should assess the impact of homophobia for each same-sex couple as individual experiences will vary widely. Same-sex couples seeking to have children and establish families will pursue adoption, donor insemination, or surrogate parenting, incurring much expense.

Several countries offer strong financial incentives to fathers to take parental leave for at least 2 months (Organization for the Economic Co-operation and Development: https://www.oecd.org/gender/Gender-Budgeting-in-OECD-countries.pdf). Finland phrases the problem differently, stating that time with fathers is in the best interest of children (Topping 2017, https://www.theguardian.com/lifeandstyle/2017/dec/04/finland-only-country-world-dad-more-time-kids-moms). Fathers in Finland spend eight minutes more a day with their school-aged children than mothers. In 2015, Germany introduced the Parental Allowance Plus and Partnership Bonus measures which provide financial incentives for both parents to work part time and share caregiving when children are very young.

DIVORCE

Both marriage and divorce rates have fallen over the past 10 years, but if the relationship has been long enough for attachment to take place (about 2 years), divorce is one of the most painful experiences in anyone's life. The ambivalence that ex-spouses feel about each other is probably more extreme than that in any other human relationship, with the possible exception of feelings about parents. The following section reviews the process and impact of separation and divorce in detail.

Marital Separation

Although separation is emotionally difficult, it is an opportunity to reassess individual and relationship goals. Separation in the early stages of a marriage may be caused by the partners moving from initial infatuation to reality and a wish to flee the task of working things out. Other motivations for separation include doubts about the wisdom of a marriage that may have occurred in response to pregnancy, marrying to get away from the parental home, or doubt about an ability to ever attract anyone else. Severe psychological problems in one or both partners, or marital affairs are also possible reasons for separation. Lastly, when children have left home and the parental role is diminished or absent, there may be little emotional or functional viability left in the marriage. For these couples, differences in individual adult development may lead to a lack of interest in maintaining the marriage.

Marital separation provides a cooling-off period and offers the opportunity for individuals to test their ability to live alone. Separation, together with new life experiences, may enable the couple to change their behavior and feelings toward each other if they desire reconciliation. Factors that indicate poor adjustment to separation, loneliness, and psychological distress are a lack of social support and an anxious attachment style. If there are children, co-parenting conflict is a common, chronic problem for many separated individuals.

Divorce

Divorce is a process, not an event, with its own developmental path. It is a series of transitions that began with marital dissatisfaction and may or may not end with a new relationship. Compared to same-race couples, mixed-race couples have a higher divorce rate.

A number of authors[1,2] have delineated four stages of the divorce process:

1. A predivorce phase involving growing disillusionment and dissatisfaction with the marriage and arrival at the consideration of divorce.
2. The separation including moving out of the house and dealing with immediate grief. For many people, this is a period of great emotional distress and confusion.
3. A period of 1 to 2 years during which the couple reorganizes the structure of their family life, parenting, finances, community status, and legal issues. Negative life stresses are most marked during the first 2 years following divorce. Parents' preoccupation with these issues will result in diminished parenting of children.
4. For each spouse, the last change is an identity change from being "part of a couple" to being a single person (i.e., the psychic divorce). Issues with children also settle down unless partners continue to use the children against each other. Parents must find ways to remain connected as parents, while separating as partners. The legal divorce may take 3 months in states with an uncontested divorce to several years, if there is conflict and persistent fighting.

In most couples, the divorce process is driven by one member. In these cases, the rejected person feels wounded and hurt. The rejecter often reacts with guilt and is unable to mourn the very real losses. Both partners may feel a strong sense of narcissistic injury. Fierce fighting over custody, money, or the story of what went wrong, serves the purpose of punishment or revenge, or a way of staying connected to the spouse. Attachment may last long after love or respect is gone, leading to confusing attempts to reconnect. The process of coming to grips with the self, recognizing one's own part in the marital dissolution, and beginning to date again often provokes anxiety. Regardless of how bad the marriage was, the transition to living alone is painful.

Children and Divorce

The majority of children of divorced parents experience distress. However, the consequences of remaining in homes where there is conflict or hostility must be contrasted with the impact of divorce. As with any other crisis, divorce offers the potential for growth. Children may be forced to cope with parental distress and economic uncertainty, which results in personal growth and maturation. Parental fighting including custody battles, disappearance of or irregular contact with the noncustodial parent, poverty, or the unavailability of parental supervision is very stressful for children. Family therapists can assist parents in making choices that benefit children and future parent–child relationships.

When children are involved, divorce mediation is more constructive than Family Court. Family Court purports to focus on the children's "best interests," but often fuels parental conflict due to the adversarial nature of the process. Although less than 5% of custody disputes go to trial, the years preceding the trial are frequently economically and emotionally destructive. Alternative interventions such as divorce education programs increase parental awareness of their children's needs as separate from adult needs, promote a greater willingness among residential parents to have their children spend time with the nonresident parent, reduce parental behaviors that put children in the middle of disputes, improve communication and result in greater willingness to settle custody and access disputes with their former partner.

In the 21st century, shifting attitudes and parenting practices has resulted in courts increasingly awarding joint custody to both parents, and more frequent visitation with fathers.

Family therapists are frequently concerned about helping the family maintain the father's involvement. Fathers may be uninvolved for several reasons. These reasons range from fathers who may have been minimal or no-contact fathers during the marriage, to fathers who experience the pain of rejection and loss and therefore avoid contact. Mothers also have a role in facilitating or limiting fathers' opportunities to parent and develop close relationships with their children. Following separation, the more mothers perceive fathers to be incompetent, the more they limit access. Fathers who pay higher levels of child support are given more access. Chronic high conflict occurs in up to 20% of divorced couples, resulting in less paternal involvement, more difficulties in the father–child relationship, and deterioration in father–child relationships over the long term.[3]

BINUCLEAR FAMILIES

The binuclear family exists when there is parental joint custody. The binuclear family consists of two separate households with a co-parenting bond. There are three main types of co-parenting. Cooperative co-parenting which is characterized by joint planning for children's lives, coordination and flexibility in arranging schedules, and mutual parental support. Children receive adequate parenting in both homes, well-articulated parenting agreements, and joint parental decision-making (http://www.apa.org/practice/guidelines/parenting-coordination.aspx). Cooperative co-parenting promotes resiliency in children.

The other two types of co-parenting, conflicted co-parental and parallel co-parenting, result in negative outcomes for children. Conflictual co-parenting is characterized by frequent conflict, poor communication, the failure of one or both of former partners to disengage emotionally, lack of focus on the children's needs, and the use of children in disputes. Parallel co-parenting is emotionally disengaged, low conflict, low communication, with separate parenting.

Children experience multiple transitions in the first 2 years after separation as a result of changes in their parents' lives. Although the majority of children appear to approve of their parents' dating, one-third of children found it highly stressful.[4] Remarriage within 1 year is more stressful to children compared with marrying 3 or 5 years postdivorce.[5] Children report the loss of the nonresident parent as the most negative aspect of divorce, and half of children and adolescents want more contact with their fathers.

Impact of Divorce Based on the Age of the Child

Babies require consistency and routine, and they're comforted by familiarity. Therefore, it's helpful to maintain normal daily routines, particularly regarding sleep and meals, during and after the divorce.

Toddlers and preschoolers may think that they are responsible for their parents' break-up. They'll often cry and want more attention than usual, regress, develop a fear of being abandoned, or have trouble going to sleep or sleeping alone.

School-age children also struggle with feelings of abandonment and may worry about losing one of their parents, or fantasize that their parents will get back together. They may believe they can rescue their parents' marriage. They may blame one parent for the separation, accuse their parents of being mean or selfish, expressing their anger in various ways such as fighting with classmates, or becoming anxious, withdrawn, or depressed.

In summary, the risk of adjustment, social, and academic problems is greater for children of divorce, compared with those in married families. However, protective factors exist.

The most protective factors are competent and warm parenting, absence of depression and other psychological disorders in parents, lower conflict, acceptable living arrangements after separation, close relationships with their fathers, and more involved fathers. Low father involvement after divorce has been linked to more conduct problems, particularly for boys. Children with vulnerabilities such as a difficult temperament or poor cognitive competence will have more trouble in a stressful situation such as that associated with divorce; temperamentally easy children with some supports already in place may experience growth and social competence.

The Functional Single-Parent Family

Single-parent families are defined as units in which only one parent is available and most single-parent families are headed by mothers. Single mothers with dependent children have the highest rate of poverty across all demographic groups (see Fig. 4.1; https://www.census.gov/library/publications/2022/demo/p60-277.html). Poverty is the single most important factor in accounting for the differences in the outcomes of children, regardless of family form.[6] Poor, single, and working parents may only be able to afford low-quality child caregivers or caregivers who are supervising too many children. Many parents choose not to work rather than compromise the care of their children. Long-term unemployment markedly increases the likelihood of poverty, and exposure to chronic, stressful conditions, such as inadequate housing and deprived neighborhoods. The chronic strains of poverty combined with task overload significantly increases vulnerability to new life stressors. Poor single mothers often experience a cycle of hopelessness and despair.

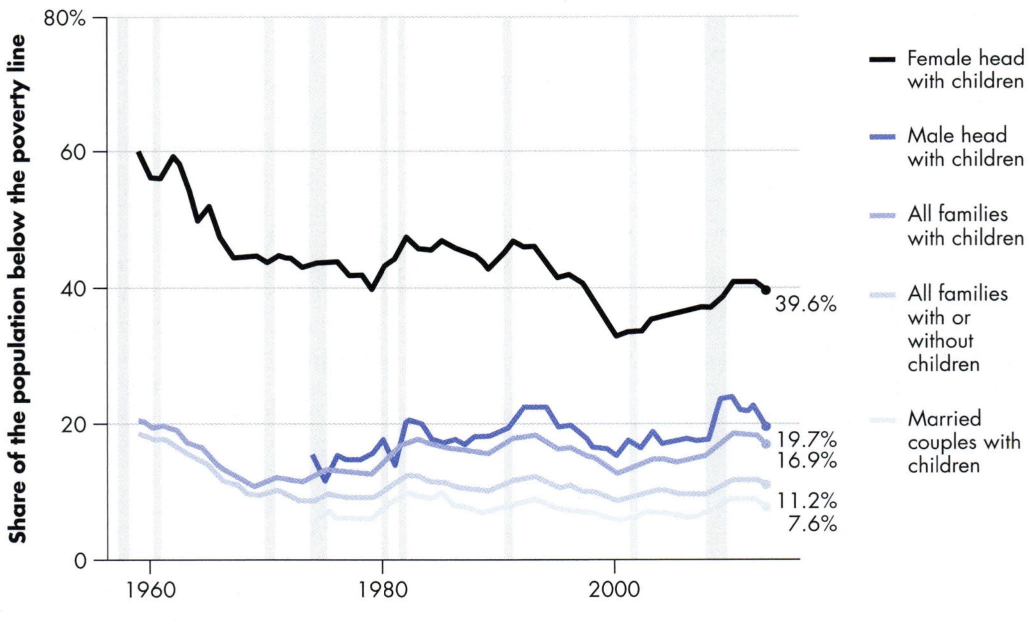

Note: Data for married couples with children and male-headed families with children are only available beginning in 1974. Shaded areas denote recessions.

Figure 4.1 Poverty rates of various types of families, 1959–2013. [*Source:* Authors' analysis of Current Population Survey Annual Social and Economic Supplement *Historical Poverty Tables* (Table 4).]

Despite these challenges, many single-parent families function well. Successful single-parent families have more available personal resources, good family organization, positive family concept, the ability to highlight positive events and place less emphasis on negative aspects of stressful events, and supportive social networks. Adaptive families possess a sense of control and perceive themselves as being more effective.

Single parents may give more power to their children. This can stimulate a sense of responsibility and maturity but only if the power is commensurate with their developmental level. As the sole parent, the bond with children may be stronger. However, particularly for mothers with no financial or family support, the need to work full time and have an adult social life can cut into child parent time. Single-parent families do equally well with either a maternal or paternal head of household. Aside from the impact of poverty, the effectiveness of parenting depends on the qualities of the specific parent.

Being the only parent creates family issues that may include the following:

1. Social isolation or loneliness of the parent
2. Awkwardness in dating and jealousy from the children
3. Demands from small children for the continuous presence of the sole parent
4. Children fending for themselves and carrying a greater share of the domestic responsibilities because the sole parent is working
5. Children feeling different because they live in a single-parent family
6. Decision-making is constrained, with less opportunity to talk things through
7. Crises and shifts if trying to introduce a new companion

Mother-Headed Single-Parent Families

Mother-headed single-parent families may be those in which the other parent is uninvolved after the divorce, or has never been present. If the partner is involved, the family should be considered binuclear (see next section).

Some noncustodial fathers fail to make complete child support payments and become distant from their children. This leads to great frustration for the mother and child. Several studies have suggested that inconsistent or absent fathers make a number of developmental issues more problematic.

Having another adult to share the tasks and responsibilities of childrearing is beneficial to child development. Many single-parent families without a second live-in adult create a network of friends and relatives to provide support. A strength of the African-American community is the involvement of extended family members in childrearing. A range of family members and other adults actively participate in childrearing in African-American single-mother families as co-parents. The concept of "other mothering" is common in poor inner-city minority families.[7] In these families, other women in the community take on the role of helping out to parent the children of the community. The family therapist can ask who in the community provides parental guidance for the children.

Father-Headed Single-Parent Families

Although classified as single fathers, many are cohabiting with a partner. More divorced men are now being given joint custody of their children than in the past. Compared to noncustodial fathers, noncustodial mothers are more apt to maintain contact with their children.

REMARRIAGE AND BLENDED FAMILIES

Four out of five divorced people remarry. The remarried family system is created by the new couple, one or both of whom had been married before, with or without children who visit or reside with them. The suprafamily system is composed of the remarried family plus former spouses, grandparents, aunts, uncles, etc. The children are part of each of their biologic parents' household systems as well as the new blended family system.

Becoming a remarried family requires a series of developmental adjustments.[8] The first issue to assess is the presence of several individual life cycles that all need to be merged with the new family life cycle. The new or blended family must complete the following tasks: form a new parental coalition, establish new traditions, acknowledge and honor each person's individual developmental needs, agree on the boundaries between "prior" families and the "new" family, and negotiate new ways of problem solving, communication, and ways of being together as a family.

Establishing the suprasystem means deciding the boundaries of the new blended family. Are the parents of the ex-wife, who are still grandparents to the children of the father, part of the blended family system? Some family members may belong in two families or may feel they do not belong in any family. If the system has permeable, open boundaries, then input is accepted from the suprafamily, from former spouses, grandparents, and children. The sheer number of people at widely differing life stages who are involved in blended families adds complexity as well as opportunity.

Remarried Couple

In the midst of this transition, the new couple must find a space to define themselves as a new couple and as lovers. They must also find the emotional energy to connect with the children and to continue to take primary responsibility for their own biologic children rather than assuming the stepparent will act like a biologic parent.[9]

Some individuals are more likely to remarry than others; those who choose not to remarry may prefer alternative arrangements like cohabitation or living apart together (LAT). LAT is a form of intimate ongoing companionship that allows each partner to maintain autonomy and independent households.

In recent years, remarriage rates in the United States have dropped. Remarriage occurs more quickly in younger adults and men remarry more often than women, especially from urban areas. Remarriage rates also differ by ethnicity; remarriage is most common among White women. Non-White women from communities with high unemployment and poverty are less likely to remarry. Having children is associated with higher rates of remarriage for both men and women.

Some women enter cohabiting relationships after a divorce instead of remarrying. This pattern of cohabiting after a divorce is more likely for White than Black women, for women without religious affiliation, with few or no children, and who live in more economically stable communities.

Compared to remaining single, remarriages are associated with greater socioeconomic security and life satisfaction. Second marriages overall do consistently better than first marriages. Rates of divorce decline as age at the time of second marriage increases. Those who enter their second marriage with no children are more likely to sustain their marriages.

Partners who bring the same problematic personal qualities to their subsequent marriage as they had during the first, will likely run into the same marital problems. People who divorce and remarry multiple times tend to be impulsive. People who are already familiar with divorce tend to be more accepting of it than people who have stayed married.

Stepfamilies (Blended Families)

The couple must decide if they are going to combine their finances and where they will live. Couples who combine their finances report higher family satisfaction and often couples report that moving into a new home works better because the new home becomes their "new family" home. For children, the remarriage of their parent might mean that the fantasy that their parents would reunite is finally over. Couples must agree on what role the stepparent will have in raising the children.

There is an innate bond between the child and their primary parents. Stepparents need to consciously develop their own bond with their stepchildren, and usually a different type of bond. The presence of a biologic parent elsewhere, in actuality or memory, brings up uncomfortable feelings about loyalty for the child. The stepparent's goal is to become an "intimate outsider." A stepparent can develop multiple types of relationships with a stepchild: friend, aunt, or uncle, or may develop a true parental connection. For stepparents and children, being able to master difficult interpersonal situations results in increased self-esteem. When children are members of two households, everyone must avoid involving children in loyalty conflicts. Lastly, if there is no legal relationship between the stepparent and the child, there is a perceived risk of abandonment in forming a new relationship.

The dynamics of stepfamilies are unique. Uninformed stepfamilies may decide prematurely to dissolve their new relationship before the rewards and satisfactions of stepfamily life can become apparent. Forming new relationships and finding solutions to stepfamily challenges take time, and family members typically go through predictable emotional stages before achieving integration.[10] Teenagers take longer than do younger children to accept the blended family. Often the adults in stepfamilies expect everything to go smoothly, the fantasy stage. When the adults fail to make the fantasy come true, they start to feel that something is wrong with them. When conflict and pressures build, the family then tends to split along biologic lines. A typical situation is when the stepparent feels left out, with the parent–child coalition as the primary alliance. The parent who has remarried feels caught in the middle between their partner and their children. Children may exploit the adult split for their own benefit. The stepparent may look for support outside the household and then becomes more vocal about their dissatisfaction. The blended family often presents for treatment at this stage. Resolving these issues is critical but takes time and understanding. As the two adults begin to work together as a parenting team, changes take place in the household so that biologic divisions blur and the blended family begins to function as a family.

Over time, typical situations rooted in the structure of stepfamilies tend to arise, especially around family events such as graduations, marriages, holidays, or deaths. The blended family may experience old feelings and behaviors, but can work them out quickly and return to a family equilibrium.

A major hurdle for stepfamily members is meeting basic human needs: to belong, be supported by someone who loves you, and have some control over your life. Families that work out ways of satisfying these needs will become more quickly blended. Most of those involved in stepfamily life eventually achieve satisfaction and find the experience rewarding. Many blended families seek out support groups, pastors, and, of course, family therapy.

GRANDPARENT-HEADED FAMILIES

When both parents have died or when a single parent has become incapacitated by illness or substance abuse, or is incarcerated, children are often cared for by grandparents. The incongruent developmental needs of an aging person and an active young child, plus grief for the lost parent, make this family system more difficult. Therapy tasks include determining the role of the parent(s) in the child's life and looking for extra family support. It is important to determine if the biologic parent is maintaining emotional and financial support for the child and the grandparents.

LESBIAN, GAY, AND TRANSGENDER FAMILIES

As of 2020, 37 U.S. states and the District of Columbia have legalized same-sex marriage. Thirteen U.S. states have a ban on same-sex marriage; however, eight of these states have court rulings in favor of allowing same-sex marriage.

The family therapist can help the family understand the stages of coming out.

- Stage 1—Identity Question: When the person begins to question their heterosexual identity. Some people never move on from this stage and live their lives as heterosexuals.
- Stage 2—Internal Identity Acceptance and Education. Accepting one's sexuality means change. Feeling scared of how family will react is a natural reaction.
- Stage 3—Typically people begin to first come out to a selective group of close friends.
- Stage 4—Pride. Depression, sadness, fear, etc. are common in the earlier stages, however, this is the stage where those feelings start to disappear. Being happy about who you are, sexuality included, is important in order to lead a happy and fulfilled life.
- Stage 5—Relationships. Same-sex couples may have a desire for commitment and families.
- Stage 6—Coming out to your family can be difficult. When parents first learn of a child's gender dysphoria, they may experience a sense of loss. Soon they realize that they haven't lost anything and that marriage and children are still possible. If the adult child's sexuality is still a secret, there will be a sense of distance from parents. Some parents may react harshly by cutting off communication and support. In most cases, parents need time to deal with the news. During that time, some refuse to talk to their children, while others ignore the sexuality issue hoping that it will go away. How parents and family are informed are crucial to consider.
- Stage 7—Balance. In this stage, being lesbian, gay or bisexual becomes just another part of who you are.

Children are increasingly being raised by lesbian, gay, and transgender couples. Adults may bring children from a heterosexual relationship, or through adoption or with assisted reproductive technologies. In some cases, one parent is the biologic parent and the other parent the adopted parent.

In the United States, studies on the effect of gay and lesbian parenting on children were first conducted in the 1970s. The widespread pattern of children being raised from infancy in two-parent gay or lesbian homes is relatively recent. According to U.S. Census, 80% of the children being raised by same-sex couples in the United States are their biologic children. Research shows that lesbian and gay parents are as fit and capable as heterosexual parents, and their children are as psychologically healthy and well-adjusted as children reared by heterosexual parents, despite the considerable discrimination and inequity that remain significant challenges.

In 2010, the results of a 25-year ongoing longitudinal study were released. Gartrell and Bos studied 78 children conceived through donor insemination and raised by lesbian mothers. Mothers were interviewed and given clinical questionnaires during pregnancy and when their children were 2, 5, 10, and 17 years of age. The mothers' reports showed the 17-year-old daughters and sons of lesbian mothers were rated significantly higher in social, school/academic, and total competence and significantly lower in social problems, rule-breaking, aggressive, and externalizing problem behavior than their age-matched counterparts. The most important determinants of the health of the child is their relationship with their parents, their parents' sense of competence and security, and the presence of social and financial support for the family.

For years there were many unfounded fears about the gender identity of children raised in same-sex households. No evidence has been found of difficulty with gender identity. In the 21st century, gender roles have become less rigid, with men taking on more traditionally female roles, and vice versa.

Older lesbian, gay, bisexual, and transgender (LGBT) individuals rely on friends as their "chosen family" to provide support and sense of family. Families of choice form the caregiving networks that support LGBT older adults in the community. Non-kin caregivers and their care recipients experience stress due to the limited support resources available to them, however, with the increased acceptance of same-sex couples, barriers such as health care issues are getting solved.

PARENTS WITH A GENDER NONCONFORMING CHILD

Many parents accept gender variance in their child, although remaining concerned for their child's welfare and unsure how to handle the challenges. Parents may seek out family therapy for guidance. These parents are frequently familiar with the concept of gender as a fluid continuum rather than a rigid binary. They do not consider that their child has a psychological problem, rather a social problem.

Other times, parents—most often fathers—struggle to accept a child who does not fit within socially accepted gender norms. Some dread the possibility of discovering that their child might be transgender and a desire to change sex. Some react very negatively and the gender nonconformity can become a significant source of conflict between parents and a damaging source of disconnection between parent and child.

A family therapist can help parents and children move from "either/or" to "both/and." It is important to help children affirm their identity and understand the demands of a world organized around the binary of gender. Parents can be supported to nurture their child's singularity and be mediators between the child's wish and the social reality.

The family therapist's ability to move flexibly between multiple positions within the family—consultant and coach for parents, family and/or child therapist, and parent group facilitator—provides support to the system where it needs it the most.

MULTIPLE-PARTNER FERTILITY FAMILIES

Parents with children with more than one partner form multiple-partner fertility families (MPF). There is a higher rate of MPF in disadvantaged families. Parents with MPF become parents at younger ages, largely with unintended first births, and often do so outside of marriage.

ADOPTION AND FAMILIES

Many children are adopted at birth, but increasing numbers of older children are being adopted from the foster care system. These children often have been exposed to trauma and/or residential instability during critical developmental life phases.

Overall adopted children do well, however adopted children may have more adjustment problems and mental health diagnoses. Studies also find that adoptive children think about their birth families frequently, but many are uncomfortable talking with their parents because of feelings of disloyalty. Adoptive children often have adjustment problems during adolescence when their identity development is more difficult. Children adopted at older ages are more likely to have an insecure attachment relationship with their adoptive mother.[11] Family therapists may be involved when an adopted child has adjustment difficulties.

Adoption can be through private or public agencies. Although practices vary, the most common arrangement in open adoptions is for the adoptive parents to commit to sending the birth mother photos of the child (and themselves as a family) each year, and short written updates, until the child reaches the age of 18. In the United States, minority children wait longer to be adopted and there is some hesitation to allow children to be adopted into a family of a different ethnic background. Many families choose international adoption, as a quicker and easier route although this practice raises more complex ethnic and identity issues.

INTERRACIAL FAMILIES

Since the decriminalization of interracial marriage in 1967, the number of interracial unions and the number of mixed-race individuals have grown and mixed-race is the fastest growing demographic group. Developing positive self-concepts biracial and multiracial identities are associated with positive psychological functioning.

Family identity develops over time. A core theme described by Black–White couples as they negotiated the process of forming a family identity is called Coming Together.[12] Four major tasks in the construction of interracial family identity are: (a) understanding and resolving family of origin chaos and turmoil, (b) transcending Black–White racial history, (c) articulating the interracial family's racial standpoint, and (d) explaining race to biracial children, across their developmental stages.

TRENDS IN PARENTING

College-educated American parents are increasingly scheduling many enrichment activities for their children. When their offspring leave home for college, they may become helicopter parents. These activities occur at the expense of their own time, either leisure, social, or simply down time. Most children will have difficulty attaining the high-flying career and life style that their parents envision. The pressure to be successful and popular can lead to false family priorities.

One recent trend is the practice called new mothering[13] with an emphasis on the importance of women as mothers. Women of diverse backgrounds in the United States raising 2 to 4 year olds, identified four beliefs (1) mothers are more suitable caregivers than fathers, (2) mothering should be child-centered, (3) parenting consists of a set of skills that need to be learnt, and (4) that parenting is labor intensive but an emotionally fulfilling activity.[14] This ideology, regardless of social class, ethnic background, household composition, and financial situation, may contribute to women experiencing guilt for not matching up to these ideals.

Lastly, the family therapist may see more families that come from diverse cultures, and families who are refugees, many of whom may have suffered complex trauma. These families will require assessment and care that takes immigrant status, ethnicity, and associated cultural norms into account.

CLINICAL PRACTICE IMPLICATIONS

It has become increasingly clear that it is healthy family processes rather than specific family structures that determine family members and children's well-being and outcomes. Important

Table 4.1 Keys to family resilience

Belief systems
1. Making meaning of crisis and challenge
2. Positive outlook: hope
3. Transcendence and spirituality
Organizational resources
4. Flexibility/stability
5. Connectedness, leadership
6. Kin, social, and economic resources
Communication processes
7. Clear, consistent messages
8. Emotional sharing
9. Collaborative problem-solving/proaction

Source: Walsh F. *Strengthening Family Resilience*. 3rd ed. Guilford Press; 2016.

family processes include the quality of parenting, the psychosocial well-being of parents, the quality of and satisfaction with relationships within the family, and the level of cooperation and harmony between parents. Research has established that children and adolescents can do well in a variety of family forms, all other things, especially financial security, being equal.

The themes are clear. First, look at effects of the social milieu, factors such as poverty, stigmatization, and bullying. A good sense of self and identity for all, inclusion, protective factors and resilience. Regardless of form, you need the basics (Table 4.1), to have a good functioning family.

SUGGESTED READINGS

This brief article summarizes the complexities of divorce and gives shape to the concerns of clinicians.
Imber-Black E. Reflections on the special issue: divorce and its aftermath. *Fam Process*. 2007;46(1):1–2.

This book provides the reader with a comprehensive study of divorce and the family processes that support good outcome.
Hetherington EM, Kelly J. For better or for worse. *Divorce Reconsidered*. W.W. Norton & Company; 2002.

This in-depth article highlights new pair-bonding structures and normalizes divorce. The implications for social policy, family law, social science, and couples and family therapy are discussed.
Pinsof WM. The death of "till death us do part": the transformation of pair-bonding in the 20th century. *Fam Process*. 2002;41(2):135–157.

This article is necessary reading for clinicians who want to help parents with gender nonconforming children.
Malpas J. Between pink and blue: a multi-dimensional family approach to gender nonconforming children and their families. *Fam Process* 2011;50(4):453–470.

This is a comprehensive test book on family resilience, describing a clinical framework for practice as well as research findings.
Stolley KS. Statistics on adoption in the United States. *Future of Children*. 1993;3(1):26–42.
Walsh F. *Strengthening Family Resilience*. 2nd ed. Guilford Press; 2006.

REFERENCES

1. Kessler S. *The American Way of Divorce: Prescription for Change*. Nelson-Hall; 1975.
2. Salts CJ. Divorce process: integration of theory. *J Divorce*. 1979;2:233–240.
3. Kelly JB. Children's living arrangements following separation and divorce: insights from empirical and clinical research. *Fam Process*. 2007;46(1):35–52.
4. Hetherington EM, Kelly J. For better or for worse. *Divorce Reconsidered*. W.W. Norton & Company; 2002.
5. Ahrons CR, Tanner JL. Adult children and their fathers: Relationship changes 20 years after parental divorce. *Fam Relat*. 2003;52:340–351.
6. Amato PR, Keith B. Parental divorce and the well-being of children: a meta-analysis. *Psychol Bull*. 1991; 110(1):26–46.
7. Burton LM, Hardaway CR. Low-income mothers as "othermothers" to their romantic partners' children: women's coparenting in multiple partner fertility relationships. *Fam Process*. 2012;51(3):343–359.
8. Visher EB, Visher JS. *Therapy With Stepfamilies*. Brunner/Mazel; 1996.
9. Glick PC. Remarried families, stepfamilies, and stepchildren; a brief demographic profile. *Fam Relat*. 1989; 38:24–27.
10. Papernow P. *Becoming a Stepfamily: Patterns of Development in Remarried Families*. Jossey-Bass; 1993.
11. Howe D. Age at placement, adoption experience and adult adopted people's contact with their adoptive and birth mothers: an attachment perspective. *Attach Hum Dev*. 2001;3(2):222–237.
12. Byrd MM, Garwick AW. Family identity: black-white interracial family health experience. *J Fam Nurs*. 2006;12(1):22–37.
13. Ruddick S. *Maternal Thinking: Towards a Politics of Peace*. Beacon Press; 1989;11:17.
14. Hays S. *Cultural Contradictions of Motherhood*. Yale University Press; 1996.

5 Problems and Dysfunction from an Integrated Family Systems Perspective

OBJECTIVES FOR THE READER

- To understand the characteristics of dysfunctional families
- To understand theories of the development of family dysfunction
- To understand theories of how one individual family member becomes the identified patient
- To obtain an overview of how symptoms and problems in a couple, family, or individual are conceptualized from a family systems perspective

For easier reading, we emphasize that the descriptors "couples" or "marital" are used nearly interchangeably in this chapter.

INTRODUCTION: THE DYSFUNCTIONAL FAMILY SYSTEM

In the preceding chapters, we described the organization and behavior of the functional family, using the concept of the family as a system with its own life cycle and tasks. In this chapter (and again in Sections IV and V) we focus on the disturbances in these areas and the ways in which families become dysfunctional. We discuss the types of disturbances manifested by dysfunctional family systems, including problematic family beliefs and myths, individual symptomatology, life cycle stressors, and the inability of the family to accomplish family tasks.

How do problems become problems? What leads to symptoms? Who begins to realize that a problem is distressing enough to require outside intervention? These are issues that intrigue family theorists (and individual theorists before them) and will preoccupy the family therapist as they begin the assessment of a couple or family.

In order to contrast systemic explanations with more traditional perspectives, it is important to briefly revisit the psychoanalytic and biologic approaches to the development of symptomatology. Freud focused on data obtained from the verbalizations of patients about their internal thoughts, feelings, and experiences. He saw psychopathology as relating both to internalized conflict between wishes and desires and to the control mechanisms within the psyche. He noted astutely that the dysfunctional patterns and defenses that hinder the life of the patient (and at times the analyst) were reenacted within the therapy in similar forms, most commonly in the form of transference toward the psychoanalyst. (Transference is the unconscious tendency of a person to assign to others in the present and immediate environment feelings and attitudes linked originally with significant figures in the person's early life.) Freud's psychoanalytic approach emphasized the individual patient, and his clinical focus was on internal experience, which was thought to have its roots in the early history of the individual.

In general, family theorists only recently incorporated psychodynamic and neurobiologic aspects of illness into their thinking. The systems perspective emphasizes what is called circular causality, in which symptomatic behavior is maintained by circular feedback loops within the family system. It is argued that with living systems, one cannot simply assign one part of the system as having a direct causal influence on another part; in other words, there may be different routes to the same endpoint, or similar events may lead to different outcomes. In this regard, the systemic perspective offers a comfortable stance for clinicians who have adopted the biopsychosocial perspective (see Chapter 1). Not only must these factors be accounted for in the assessment of a patient system, but narrow interventions must be contrasted with those that explicitly address biologic, psychological, and social dimensions.

There is a brain, a mind, a family, and a community for all of us. The family therapist must try to determine the lesions and the strengths in each of these components.

A SYSTEMS APPROACH TO PROBLEMS AND DYSFUNCTION
Historical Perspectives
Current Perspectives
Family Resilience Key Processes
Structural and Organizational Problems
The Solution as the Problem
FAMILY BELIEFS AND MYTHS
THE LARGER SOCIAL SYSTEM AND DYSFUNCTION
IMPLICATIONS FOR TREATMENT—THE DEVELOPMENT OF SYMPTOMS IN A PARTICULAR PERSON
LIFE CYCLE PROBLEMS AND DYSFUNCTION
Unresolved Grief
Toxic Secrets
TASK PERFORMANCE IN THE DYSFUNCTIONAL FAMILY
Providing for the Family's Basic Needs
Maintaining a Functional Marriage: Issues of Sex, Intimacy, and Commitment
Rearing and Socializing of Children
CLINICAL PRACTICE IMPLICATIONS

A SYSTEMS APPROACH TO PROBLEMS AND DYSFUNCTION

Just as reductionistic views have emphasized the individual's inner life and neurobiologic system, it is equally important to widen the lens and look at the same phenomena from an interpersonal and systems perspective. Because current psychoanalytic theory and practice have been moving toward an interpersonal and systems perspective steadily over the past decades, the renewed focus on context represents a larger swing within the field of psychiatry and psychotherapy.

Historical Perspectives

Freud's microscope was focused on the individual and the individual's inner life. We will not go deeply into the history of the family systems view of symptoms but simply highlight in a simplified way a few crucial steps along the way. At this point, it would be helpful to review the basic concepts of systems theory (see Chapter 1).

Systems theories of etiology, as applied to mental disorders such as schizophrenia, are now dated. For the sake of understanding these theories, we summarize them here. One of the pioneering interactional concepts about symptomatology was Bateson et al.'s[1] articulation of the double bind. The term double bind described a communication impasse between individuals in a relationship system, which hypothetically gave rise to responses in one individual that were labeled schizophrenic. Rather than being a disorder of reality testing, schizophrenia was viewed as the individual's best effort to cope with a reality of disturbed communication. In other words, schizophrenia made sense when understood in the context of disconfirming and disqualifying communications and behaviors.

Jackson began to look at family norms and values that were maintained by what he viewed as homeostatic mechanisms.[2] In his initial work, he proposed that symptoms served a homeostatic function; that is, they functioned to keep the family operating within the same narrow range of behavior. As a result, dysfunctional families used only some of the full range of behaviors available to them in order to maintain the status quo, which produced the symptomatic behavior in the first place.

At the National Institute of Mental Health, Bowen and later Wynne were also trying to understand the etiology of schizophrenia from a systems perspective. Bowen[3] who studied the families of patients with schizophrenia, concluded that two-person relationships (e.g., marriages) were intrinsically unstable. He proposed that when confronted with stress, a two-person emotional system may draw in, or triangulate, a third person. Anxiety between the original twosome is shifted to the third person. Although it is hypothesized that triangulation occurs in all families, pathology is associated with those families in which there is a rigidity about such triangles under change or stress. This triangulation process may spread to the entire family and even peripheral family members and outsiders as the emotional contagion grows.

Wynne and his colleagues attributed psychopathology to deviant family communication processes and properties of families that blocked the young person's natural development.[4] Among the processes they noted were unreal qualities of both positive and negative emotions (i.e., pseudomutuality, which masks conflict and blocks intimacy; and pseudohostility, which obscures splits and alignments), rigid family boundaries (so-called rubber fences), and distorted patterns of communication (i.e., communication deviance). Finally, Lidz[5] grounded his initial investigations in psychoanalytic theory, challenging the prevalent view (at that time) that maternal rejection was the distinguishing feature in psychopathology. He looked at the role of fathers and at problems in marital roles. In particular, marital schism was identified as the chronic failure of accommodation or role reciprocity, whereas marital skew reflected marriages in which psychopathology was present in one partner, who dominated the other. Other psychoanalytically informed pioneers (e.g., Ackerman[6]) believed that family problems arose in response to the immediate environment and to the individual psyche.

As we discuss later in this chapter, these theories aid our understanding of general couple and family dissatisfaction and of the family contribution to symptomatology. These types of family dysfunction create levels of stress in family members that can magnify and maintain psychotic processes in vulnerable individuals.

Current Perspectives

The biologic determinants of most of the major psychiatric disorders have been identified, using imaging, neuropathologic, and neurochemical methods. The idea that rearing alone, or the current family system alone, is responsible for these disorders is now outdated, much to the relief of the families that were blamed for their members' pain. However, family stress or dysfunction is often involved in the onset and maintenance of symptoms. The person with psychosis puts stress on the family, and certain types of family dysfunction, such as triangulation and rigid family boundaries, puts stress on the ill person. Levels of family dysfunction must be investigated as part of the evaluation and treatment of psychosis.

Family systems explanations for symptoms are as numerous as the schools of clinical theory and practice in the field. In this section, we define symptoms as problems that distress others in the family and, usually, the person who has them.

A "good and stable relationship buffers against the genetic vulnerability to both medical and psychiatric disorder"[7] and the following family factors have been shown to be associated with family resilience.[8]

Family Resilience Key Processes

Organizational Patterns

- Flexibility
- Connectedness
- Social and economic resources

Belief System

- Making meaning out of adversity
- Positive outlook
- Transcendence and spirituality

Communication and problem solving

- Clear and consistent messages
- Open emotional expression
- Collaborative problem solving

In the remaining sections of this chapter, we examine some of the more influential perspectives on family systems problems. Each of the following approaches may be thought of as a hypothesis that the clinician may test in approaching a new case. Evidence of family resilience, and opportunities to enhance resilience are important factors to identify. Telling a family what they do well, is a very powerful intervention.

Structural and Organizational Problems

Sometimes symptoms in an individual may be viewed as a reflection of organizational problems existing within the marriage or family. According to Minuchin,[9] (p. 51), family structure is "the invisible set of functional demands that organizes the ways in which family members interact. A family is a system that operates through transactional patterns. Repeated transactions establish patterns of how, when, and to whom to relate, and these patterns underpin the system." In Minuchin's influential structural approach, a pathologic family could be one "who in the face of stress increases the rigidity of their transactional patterns and boundaries, and avoid or resist any exploration of alternatives." As the family's range of choices narrows, family members develop predictable and stereotyped responses to one another and to the extrafamilial environment. The family then becomes a closed system, and family members experience themselves as controlled and impotent.[10] From the structural perspective, the family therapist's definition of a dysfunctional family is one whose adaptive and coping mechanisms have been exhausted.

Symptoms of unhappiness in a family member may be embedded in problematic family function when symptoms represent the family's groping for new solutions during a period of transition. Flexibility and connectedness can alleviate this stress.

As we mentioned in Chapter 3, dimensions of family structure that warrant attention are family boundaries, hierarchies, and coalitions. Minuchin considers boundaries on a continuum ranging from enmeshment to disengagement. Enmeshment refers to a style of family involvement in which boundaries within the family are highly permeable but those between the family and the outside world are usually rigid. At the extreme, this style can become a handicap in that a heightened sense of belonging may require a major yielding of autonomy. In more disengaged families, only a high level of stress (e.g., caused by serious illness or a suicide attempt) can reverberate strongly enough to activate the family's supportive systems. If the concept of boundaries addresses proximity, the dimension of hierarchy is defined in terms of authority or relative influence that family members exercise in relation to one another.

Problems in alliances or coalitions represent another facet of structural difficulties. In a three-person system, ample opportunities exist for two of the members to be allied against or to exclude the third member. Minuchin has described three different types of triangles:

1. Triangulation, in which the parents make equally strong but different demands on the child, and the child responds by being unable to choose between the parents' demands, by moving back and forth between the parents (i.e., acting as a go-between), or by being rebellious.
2. Detouring, in which parental conflict is put aside to attend to the child, either to care for the child because they are needy or ill (i.e., protective behavior) or to attack the child because they are misbehaving (i.e., hostile and blaming behavior). Detouring requires that the child continues to be problematic so that the parents can avoid the conflict.
3. Stable coalition between one parent and a child, in which the parent and child are tied closely to each other, either in response to the other parent's inadequate involvement or in order to block the other parent's involvement. Problems in family structure can be likened to structural problems in a house: Left unattended, symptoms gradually emerge and can worsen.

The Solution as the Problem

In the solution-as-the-problem approach, symptoms are explained as problems in the rules of the systems or patterns of repetitive interaction. All families are faced with everyday problems in living—for example, how to get household tasks completed, how to get children to go to school or do their homework, and how to compromise when differences occur. In addition, all families face some difficulties at some time or other in their lives. In facing a problem, each family member tends to approach the problem with characteristic ways of thinking, feeling, and acting. These initial responses may or may not be effective for the specific problem. If the family members are unable to modify their problem-solving behavior when it doesn't work, they may continue to repeat the same ineffective behavior to the point that a small or even nonexistent problem turns into a major one. Consider the following case example:

> *Mrs. B believed that children should eat specific kinds and amounts of food. When her children did not do this, she punished them. The oldest child, a compliant boy with a good appetite, responded by eating in the way she required, so Mrs. B felt like a good mother. The younger child, however, was temperamentally more of a fighter and had a very uncertain appetite. She refused to eat. Mrs. B continued to apply the same problem-solving behavior, that of punishment, and the result was a pitched battle and eventually an eating disorder—exactly what Mrs. B had not wanted to accomplish.*

This model posits that mishandling of the original problem occurs when the solution involves denying that a problem exists, and nothing is done; change is attempted for something that is unchangeable or nonexistent; or action is taken at the wrong level.[11] In the preceding case example, one could consider several possibilities:

The child's original eating behavior was not, to many observers, a problem, in that they were healthy and not losing weight. The problem was Mrs. B's belief system (see section on family belief systems later in this chapter) that to be a good mother you should feed a child well and demand discipline around eating.

If the child needed to eat more, action could have been taken at a different level—that of discussing with the child what and how she needed to eat—rather than at the level of discipline. If the child was not eating because of anxiety over her parents' quarreling, then the problem needed to be solved by treating the parents.

When Mrs. B's attempts at discipline failed, rather than change her solution (i.e., demanding obedience), she escalated her previous behavior. If, when the child developed a serious eating problem, Mrs. B refused to believe it and insisted that this was simple disobedience, the problem would continue to worsen. This outcome would illustrate our first point—symptoms occur when the solution involves denying that a problem exists.

Sometimes the problem is a conflict in problem-solving behaviors between family members. Consider the following case example:

A child stayed home for a week with the flu. She had a fine time with her mother, who was lonely and bored and was happy to have her at home. When she recovered from the flu, she protested and said she was still sick. Her mother wanted to keep her daughter home, and her father began to shout and say that the mother was spoiling the child and that the child had to go to school. This argument raised the child's anxiety and she began to throw up. She was allowed to stay home again. Eventually she developed a school phobia. If this process resulted in her forming a coalition with her mother against her father, we could say that the problem had changed the family structure.

Sometimes the problem is very real, but the solution is ineffective. Consider the following case example:

When Mrs. C's husband began drinking, she tried to protect him by covering for him, calling in sick for him, and so on. This allowed him to continue his drinking behavior and also created a new problem—she became depressed by the situation. When she no longer supported him and instead said that she would leave him if the behavior continued, she became less depressed. He also sought help and stopped drinking.

When the attempted solution becomes the problem, the way to change the situation is to do something else. In most cases it becomes the therapist's job to realize that the solution has become the problem and to help the family find alternative methods of behavior. This involves both understanding the beliefs that underlie behaviors and make it difficult to change (see next section) and conducting a careful examination of the communications of all family members to determine how and why the problem-solving behavior is failing.

When the attempted solution becomes the problem, the way to change the situation is to do something else.

FAMILY BELIEFS AND MYTHS

Individuals and families have belief systems that, in part, determine their feelings and behaviors. These subterranean structures have been referred to as family myths. They are often found to be important contributors and maintainers of family difficulty, and family therapists must be aware of them if they are to understand family behavior that might otherwise seem inexplicable. As Walsh described, family beliefs can be a strength and factor in family resilience.

For example, in the C family case example, the wife's belief that a good woman must stand by her man made it impossible for her to stop covering for her husband. Only when the wife became very depressed and her husband lost his job as a result of alcoholism was she able to change her belief to "In the end you cannot allow another person to destroy your life" and each individual has to set some limits. Ferreira[12] defined family myths as "a series of fairly well integrated beliefs shared by all family members, concerning one another and their mutual position in the family, which go unchallenged by everyone involved, in spite of the reality distortions which they may conspicuously imply." The implications of Ferreira's definition involve very personalized and specific myths for each family, in which individual family members are singled out for particular slots, roles, or self-fulfilling prophecies, such as "Mother is the emotional one in the family" or "Our son misbehaves continually."

Papp[10] and Imber-Black[13] have noted that behavioral cycles are governed by a "belief system that is composed of a combination of attitudes, basic assumptions, expectations, prejudices, convictions, and beliefs brought to the nuclear family by each parent from his/her family of origin,"[14] Some beliefs are shared, whereas others complement one another.

Beliefs, just as behavioral cycles, can be constraining of new experimentation by family members. The family's beliefs and themes,[10] constructs,[15] and myths[12] provide an added framework for the clinician who wants to go beyond interactional data to understand the ways in which family members are blocked in their accomplishment of tasks and aims. Consider the following case example:

> *A grandmother is deserted by her alcoholic husband and raises her daughter to distrust men. Her daughter marries a man who seems to provide the money and security she lacks, but he eventually has an affair. The family story, some variant of "no man can be trusted," will be passed down in different ways to male and female children. Subsequently the granddaughter may be caught in a loyalty bind—how can she trust her husband and be loyal to her mother?*

The same situation can create different myths depending on the players. For example, a family in which several members become seriously ill but survive can label itself a family of survivors or a family of failures and sick people. This will sharply affect the level of anxiety and dysfunctional behavior when the next person gets sick. This model assumes that a family's construction of the problem is as vital as its overt behaviors. It also opens the way for the therapist to construct more positive stories with the family.

In addition to specific family myths, a variety of myths are promulgated by the culture. As a result, many of these myths will be shared by family members and perhaps by the therapist. Each therapist must work out their own values with respect to these issues. The therapist must be sensitive to, and deal appropriately with, those attitudes and beliefs that seem to be deleterious to a family's functioning and, conversely, must understand that some myths aid functioning. In the next several sections, we discuss some examples of myths or beliefs that can impact functioning.

- Organization: Romantic myth. If life has not worked out well for you as an individual, getting married will make everything better. This is associated with the belief that couple and family life should be totally happy. The togetherness myth is similar, in that merely remaining in proximity or jointly carrying out all activities will lead to satisfactory family life and individual gratification. Most people need areas of separate interest to maintain a sense of self.
- Communication: Full and open frankness in feeling, action, and thought may cause at least as much harm as good. Honesty can be enlisted in the service of hostility, or it can be a constructive, problem-solving approach. It is important to approach sensitive topics with care and gentleness. Many hurtful statements, especially regarding factors that cannot be changed, are perhaps best left unspoken.
- Problem solving: A well-functioning couple or family is one in which disagreements are discussed and worked through. Many families, however, seem afraid to disagree and therefore cover up differences. In contrast, some families fight all the time about almost every issue but seemingly are unable to resolve any disagreements; instead, they seem to resort to personal attacks on one another's motives and veracity.

In successful marriages, the partners seem able to reconcile the needs of the separate individuals with those of the needs of the family unit. Some individuals, however, live as if they do not have personal needs and satisfactions but are there only to serve the larger family system. After a time, they frequently become angry or depressed. Successful family units recognize that space must be made in one's life for individual needs as well as one's role as a marital partner and a parent.

When something goes wrong in the family, each family member can be encouraged to assess their own role in the situation and in the solution to the problem. Often, one of the first jobs of the family therapist is to act as a kind of traffic cop in stopping nonproductive family interactions.

- In any relationship, positive feedback is more important than negative feedback. Many individuals have gotten out of the habit of letting their partner know when they have done something pleasing. There is often less hesitancy in commenting on something that has caused hurt or disappointment. Positive reinforcement of desired behavior usually increases its occurrence and is usually a much more effective behavior-shaping technique than is negative feedback or punishment. The therapist can model this by noticing and complimenting positive interactions.
- Separation and divorce do not necessarily represent failure, although this has been a traditional view. Individuals in a marital union, however, may be poorly matched at the outset or may grow too far apart as each person changes over time. Separation, divorce, or both may represent a creative and positive step rather than a failure for the partners, although it may increase the stress on the children.

The important things to remember are that everyone needs positive feedback, and no one can read minds well enough to substitute for clear communication.

THE LARGER SOCIAL SYSTEM AND DYSFUNCTION

Systems theory encompasses not only the family but also the wider community. The family is basically a subsystem of the community and of the culture in which it is embedded. Families do not live in a vacuum. Often the culture around them puts enormous pressure on the family system. The fit between the family and the culture, in certain locations or in cases of immigration, may be problematic.

For example, the only Jewish family living in an anti-Semitic small town may develop boundaries that in another situation would be called enmeshed but in this case are necessary to protect the children. A couple in an arranged marriage with a very traditional role structure who come to the United States can be torn apart if only the woman is able to get a job and be exposed to the new culture, thereby turning the family hierarchy upside down.

Traditional gender roles strongly affect the direction of family life. For example, a family with an overinvolved mother and a distant father is not just a family with problems; it is the end result of a historical and cultural pattern in which husbands are encouraged to see their worth as economic and wives are seen as the children's caretakers and keepers of hearth and home. In rigid or vulnerable families, this will create a huge gulf between the partners.

IMPLICATIONS FOR TREATMENT—THE DEVELOPMENT OF SYMPTOMS IN A PARTICULAR PERSON

Marital and family systems, like individuals, have characteristic patterns of coping with stress. The family's first line of defense is usually to evoke, strengthen, and emphasize characteristic adaptive patterns that the family unit has used in the past. If these patterns are inappropriate or maladaptive, the type of disturbance resulting in the family may be similar to the rigid inflexible character of an individual with a personality disorder.

If characteristic adaptive mechanisms are not available or fail to deal adequately with the situation, one or another family member may also develop overt symptoms. These symptoms in the family member may cause the individual to be labeled as being bad or sick. The appropriate social institutions (police, child welfare, community mental health centers) may become involved with that individual in an attempt to deal with the particular symptomatic expression. The individual then takes on the role of the identified patient. More often than not, the family context from which the individual's symptoms emanate will be overlooked entirely, deemphasized, or inadequately attended to. The so-called bad, sick, stupid, or crazy individual family member will be treated and will be found either intractable or improved.

If improved, they may soon become symptomatic again when returned to the family context or may cause another family member to become symptomatic. The underlying family disturbance will have to be treated. Often the symptom bearer is biologically vulnerable.

A major tenet of family therapy is that the symptomatic family member may be indicative of disturbance in the entire family system. If the therapist overlooks or deals inadequately with the more general family disturbance, family members are likely to continue to be symptomatic.

Consider the following case examples:

Mr. and Mrs. D found that over the course of 12 years of marriage their sexual relationship had become more and more unsatisfactory. They contemplated divorce. At about the same time, their son began to do poorly in school, and they sought help for this problem. Concurrently they felt less concerned about the dysfunctional nature of their marriage. As their son's schoolwork improved, the marital problem returned to the foreground.

Dr. E brought Mrs. E for individual psychotherapy because she had "headaches and depression." Her headaches always occurred after he had problems with his patients. Dr. E was a hardworking but rigid person who believed firmly in male superiority. Things had gone well for the couple in the early years of their marriage, until Mrs. E became dissatisfied with the role of number two in the marriage and pressed for equality. At that point, Dr. E intensified his authoritarian approach, especially when he felt helpless or unsuccessful at work, and rather than fighting back, Mrs. E became depressed.

The patterns of interaction within a family cannot always be clearly related to any specific dysfunction. The reasons that a specific type of disturbance is manifested in a family system or family member are not understood clearly, but certain innate tendencies and life circumstances probably favor the development of one or another symptomatic expression in a particular instance. Similarly, the reasons why one family member rather than another becomes symptomatic have not been definitively settled, although several reasons have been suggested to account for this phenomenon:

- Individual susceptibility, biologic disposition to disorder such as schizophrenia, bipolar disorder, or attention-deficit/hyperactivity disorder, or a learning disability in a child, creates an increased vulnerability to psychiatric illness. Inborn temperamental differences may also contribute.[16]
- The situation in the family at the time of birth. For example, a parent whose own parent died around the time of the birth of a sibling might feel helpless about parenting.
- Physical illness of the child. Family problems may be projected onto a child who is chronically ill whenever they have an acute episode. In addition, the amount of care needed by the ill child may skew family function, leading to infantilization of the ill child and to anger and resentment in well siblings.
- Precipitant in the extended family. An accident or a death that relates somehow to one child more than another (e.g., an eldest daughter who was with her grandmother the day the grandmother had a heart attack) may make one family member the focus for family problems.

- Sex of a child. A child's sex may correspond to a particular difficulty of the parent. For example, if a father feels particularly inadequate with other males, his son may become symptomatic.
- Birth order of siblings. The eldest child may receive the major parental pressure to mature quickly and perform well, whereas the youngest child is often babied and kept dependent.
- Family myth attached to a specific individual. Certain family members may be known as the stupid one, the smart one, the lazy one, the good-looking one, or the ugly one. First names of children and nicknames may reveal these myths. Children are sometimes named after god-parents or other people significant in the parents' past, and these children may carry along a myth attached to their namesake.

The symptomatic family member may be the family scapegoat, with family difficulties displaced on them, or this family member may be psychologically or constitutionally the weakest, the youngest, or the most sensitive family member, unable to cope with the generalized family disturbance. The identified patient may be the family member most interested or involved in the process of changing the family. For example, some teenagers want to "save" their parents because they are not getting along with each other. One hypothesis about family functioning is that these children may begin to get in trouble in order to get caught, so that the entire family can be referred for help.

LIFE CYCLE PROBLEMS AND DYSFUNCTION

Although some families may struggle with problems continually over their lives, others will experience difficulties only at specific life cycle periods. A family is subject to inner pressure coming from developmental changes in its own members and subsystems, and to outer pressure coming from demands to accommodate to the significant social institutions that affect family members.

Episodic family problems may be related to (1) an inability to cope adequately with the tasks of the current family phase; (2) the need to move on to a new family phase; (3) the stress of unexpected, idiosyncratic events; or (4) all of these problems.

In the case of normative, expectable family life transitions, a family's inability to master the present tasks may be cause for the expression of symptoms. For example, two people optimally need to reach a certain stage in their own personal development, and in their relationships with their families of origin, before being ready as two independent individuals to consider marriage. To the extent that this and other prior stages are not mastered, the individuals and the marital unit will be hampered in dealing with current challenges. This same hypothesis can be applied to each of the family phases, wherein a family's skill at a particular stage may not necessarily transfer to similar capacities at the next developmental stage (e.g., a couple competent with younger children may find themselves overwhelmed and inadequately prepared for the challenges of adolescence).

Although expected developmental transitions may be stressful for family members, unexpected or idiosyncratic changes can be more difficult to handle. Unusual events in the family life cycle may overwhelm the coping capacities of family systems to handle developmental changes. Common examples of such events include unemployment, catastrophic illness, accidents, violent crime, or a death in the family. Any of these events may require the family to explore new ways of organizing itself temporarily to manage the additional strains posed by the event. Marital and family systems, like individuals, have characteristic patterns of coping with stress. As we have said, the family's first line of defense is usually to evoke, strengthen, and emphasize characteristic adaptive patterns that the family unit has used in the past. However, if these do not work, the family patterns may disorganize. From this may come serious dysfunction or a creative new solution.

Whatever the particulars of a family's dysfunction, by outlining the family's individual life cycle, the therapist helps in elucidating the family's idiosyncrasies and provides a framework from which successful therapy can begin.[17]

Unresolved Grief

The death of a parent or a child, especially when mourning does not occur, commonly leads to family problems. Often the family development stops at the point of the death and the family remains in limbo, unable to move on or to truly grieve. This is often expressed in family ritual—for example, if a child died near Christmas, the family may be unable to celebrate for years to come, or the family may insist that the Christmas ritual be exactly the same as before the child died, long past the point at which the ritual would have changed to accommodate the other children. Death from stillbirth or miscarriage may have the same effect. Most often, the family needs help to talk about the death and to find some way to grieve and continue living.

Toxic Secrets

Families may have secrets that some members know but others don't (e.g., the mother and daughter, but not the father, may know the daughter had an abortion), secrets that everyone knows but no one admits (e.g., the father has a substance use disorder), or secrets that most family members suspect but don't want to know about (e.g., the mother is having an affair). Secrets prevent clear communication, skew coalitions, and mystify children who know something is wrong but not what. Secrets contribute an air of unreality to the family, which is bad for children's development and reality testing. Thus, as part of life cycle problems at a certain point in time, a secret may result in dysfunction.

The therapist must find a way to uncover the secret carefully, giving time to support everyone in the family. It is seldom in the family's best interest for people to keep a major family secret. We return to this topic in Chapter 13 (on the subject of resistance) and again in Chapter 25 (in the context of ethics).

TASK PERFORMANCE IN THE DYSFUNCTIONAL FAMILY

Various deficiencies in carrying out the family's functions will lead to strains and distortions, problems, and symptoms in family life. The three major family tasks, as we discussed in Chapter 3, are (1) to provide for basic needs, (2) to develop a working marital coalition, and (3) to rear and socialize the offspring.

In the dysfunctional family, these tasks either are not handled or are handled differently and less adaptively than in healthy families. In Chapter 3, we detailed some of these processes and outcomes for both functional and dysfunctional families.

Task performance in the family may be compromised by an unendurable environment, by the individual physical or mental illness of one or more family members, or by serious conflict among family members, particularly the marital dyad or adult caretakers.

Providing for the Family's Basic Needs

An inability to provide for the family's basic needs is common in times of war, poverty, or economic depression. Families fleeing from trauma, being subjected to cruel immigration policies and family separation create additional burdens. Maintaining family integrity in the face of severe poverty requires ingenuity and endurance, which are hard to maintain on a daily basis if the adults become incapacitated or depressed. However, inability to provide for basic needs may occur in the face of adequate finances if the caretaking adults (especially the mother, who is most often left in charge of daily family functioning, even when ill) are absent due to substance use disorders, psychosis, or violence or are so caught up in their own concerns as to be oblivious to those in their care.

Maintaining a Functional Marriage: Issues of Sex, Intimacy, and Commitment

Marriage is one of the few human relationships that functions profoundly on two levels: as an intense love relationship and as a functional, daily economic partnership or small business. It requires a complex set of skills and feelings and the ability to switch from one functioning mode to another. It is possible, although not pleasant, to have a marriage in which intimacy has gone but the couple functions well on a "roommate" level to parent and keep the home going.

In these couples, problem-solving skills and communication may be clear, but intimate contact is absent. These marriages often break up when the children leave. It is also possible to have a marriage in which sex and passion are very much present, but fierce battles over power and control issues make it very hard to get much done. As the couple becomes more dysfunctional, anger and rage overwhelm positive feelings, communication, and task completion, leaving the couple in a constant battle, isolated and silent, or with one spouse completely dominating the other. These couples are likely to triangle in a child, parent, or lover to deal with the stress.

Rearing and Socializing of Children

It is difficult to deal with the constant needs of children when one is overwhelmed by marital strife, individual illness, racism, or poverty. The more parents are disconnected from the part of themselves that is capable of nurturing, the more the children are neglected or become used to taking care of the parents—by being responsible for household tasks, providing emotional support to the parents, or by supporting one parent against the other. The ultimate form of using the child is incest, in which the child becomes a substitute sexual object. Children as young as 4 or 5 years can be inducted into trying to cheer up a depressed parent, making their own food because the parents have forgotten, or trying to shield a younger child from abuse.

Members of very troubled families may demonstrate styles of thinking and communication that are particularly difficult for children to understand, including intrusive, projective, or bizarre thinking. In some families the children's emotions are consistently denied, contradicted, ignored, or punished, leading to depression, rage, or numbing in the children.

It needs to be said, however, that some children are very difficult to deal with and make the task of childrearing formidable. Children with a difficult temperament, attention-deficit/hyperactivity disorder, or some forms of child psychosis require their parents extraordinary reserves of patience and attention and have little ability to maintain impulse control or soothe themselves. The parents must maintain a calm, structured environment in the face of constant testing. If the parents do not share a commitment to put in extra time, or if they cannot reach an agreement on ways to deal with the child, these children can cause major rifts in marriages that otherwise would function within the normal range.

Other children might not be difficult for every parent but temperamentally are a bad fit with a particular parent. For example, a very active, mischievous boy might be a bad match for a fearful and depressed mother, who might have done better with a more docile and quiet child. Or, a young boy who is shy and retiring might be a great disappointment to a tough, demanding, athletic father, who may try to toughen him up by being harsh in a way that leaves permanent emotional scars.

CLINICAL PRACTICE IMPLICATIONS

In this chapter, we described (1) the process of how a family can become dysfunctional, (2) the systems perspective, and (3) how an inability to negotiate life cycle transitions or perform family tasks causes problems or symptoms. We also emphasized factors that contribute to family resilience.

A member of the family may ask for external help for themselves or another family member may try to harm themselves, someone, or something and thus come to the attention of an external agency. To take the identified patient at face value and to deal only with that person, without seeing the rest of the family, would represent a distorted and limited perspective of the dysfunction inherent in the family.

A functional family is like an orchestra playing a beautiful symphony: Each of its members plays a different instrument, but together they add up to an overall configuration of harmony that is effective and fulfilling. Conversely, a dysfunctional family is like a poker game in which each player holds certain cards, yet no one will put them on the table. As a result, the same old game keeps being played. Because no one will risk losing (or winning) by playing a new card, in effect, no one wins and no one loses, and the game becomes a pointless exercise. Alternatively, one player may win the same hollow victory repeatedly, and another may always be identified as the loser. These sequences characterize a couple or family in distress.

SUGGESTED READING

This is an excellent guide on how to make marriage work. This is also applicable to couples.

Karasu SR, Karasu TB. *The Art of Marriage Maintenance.* Jason Aronson; 2005.

REFERENCES

1. Bateson G, Jackson D, Haley J, et al. Toward a theory of schizophrenia. *Behav Sci.* 1956;1:251–254.
2. Jackson DD, Yalom I. Family homeostasis and patient change. In: Masserman J, ed. *Current Psychiatric Therapies.* Grune & Stratton; 1965:155–165.
3. Bowen M. *Family Therapy in Clinical Practice.* Jason Aronson; 1978.
4. Wynne LC, Gurman A, Ravich R, et al. The family and marital therapies. In: Lewis JF, Usdin G, eds. *Treatment Planning in Psychiatry.* American Psychiatric Association; 1982:225–286.
5. Lidz T. *The Family and Human Adaptation.* International Universities Press; 1963.
6. Ackerman N. *Psychodynamics of Family Life, Diagnosis and Treatment in Family Relationships.* Basic Books; 1958.
7. Lewis JW. For better or worse: interpersonal relationships and individual outcome. *Am J Psychiatry.* 1998; 155:582–589.
8. Walsh F. Family resilience: a framework for clinical practice 2003. *Fam Process.* 2003;42(1):1–18.
9. Minuchin S. *Families and Family Therapy.* Harvard University Press; 1974.
10. Papp P. *The Process of Change.* Guilford; 1980.
11. Watzlawick P, Weakland J, Fisch R. *Change: Principles of Problem Formation and Problem Resolution.* WW Norton; 1974.
12. Ferreira AJ. Family myths and homeostasis. *Arch Gen Psychiatry.* 1963;9:457–463.
13. Imber-Black E. A family larger system perspective. In: Gurman A, Kniskern D, eds. *Handbook of Family Therapy.* Vol 11. Brunner/Mazel; 1991:583–605.
14. Carroll EJ. Treatment of the family as a unit. *Pa Med J.* 1960;63:57–62.
15. Reiss D. The working family: a researcher's view of health in the household. *Am J Psychiatry.* 1981;139:11–22.
16. Thomas A, Chess S. *Temperament and Development.* Guilford; 1985.
17. Carter B, McGoldrick M. Conceptual overview. In: Carter B, McGoldrick M, eds. *The Changing Family Life Cycle: A Framework for Family Therapy.* 2nd ed. Gardner; 1988:3–25.

The family therapist's first task is to evaluate the couple or family's areas of healthy functioning and dysfunction. Next, the family therapist should formulate an evaluation of what is wrong and what can be done about it. In Chapter 6, we examine the *process* of conducting the family evaluation. In Chapter 7, we look at the *content* of the evaluation (i.e., what areas to cover). In Chapter 8, we discuss how to formulate the case, plan the therapeutic approach, and establish a treatment contract. In Chapter 8, we include a case example illustrating the process. The purpose in crafting such a formulation is to create a succinct and focused case conceptualization that can guide family treatment and anticipate possible outcomes.

Section

III Family Evaluation

6 The Process of Evaluation 85

7 The Content of Evaluation 94

8 Formulating an Understanding of the Family Problem Areas 102

6 The Process of Evaluation

OBJECTIVES FOR THE READER

- To identify the premises of systemic assessment
- To be able to gather historical data
- To be cognizant of the progression and choice points of the evaluation interview
- To understand the role of individual and family diagnoses in gathering data

For easier reading, we emphasize that the descriptors "couples" or "marital" are used nearly interchangeably in this chapter.

INTRODUCTION

The evaluation of a couple or family should be understood as a continuing process, which begins at the first contact but is not necessarily completed at any particular point. Some initial formulation (i.e., an understanding of what is wrong) can help the therapist gather data and form hypotheses, but in a larger sense the evaluation is often an inextricable part of the therapy itself. Oftentimes, if patients can hear and analyze their histories then their present situations will change.

As data are gathered, the therapist forms hypotheses based on a conceptual frame of reference. The therapist should assign priorities and weights to the contributory variables, while setting up an overall intervention strategy.

It is hoped that the particular interventions will lead to desired therapy goals. In this process, data are used to confirm, modify, or negate the original hypotheses, strategies, or tactics. These later formulations are then tested in the matrix of the family sessions as further data is obtained. We describe details of this strategy and its tactics in Section IV, which explores in more depth various family therapy techniques.

WHO TO INCLUDE IN THE FAMILY EVALUATION
PROGRESSION OF THE FAMILY EVALUATION INTERVIEW
DIMENSIONS OF COUPLE AND FAMILY ASSESSMENT
  Joining with the Couple or Family
  Seeing Systemic Patterns
  Recognizing Family Developmental Stage, History, and Culture
  Identifying Family Structure

WORKING WITH A SYSTEMIC MODEL OF CHANGE
ROLE OF HISTORICAL MATERIAL
ROLE OF INDIVIDUAL AND FAMILY DIAGNOSES
CLINICAL PRACTICE IMPLICATIONS

WHO TO INCLUDE IN THE FAMILY EVALUATION

An early and strategic question involves which members of the family should be included in the evaluation sessions. From the very first contact, usually by telephone call, the therapist often talks to one individual who represents the family and presents the problem. Sometimes the problem is presented as a family problem; other times the problem is presented as an individual's problem that is disturbing the other family members. Here, we will assume that from the first telephone call or contact by a family member the therapist is considering the possibility of family intervention. Thus, the question arises of who to include in the evaluation sessions. **Most family therapists would agree that it is important, from the first session, to include all members of the family in the evaluation sessions.** This usually means all members of a nuclear family, that is, all family members who reside under the same roof. Relatives living with the family should probably also be included at some point. It is obviously impractical and often unnecessary to include, for example, an adult child who lives 2,000 miles away from their parents, at least for the initial sessions. In addition to nuclear family members, significant others must be included if they are living with or deeply involved with the children. This is especially true in single-parent or blended families. Therapists seeing a custodial parent and child need to make a very serious effort to include the noncustodial parent at some point early in therapy.

Clinical experience suggests that it is easier to include all family members for evaluation sessions at the beginning than it is to wait to do so later. This provides a clearer picture of family dynamics and allows better evaluation of family problems. If the therapist begins with all family members, then they can hold subsequent sessions with one subsystem alone.

Particular circumstances may cause the therapist to not want to include the entire family in the evaluation sessions. For example, a couple that is having sexual difficulties should be seen as a couple without their children. Likewise, the couple may be seen alone for marital difficulties without involving the children, although the children may be included later if appropriate. Some therapists will see both spouses together in an initial evaluation session, followed by an individual session with each spouse alone. Although some leading clinicians say that such a situation allows one spouse to tell secrets to the therapist, others suggest that the only way for a therapist to proceed is to have all information at the beginning.

Some therapists hold individual sessions with each spouse but indicate before the session that it is not confidential to the couple sessions, thus precluding the forming of coalitions, but yet possibly discouraging full disclosure of information. Some parents will insist on "checking out" the therapist before bringing the children in that is comfortable working with the clinician.

A practical consideration for the evaluation sessions arises when one or more central family members are absent. **Missing family members often have crucial roles in the problem. Their absence must be discussed and their presence brought about**. Napier and Whitaker[1] provide an interesting clinical illustration of a family in which the initial evaluation session is stopped because of a missing son, and the family's task becomes insisting on his participation. It is probably not an uncommon practice of family therapists to refuse to proceed with the evaluation until the missing member is present; however, some therapists will do a few sessions without a missing member, focusing on how the missing member could be convinced to come in as one of the treatment issues. If, for example, a major family problem has been a couple's inability to put limits on their 16-year-old son, then refusing to treat the family until they bring the son in may result in their giving up on treatment. It may be better to focus treatment on the couple with a discussion of how they can set limits that will encourage their son to come to treatment.

PROGRESSION OF THE FAMILY EVALUATION INTERVIEW

Several authors have discussed the sequential progression of the family evaluation interview. Most would suggest that the first interview task is to greet each of the family members and to begin to accommodate to the family. **Next, the interview can proceed with the narrative describing the family problem as each family member sees it.**

Reiss[2] has provided a helpful analysis of the choice points that a clinician faces in the initial assessment of a family. He distinguishes substantive and theoretical choice points from technical choice points.

The first substantive choice point is whether to focus on the cross-sectional view (i.e., current functioning of the family), or to give more attention to the longitudinal developmental history of the family unit and its individuals. A second choice point is whether to focus on the family as the central shaping force, or to focus on the extended family system or larger community/social systems that influence the family. The latter would include focus on the network of extended family, friends, school, and so on. A third choice point concerns crisis versus character orientation. The former focused on the current immediate concrete problem or symptom that brings the family in, whereas the latter focuses on the more enduring patterns of self-protection, cognitive, and affective style, as well as the deficits the family manifests. Another choice point is whether to focus on the pathology or the functional competence of the family unit. A fifth choice point concerns the basic theoretical understanding of the evaluator and their emphasis on finding family themes versus looking at concrete behaviors and their consequences.

The first technical choice point concerns the pacing of the assessment. Some authors advocate a thorough assessment before beginning treatment, with a clear marker between the assessment and the treatment; others emphasize that assessment and treatment merge, especially because assessment involves intervening and assessing how the family responds. A second technical choice point involves individualized measurement of the family (emphasizing the uniqueness of the family), or standardized measurement of the family (focusing on major dimensions relevant to all families). In Chapter 8, we discuss another choice point involving assessment: the issue of dimensionalizing the data (e.g., how does the family rate on communication), focusing on the typology of the family (e.g., the enmeshed family). Another choice point is the clinician's perspective of being "inside," emphatically feeling what it is like to be with this family, versus observing as objectively as possible (as an outsider) how the family performs and carries out functions. A final choice point is whether to focus on the children or adults, and whether the method should involve talking or an activity.

These choice points are not either–or situations. Depending on the situation, the evaluation will emphasize different areas. But these choice points must be faced (in the time-limited setting of conducting evaluations). For those fortunate enough to work in training centers or non-solo practices, an effective way of evaluating families is with a team behind a one-way mirror. The experience of being behind a mirror and watching is fundamentally different from being in the room. Although subtle emotional cues, anxiety, or connection is often missed by not being in the room, the overall pattern, including the relationship of the therapist to the family, is more clear. With a team, one can obtain many differing viewpoints. It is humbling but invaluable to see how the understanding of a family is affected by the personality, age, and gender of the viewer and the process opens up many different realities for the therapist.

DIMENSIONS OF COUPLE AND FAMILY ASSESSMENT

We emphasize five important conceptual and practical features of couples and family assessment: (1) joining with the couple or family; (2) seeing systemic patterns that maintain maladaptive behaviors, thoughts, and feelings; (3) recognizing the importance of family developmental stage, history, and culture; (4) identifying the family structure; and (5) understanding and using a systemic model of change.[3] These skills are taught in the broader context of the biopsychosocial model embedded in most training programs, as opposed to the more specialized models of many couples and family therapy institutes.

Joining with the Couple or Family

One of the most difficult challenges that therapists face is learning how to manage therapeutic relationships with couples or multiple family members in an environment characterized by conflict, emotionality, vulnerability, and threat. To new and experienced clinicians alike, there appear to be so many ways to fail: by overidentifying with one family member, overprotecting another, or sharing in the family's experience of helplessness.

Not surprisingly, the dropout rate in couples and family therapy is higher than in individual treatment.[4] It is easy to take a wrong step, inadvertently take sides, and disappoint a patient whose relationship is foundering. The family therapist must actively understand the family's predicament, recognize that they will be able to repair even the most problematic relationships, and instill hope that the couple or family's circumstances can change.

Minuchin and Fishman[5] describe the family and clinician as forming a time-limited partnership that will support the process of exploration and transformation. From the structural family therapy perspective, "joining" is considered to be the glue that holds together the therapeutic system. Virtually every model of family therapy highlights the importance of developing a strong initial bond with the couple or family and its members, as the therapeutic work requires alliances sturdy enough and flexible enough to support challenges to the couple's or family's preferred patterns of interaction. As any clinician walking the tightrope between battling family members or competing coalitions knows, the most formidable clinical task involves not simply building these alliances, but sustaining them over the course of therapy.[3]

Seeing Systemic Patterns

Therapists subsequently consider how various forms of individual psychopathology elicit recognizable interpersonal patterns that reinforce signs and symptoms of the disorders. In particular, the regularities that link the biologic, intergenerational, and sociocultural contexts of family life are explored. Because problems from a systemic perspective are situated in their interpersonal contexts, a new vocabulary is needed to characterize them. Therapists come to appreciate how complementarity functions as a defining principle in every relationship. The importance of this conceptual shift cannot be underestimated. Minuchin and Nichols[6] observe, "In any couple, one person's behavior is yoked to the other's … it means that a couple's actions are not independent but codetermined, reciprocal forces" (p. 63).

Consequently, the family therapist begins with a microscopic focus on the individual, their illness, and its treatment and then adds a wide-angle lens to better perceive the powerful social factors that influence, and are affected by, the sick person's experience. Seeing these complementary relationships between self and system, between the individual's behaviors and the system's responses that maintain them, stands as the linchpin of systemic thinking.

Recognizing Family Developmental Stage, History, and Culture

It is difficult to overestimate the importance of identifying the family's developmental stage. Just as in individual treatment, therapists must recognize the normal developmental tasks and transitions, beginning with couple formation and ending with death, that couples and families routinely encounter. Therapists soon appreciate that both centripetal (couple formation, marriage, birth of a child, birth of grandchildren, death) and centrifugal stages (going to school, adolescence, leaving home) occur and recur throughout the family life cycle, presenting new challenges that require reorganization at each step (Table 6.1).

Table 6.1 Family life cycle

Centripetal stages	Centrifugal stages
Marriage	
Birth of first child	
Family with young children	
	Child enters elementary school
	School-aged children
	Entry into adolescence
	Leaving home
Birth of grandchildren	
Retirement and older age	
Dying and death	

Source: Reprinted by permission of Springer: Rait D, Glick I. A model for reintegrating couples and family therapy training in psychiatric residency programs. *Acad Psychiatry.* 2008;32(2):81–86. Copyright © 2008 Academic Psychiatry.

At the same time, members of a couple bring with them idiosyncratic histories that serve as blueprints against which current situations are appraised. Therapists learn to construct three-generational genograms, or family trees, that identify family patterns and themes as well as highlight connections between present family events and prior experience.

The genogram is a useful tool because "a picture is worth a thousand words," and therapists soon recognize its value in efficiently gathering family historical information visually rather than in the traditional narrative form. Most couples and families enjoy the process of generating a genogram, as they see patterns emerge in their family histories in a way that is accessible and clarifying (Fig. 6.1).

Finally, therapists must develop cultural competence in their work with couples and families. By recognizing how each family member's distinctive sociocultural background provides

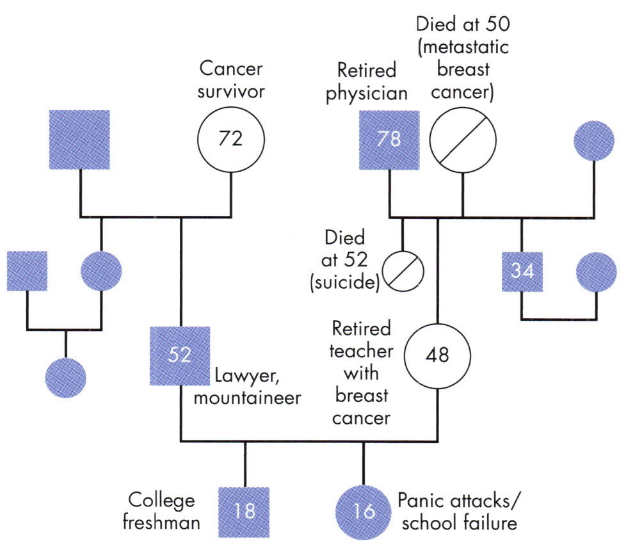

Figure 6.1 Genogram showing family with a symptomatic daughter. (*Source:* Reprinted by permission of Springer: Rait D, Glick I. A model for reintegrating couples and family therapy training in psychiatric residency programs. *Acad Psychiatry.* 2008;32(2):81–86. Copyright © 2008 Academic Psychiatry.)

context and meaning for a family's traditions, choices, and preferences, trainees can tailor both clinical formulations and strategies for change. Therapists frequently comment that they receive far too little training in appreciating the strengths and differences among patients and families from different cultural and ethnic groups. In all cases, identifying critical influences such as gender, culture, class, race, religion, disability, and sexual orientation contributes to the development of culturally sensitive practices that address the distinctive aspects of each family's idiosyncratic culture.

Identifying Family Structure

If genograms map the family's history over time, the structural map represents the family's present organization with special attention paid to proximity and affiliation, hierarchy and power, and boundaries and subsystems. Family structure, most notably associated with Minuchin,[7] represents an inference drawn from redundant pieces of family process that identify preferred patterns and available alternatives: therapists learn to see the couple or family in terms of its structure—instead of seeing only individuals, they begin to notice hierarchical imbalances in couples, coalitions and alliances, and relationship triangles (Fig. 6.2).

Over time, therapists begin to understand the couple or family's preferred patterns and available alternatives. They practice diagramming couples and families, looking at patterns of closeness and distance, power, boundaries, coalitions, and alliances. In Families and Family Therapy, Minuchin[7] writes:

> *A family map is an organizational scheme. It does not represent the richness of family transactions any more than any map represents the richness of a territory. It is static, whereas the family is constantly in motion. But the family map is a powerful simplification device, which allows the therapist to organize the diverse material that he is getting* (p. 90).

These structural maps serve as the basis for family assessment, goal setting, and the determination of therapeutic progress.

WORKING WITH A SYSTEMIC MODEL OF CHANGE

Therapists learning about systemic change can initially find it disorienting to find that the shortest distance between the point of assessment and intervention is not necessarily a straight line. Rather than targeting problematic individual behaviors, the wider systemic view recognizes that

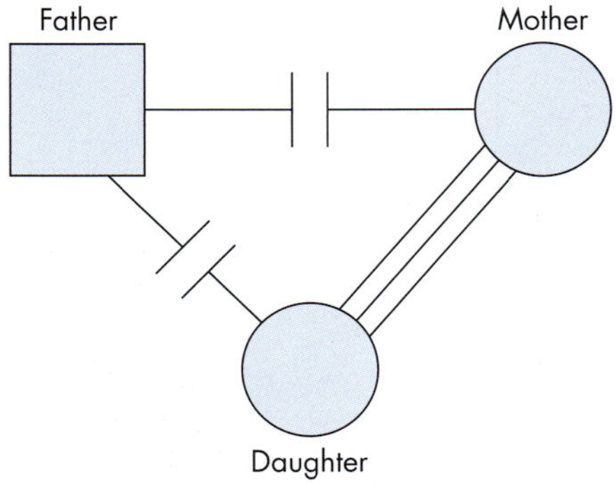

Figure 6.2 Structural map showing same family in therapy. (*Source:* Reprinted by permission of Springer: Rait D, Glick I. A model for reintegrating couples and family therapy training in psychiatric residency programs. *Acad Psychiatry.* 2008;32(2):81–86. Copyright © 2008 Academic Psychiatry.)

Table 6.2 Thinking family and working systemically

Join with the family
Focus on patterns and process rather than content
Consider family developmental stage, history, and culture identify family structure
Devise systemic interventions that encourage systemic/structural change
Support the couple/family and highlight their strengths

Source: Reprinted by permission of Springer: Rait D, Glick I. A model for reintegrating couples and family therapy training in psychiatric residency programs. *Acad Psychiatry*. 2008;32(2):81–86. Copyright © 2008 Academic Psychiatry.

intervening in relationships that support these behaviors can be quite powerful. In this regard, therapists must experience a figure-ground shift, in that the individual "problem" can best be understood and treated by bringing these contextual factors into the foreground. The aim of systemic therapy is to disrupt dysfunctional patterns, to introduce alternative rules, and in doing so, to provoke systemic change. In this regard, the trainees begin to recognize the significant difference between "first-order" or technical change (such as improving communication skills) and "second-order" or systemic change (whereby the "rules of the game" are modified).

An integrative perspective allows for both an active here-and-now focus that therapists appreciate with the added richness of a family-of-origin historical approach to data gathering. Specifically, therapists learn the premises for a treatment model in which the therapeutic task is to help the family move from one stage of development to a new stage where members' developmental needs are better met; the therapist joins with the family by entering into their reality and becoming involved in the repeated interactions that form the family's structure; the therapist expands the family's range by challenging family rules, fostering boundary reorganization, promoting communication and conflict resolution, and supporting greater individuation of family members; and the therapist monitors change process by helping family members integrate emerging patterns into a new level of functioning. These steps, originally developed by staff at the Philadelphia Child Guidance Clinic, serve as a guide for a flexible approach to working with couples and families (Table 6.2).

It has been said that the only way to learn to ride a bicycle is to climb on a bicycle and ride. In some regards, this analogy applies to learning psychotherapy as well, and there is no substitute for actually working with a couple or family. Therapists working with couples and families should be competent to form an alliance with, assess, educate, and support families. In addition, they should be able to see a presenting problem through a systemic or an individual basis. While adopting a systemic perspective can be challenging, learning how to intervene systemically requires practice, reflection, and careful attention.

ROLE OF HISTORICAL MATERIAL

Several points of view exist regarding the type and quantity of historical data that should be gathered. Some family therapists begin with a specific and detailed longitudinal history of the family unit and its constituent members, that is, the *genogram*, which may span three or more generations (see Chapter 7). This method permits the family and the therapist to review together the complex background of the present situation. The therapist will begin to understand unresolved past and present issues, and will usually gain a sense of rapport and identification with the family and its members. The therapist may then feel more comfortable defining problem areas and planning strategy. The family also benefits by reviewing together the source and evolution of its current condition, which may be a clarifying and empathy-building process for them. The good and the bad are brought into focus, and the immediate distress is placed in a broader perspective. For a family in crisis that is too impatient to tolerate exhaustive history gathering, lengthy data gathering must be curtailed.

Some therapists do not rely heavily on the longitudinal approach. Instead, they prefer to begin with a cross-sectional view of family functioning, delineating the situation that led the family to seek treatment at the present time. This cross-sectional view attempts to understand the current problem and to obtain a cross-sectional view of the family's present functioning. This procedure has the advantage of starting with the problems about which the family is most concerned, and is not as potentially time-consuming or seemingly remote from the present realities as the longitudinal method. The therapist, however, may not emerge with as sharp a focus on important family patterns, because much of the discussion may be negatively tinged because of the family's preoccupation with its current difficulty.

A minority of therapists may severely curtail history gathering and minimize formalized discussions of the family's current situation. They may begin instead by dealing with the family's important characteristic patterns of interaction as they are manifested in the interview setting. To do this, they may primarily or exclusively use the immediate here-and-now observable family transactions, interpreting these to be characteristic of the family. They may clarify and comment on these transactions, intervening in a variety of ways. Observation of the interactions among family members provides the therapist with raw data rather than historical reconstruction.

A family's biography is an altered history bent through the prism of the person telling the story. History reported by involved individuals must be considered as potentially biased secondhand information because the therapist is not witnessing the dysfunction described. The information will vary sharply among historians, and key pieces of information may be omitted.

A present-oriented approach has the advantage of initiating treatment immediately, without the usual delay of history gathering. With this approach, there is often a heightened sense of emotional involvement, which may cause more rapid changes to occur. However, sometimes families are overwhelmed by such an approach and may feel threatened and defensive. When specific information and patterns are allowed to emerge in this random fashion, the therapist does not always have the same degree of certainty as to whether the emerging family patterns are indeed relevant and important. As a result, such an approach is not usually recommended for beginning therapists.

To a considerable extent, these differences in technique may mirror differences in therapists' training, theoretical beliefs, and individual temperaments. Most therapists likely use a combination of these approaches depending on the situation, for there is no evidence that one technique is better than another. We strongly recommend reviewing *both* past history and presenting complaints while gathering a three- or four-generation genogram.

ROLE OF INDIVIDUAL AND FAMILY DIAGNOSES

In deciding who to include in the family assessment, the question must be expanded to consider the purpose for which an individual is included in the assessment. In this text, our bias is that both the family and the individuals in the family unit are important in the diagnostic equation.

In psychiatry, an imperfect relationship exists between individual diagnosis and treatment planning because often the diagnosis itself does not give enough information to plan the interventions. This imperfect relationship between diagnosis and treatment planning is compounded in the area of family therapy, where one must have enough information to give an individual diagnosis (especially if there is a clearly identified patient) and also make a family diagnostic statement.

The first implication is that in assessing families one must obtain enough individual information to be able to give individual diagnoses to members exhibiting pathologies that meet the diagnostic criteria in *The Diagnostic and Statistical Manual of Mental Disorders, Fifth Edition* (*DSM*-5),[8] to members exhibiting pathologies that meet the diagnostic criteria. New to DSM-5 are codes that identify relational problems if a nonmental disorder is the reason for the current visit, or that help explain the need for an intervention or treatment. Examples include:

- Problems related to family upbringing (e.g., parent–child relational problem, sibling relational problem, upbringing away from parents, child affected by parental relationship distress)
- Problems related to primary support group (e.g., relationship distress with spouse or intimate partner, high expressed emotion level within the family, disruption of family by separation or divorce, uncomplicated bereavement)

CLINICAL PRACTICE IMPLICATIONS

We discuss these issues as they relate to case formulation in Chapter 8 and in the context of the relationship between the family and individual psychiatric disorders in Chapter 18. For now, let us emphasize that while not all family therapists use DSM-5 criteria, we believe that family members must be assessed to determine the presence of serious psychopathology and the need for medication. In considering the couple or family, and its constituent members, a comprehensive evaluation will account for individual, family, and larger systemic variables that not only inform a view of the family's problems, but also its strengths, resources, and ability to change.

REFERENCES

1. Napier A, Whitaker C. *The Family Crucible*. Harper & Row; 1978.
2. Reiss D. *The Family's Construction of Reality*. Harvard University Press; 1981.
3. Rait D, Glick I. A model for reintegrating family therapy training in psychiatric residency programs. *Acad Psychiatry*. 2008;32:81–86.
4. Bischoff R, Sprenkle D. Dropping out of marriage and family therapy: a critical review of the research. *Fam Process*. 1993;32:353–375.
5. Minuchin S, Fishman C. *Family Therapy Techniques*. Harvard Press; 1981:30.
6. Minuchin S, Nichols M. *Family Healing: Strategies for Hope and Understanding*. Simon and Schuster; 1984:63.
7. Minuchin S. *Families and Family Therapy*. Harvard University Press; 1974.
8. American Psychiatric Association. *Diagnostic and Statistical Manual of Mental Disorders*. 5th ed. American Psychiatric Association; 2013.
9. Rait D, Glick I. Reintegrating family therapy training in psychiatric residency programs: making the case. *Acad Psychiatry*. 2008;32:76–80.

7 The Content of Evaluation

OBJECTIVES FOR THE READER

- To be aware of the information needed (i.e., the dimensions for each category in the family evaluation outline)
- To be aware of the salient content areas of family evaluation

For easier reading, we emphasize that the descriptors "couples" or "marital" are used nearly interchangeably in this chapter.

INTRODUCTION

In Chapter 6, we indicated that there is more than one potentially useful way to evaluate a family, depending on the situation. The procedure we offer in this chapter combines useful aspects of the longitudinal and cross-sectional approaches we discussed in Chapter 6. These approaches combine both verbal and nonverbal techniques for obtaining information. In Chapter 12, we discuss in greater detail the process of gathering information over the course of therapy. Because one cannot evaluate everything about a family without getting lost in the details, both the trainee and the experienced family therapist need an outline that indicates not only what to evaluate but also the priorities of evaluation.

Such an outline is analogous to the outline used for assessing individual patients (i.e., chief complaint, present illness, and so on), which every medical student and resident has committed to memory. The theory of family functioning and its relationship to the cause and maintenance of pathology in an individual family member should in part guide and prioritize such an evaluation.

DIMENSIONS OF FAMILY FUNCTION
FAMILY EVALUATION OUTLINE
Gathering Identifying Data and Establishing Current Phase of Family Life Cycle
Gathering Explicit Interview Data
What Is the Background of the Family Problem?
What is the History of Past Treatment Attempts?
What Are the Family's Goals and Expectations of the Treatment?
THE FAMILY GENOGRAM
CLINICAL PRACTICE IMPLICATIONS

DIMENSIONS OF FAMILY FUNCTION

Because of its thoroughness, operational definitions, congruence with the major areas of family functioning or dysfunction mentioned in Chapters 3 to 5, teachableness, and relevance to treatment planning, we recommend a modified version of the McMaster model of family evaluation.[1] According to this model, five dimensions of family functioning must be assessed. These dimensions are congruent with the concepts of functional and dysfunctional families (enumerated in Chapters 3 to 5) and are congruent with the consensus areas of importance across family models. These dimensions are communication, problem solving, roles and coalitions, affective responsiveness and involvement, and behavior control. The therapist must also carefully evaluate the family members' beliefs about themselves and about the problem. Finally, the family's cultural background and its patterns of beliefs and values must be assessed.

FAMILY EVALUATION OUTLINE

Drawing heavily from the McMaster model and integrating other aspects, we developed the evaluation outline presented in Table 7.1. This outline offers a practical alternative to either gathering an extensive history or plunging into the middle of the family interaction. Although far from exhaustive in scope, this outline provides some anchoring points for initial understanding and planning. It is not meant to be inflexible or unchangeable, and it certainly can be expanded or contracted as the situation warrants. We cover the first two outline topics in this chapter and the third topic (i.e., formulating the family problem areas) in Chapter 8. In Section IV, we discuss the last topic relating to treatment.

Gathering Identifying Data and Establishing Current Phase of Family Life Cycle

Family members' names, ages, and relationships and the family's composition, race, ethnicity, socioeconomic status, and living arrangements should be obtained early. To identify the current phase of the family life cycle, the therapist will ascertain the ages and relationships of those family members living under one roof, adult children living separately, and ages of grandparents.

Table 7.1 Family evaluation outline

I. Gathering identifying data and establishing current phase of family life cycle
II. Gathering explicit interview data:
   A. What is the current family problem?
   B. Why does the family come for treatment at the present time?
      1. Recent family events and stresses
   C. What is the background of the family problem?
   D. What is the history of past treatment attempts or other attempts at problem solving in the family? What other problems has the family had?
   E. What are the family's goals and expectations of the treatment? What are its strengths, motivations, and resistances?
III. Formulating the family problem areas:
   A. Rating important dimensions of family functioning:
      1. Communication
      2. Problem solving
      3. Roles and coalitions
      4. Affective responsiveness and involvement
      5. Behavior control
      6. Operative family beliefs and stories
   B. Family classification and diagnosis
IV. Planning the therapeutic approach and establishing the treatment contract

Source: Adapted from Epstein and Bishop (2007),[2] Gill et al. (1954),[3] and Group for the Advancement of Psychiatry (1970).[4]

An important criterion for understanding the family's structure is knowing each phase the family has reached in its developmental cycle. Each phase is associated with unique stresses, challenges, opportunities, and pitfalls. By being alert to these, the therapist is in a position to observe and explore phase-specific tasks, roles, and relationships for the family. The therapist can also discover to what extent the family members clearly recognize and are attempting to cope with issues relevant to the family's current developmental phase. For many married couples and families, the basic difficulty underlying the need for professional help can be related to their inability to cope satisfactorily with their current developmental phase or with the transition into the next phase. The A family (see the first case example in this chapter) is a good example of the type of problem arising in a later stage of marriage—the empty-nest syndrome—in which the parents could not cope with the separation of their child from the home, in part because of their fears of not being able to relate to each other as husband and wife.

One or both parents may be going through an individual developmental phase that powerfully affects the family life cycle. For example, the birth of a baby to a 40-year-old mother and a 60-year-old father may be in conflict with the father's sense of aging and his thoughts of ease and retirement. Alternatively, it might bring both parents a sense of renewed youth and empowerment.

Gathering Explicit Interview Data

What is the current family problem? The interviewer asks this question to each family member, in turn, with all family members present. The interviewer attempts to maintain the focus on the current family problem, rather than on one or another individual, or on past difficulties. Each family member receives an equal opportunity to be heard, without interruption, and to feel that their opinions and views are worthwhile, important, and acknowledged.

The interviewer will begin to note what frames of reference the family members use in discussing their difficulties. By *frames of reference* we mean whether there exists a family or an individual problem, which individuals seem to be bearing the brunt of the blame, how the identified problem members deal with their role, who has overt power in the family, where the alliances exist in the family, who seems to get interrupted by whom, who speaks for whom, who seems fearful or troubled about expressing an opinion, who sits next to whom, and so forth. A family's nonverbal communication is a key to family patterning. It is also often more difficult to follow and interpret than verbal communication. Videotaping a family interaction is one way to closely observe nonverbal communication, which may be expressed by a child who twiddles his thumbs in the same way as his mother, a father whose facial expression and bodily movements indicate the opposite of what he is saying, or a parent who stares off into space when his adolescent daughter yells. All of these observations are as valuable as some of the verbal comments that the family may make to the interviewer.

Why does the family come for treatment at the present time? The answer to this question helps to shift the focus of difficulty closer to the current situation and also provides an opportunity for further specifying the factors that led to family distress. Various types of last-straw situations usually present the important patterns of family interaction in a microcosm (i.e., what may have been going on for long periods).

Consider the following case example:

Mr. and Mrs. A's son, age 25 years, has had symptoms of schizophrenia for many years. His parents allowed him to sleep in their bedroom at night. On the day after he moved out to his own apartment, Mr. and Mrs. A began to blame each other for their son's behavior and sought attention because their son was "out on the streets where anything could happen." Their son had maintained an uneasy balance between the parents by staying in the parental bedroom at night, thus obviating their need for intimacy or sex. It was only when he moved out that the parents' problem came into sharp focus.

The clarification of why the family is seeking treatment *now* also helps alert the therapist to any acute crisis situation that may need either the therapist's or the family's immediate intervention. The answer will be relevant, too, in assessing the goals the family has in mind for the therapy and the degree to which it is motivated to seek help.

Most often it is the wife who requests psychotherapy for herself or who brings the family under protest. This most commonly reflects the wife's greater sense of responsibility for the family's emotional functioning, her willingness to accept blame or guilt, and her willingness to seek and accept expert help, rather than being a reflection of a greater degree of intrapsychic disturbance. With the popularization of therapy and family therapy, in particular since the 1970s, men have become more attuned to family issues and more comfortable with therapy as a possible solution. The therapist must understand that there are usually very different levels of motivation in different family members, whether split on gender or other lines.

The therapist must be sure to determine the referral context and history. This includes referral source(s), conflict and agreement among family members or referral source(s), current involvement in other treatment (including medical), history of treatment (type, hospitalization, outcome, and satisfaction), and presence of other informal advisors such as extended family members or clergy.

What Is the Background of the Family Problem?

1. **Composition and characteristics of the nuclear and extended family, such as age, sex, occupation, financial status (including differences between spousal income, and joint financial status), race, class, and ethnicity.** Couples from ethnic groups with widely differing traditions or communication styles will often have communication problems. If the couple has moved up or down a social class from their parents' generation, this is important to note. The therapist can use a three-generation genogram (see section "The Family Genogram" later in this chapter, where genograms are discussed and are shown in Figs. 7.1 and 7.2).
2. **Developmental history and patterns of each family member.** The therapist should evaluate individual family members' life histories in terms of patterns of adaptation, including an impression of how the individual manages affects, frustration, and identity outside the family. Although somewhat outside the scope of a family therapy text, our bias is that the evaluator should not underestimate the importance of individual styles of adaptation, the use of defenses and resistances, tolerance of stress and ego strengths, signs and symptoms of any mental disorder, and the capacity of each person to be supportive and empathic to their partner.
3. **Developmental history and patterns of the nuclear family unit.** The therapist should explore the longitudinal course of the family unit with reference to the role of the spouses' individual expectations, values, goals, and conflicts in their relationship; the effect of each partner's adaptive patterns on the other partner; how gender roles have been expressed over time in the family; the need for control by one partner or the other, including how control is obtained and maintained; the existence of mutual trust and ability to share; the importance of individual and mutual dependence issues; and the family's ability to deal effectively with its earlier life phases (in the family's life cycle).
4. **Current family interactional patterns (internal and external).** Here the therapist considers and rates dimensions of family function by observation. The therapist also questions the family about their sense of these patterns. Is the power structure flexible, rigid, or chaotic? Are the generation boundaries intact, blurred, or broken? Is there an affiliative or oppositional style? What degree of individuation is noted? Is there clarity of communication, tolerance for ambivalence and disagreement, respect for others' differentness versus attempts at control or intrusiveness, responsiveness to others, ability to deal realistically with separation and loss? Do the family beliefs seem congruent to the situation? What is the overall family affect: that of warmth, humor, caring, hope, tenderness, and the ability to tolerate open conflicts, or that of constricted, unpleasant, hostile, depressive, or resentful behavior?

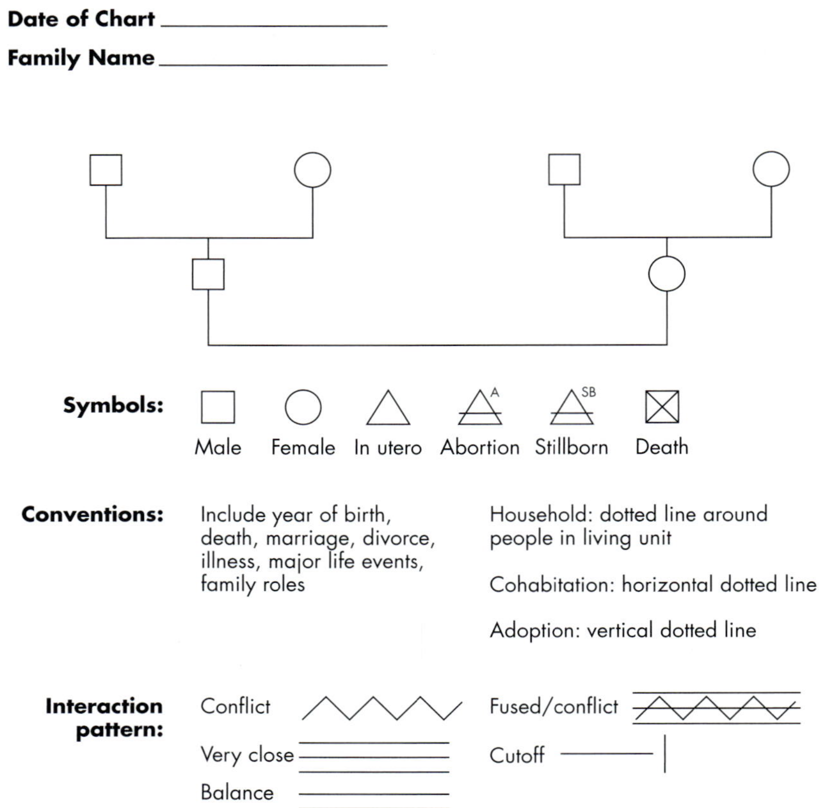

Figure 7.1 The family genogram and symbols.

This part of the evaluation—the background of the family problem—lends itself to expansion or contraction, depending on the circumstances. For example, a very specific examination of a particular part of the family's current functioning or history might be thought relevant in a particular instance. In another situation, only a brief amount of background data might be gathered initially, with the feeling that more would come out as the treatment sessions proceed. In any event, the therapist would always want to identify the important participants in the family's current interactions, the quality of the relationships, and the developmental patterns of the family unit over a period of time.

What Is the History of Past Treatment Attempts?

It usually is illuminating to understand the circumstances that have led a married couple or a family to seek assistance in the past, from what sort of helpers this assistance was elicited, and the outcome of the assistance. Experience in previous help-seeking efforts illuminates more clearly the family processes and possible therapist traps, and it delineates useful strategies. **Past help-seeking patterns are often useful predictors of what the present experience will be both in family therapy and in other therapies.**

Mr. and Mrs. B presented for treatment with the complaint that they could not get along with each other and were contemplating divorce. They gave a history of being in family therapy several years earlier. They had some 20 sessions, which "of course led to nothing." In discussion with the couple and the former therapist, the present therapist discovered that the couple had

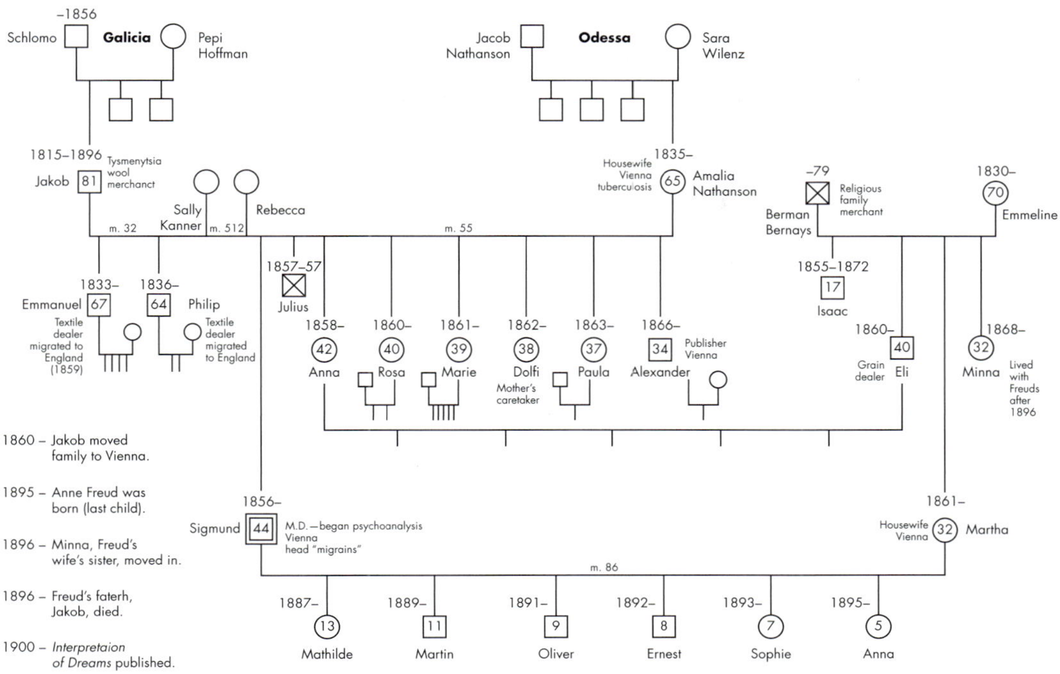

Figure 7.2 Example of a genogram (Sigmund Freud's family) with demographic, functioning, and critical event information.

spent most of the sessions blaming each other and attempting to change each other, rather than making any change in their relationship or in themselves. In addition, Mr. B, who was quite authoritarian, had persuaded the former therapist to line up on his side and say that his wife was quite unreasonable. This treatment had been unsuccessful. The strategy in this case was to go over, in detail, the past problems in treatment, suggest that the present therapist would not be a judge, and explain that the focus was to be on the couple's relationship and on each partner's own responsibility for change in the self rather than on what the other partner would have to do.

Often one spouse has been in intensive individual psychotherapy to seek help with the marital relationship. When this therapy has been unsuccessful, both therapist and patient may blame the failure on the spouse not in treatment. This situation may exacerbate the difficulty and lead to separation or divorce.

Mrs. C sought individual therapy because she felt her husband was inadequate. Her own life had been replete with difficulties, starting from the time her parents had died in an automobile accident when she was 2 years old. She had lived in various orphanages, had been married twice by the time she was 22 years old, and experienced periodic bouts of alcoholism and depression. She felt that her present marriage of 5 years was acceptable until she had children. She felt that although she had some difficulty in raising the children, the real problem was with her husband. She went into individual psychotherapy three times a week and in the course of this therapy began to "see quite clearly what a loser he was." Although Mrs. C's therapist struggled valiantly to point out her own difficulties at first, he, too, began to see the difficulties in the husband. The husband himself was never called into therapy, and after 2 years of treatment the couple was still experiencing the same problems and was contemplating divorce. A consultant suggested marital therapy.

What Are the Family's Goals and Expectations of the Treatment?

Some families come to treatment with short-term goals, such as finalizing a fairly well-thoughtout separation between husband and wife. Others come with more long-term goals, such as making a basic change in how the family functions. Other families come because of an individual-oriented goal (e.g., mother is depressed; they are there to help her), whereas still others come because of a family goal (e.g., "the family isn't functioning right"). If the goals are individual oriented, the therapist's task is to translate for the family the relationship between the symptoms and the family process. Initial goals may be at times unclear or unrealistic. In such instances, the therapist and the family must work out from the beginning of an appropriate and clear set of goals (see Chapter 10).

The married couple or the family presumably will have certain types of positive hopes and motivations for seeking help but at the same time will have some hesitations, doubts, and fears. One of the therapist's tasks is to explore and reinforce the positive motivations, to clarify them, and to keep them readily available throughout the process of therapy, which at times may be stormy and stressful. In marital therapy, the motivation of each partner for conjoint therapy should be evaluated. The evaluation should include the partners' stated commitment to the marriage, the evaluator's opinion of their commitment to therapy, the reality of their treatment expectations, and the opinions of other interested parties (e.g., parents, friends, and sometimes lovers), as related by the pair.

The positive expectations, goals, and motivations keep the family members in treatment, and every effort should be made to ensure that each family member will benefit from the family therapy sessions both as individuals and as concerned members of the family. It is helpful for family members and the therapist to work out these expectations explicitly.

Ideally, each involved family member will understand the positive reasons for their own participation and understand the more general family system goals. At the same time the therapist must be aware of individual and family resistance before they undermine the successful implementation or continuation of treatment. The therapist's clinical judgment will suggest when such fears and resistances need immediate attention and when they only need to be kept in mind as potentially major obstacles. Such resistances may be of various sorts. Although some may be specific to particular families, many are general concerns. Among these is the feeling that the situation may be made worse by treatment; that some member of the family will become guilty, depressed, angry, or fearful as a result of the treatment; that a family member may go crazy; that the family may split up; that there is no hope for change and it is already too late for help; that shameful or damaging family secrets may have to be revealed; or that perhaps it would be better to stick to familiar patterns of family interaction, no matter how unsatisfying they may be, rather than attempt to change them in new and therefore frightening directions. (Chapter 13 is devoted to a more detailed review of resistance to treatment.) **Family formulation, therapeutic approach, and treatment contracts will be discussed in Chapter 8, which is essential reading for every clinician working with families.**

Mrs. D felt that to continue in marital treatment after her recovery from an acute psychotic episode might mean that she would go crazy again. She believed that she and her husband would have to explore their unsatisfactory marriage and that this might lead to separation or divorce. She also felt that she would have to be strong and powerful to prevent her husband from committing suicide as his father had done. Mr. D, for his part, had a very obsessional personality structure with little interpersonal sensitivity or emotional awareness. He felt angry at psychiatrists and was insecure and threatened by the therapist as a male role model. The therapist working with this couple would need to look for and stress the couple's strengths and allow them to avoid discussing areas of maximal sensitivity before they were ready.

THE FAMILY GENOGRAM

Even in the absence of a comprehensive assessment scheme such as our family evaluation outline, the family genogram remains an extremely useful tool for the assessment of couples and families. The genogram, developed by Bowen,[5] is a graphic depiction of the patient and several generations of their family, noting important dates (e.g., births, deaths, marriages, separations), occupational roles, and major life events such as illness. The genogram uses symbols and conventions to note the important information, as shown in Figure 7.1. A good example of a genogram is shown in Figure 7.2. For the sake of clarity, the example is drawn without symbols. Usually, the genogram is completed during the beginning phases of treatment and serves many purposes, related to both process and content:

1. It provides the patient, family, and family therapist with a structure with which to explore current difficulties and their background.
2. It gives the therapist background information with which to put current difficulties in context.
3. The process of gathering the information, may give the patient some conception, distance, and control over the emotional tugs and pulls created by the family.
4. It can be used later in the therapy to set realistic goals for dealing with the emotional strains of the family system in the future.

The genogram displays information about the family in an accessible graphic fashion so that the therapist and family can begin to understand how present family circumstances may be linked to the family's evolving context of relationships. McGoldrick and Gerson[6] have written the most comprehensive text to date on using the genogram. They provide a format for the standard genogram symbols and outline the principles underlying the effective application and interpretation of the genogram. Figure 7.1 shows the genogram form used in the Couples and Family Therapy Clinic at Stanford University Medical Center. Therapists routinely collect this information from the couple or family, often on a whiteboard, so that family members can observe it unfolding and make additional contributions. Clinicians then transcribe the data onto the form shown in the figure and include them in the patient's clinical chart. Genograms should be a routine part of any assessment.

CLINICAL PRACTICE IMPLICATIONS

A family therapist must be competent and knowledgeable about a variety of evaluation techniques while remaining maximally flexible and comfortable in adjusting their methods to make an evaluation work for the individual family. Remember who the identified patient is, and what the family problem is and that family problem often changes over time. As such, the clinician will need to update "content" of the evaluation as circumstances dictate.

REFERENCES

1. Keitner IK, Heru AM, Glick ID. *Clinical Manual of Couples and Family Therapy*. American Psychiatric Publishing, Inc.; 2012.
2. Epstein NB, Bishop DS. Problem-centered systems therapy of the family. In: Gurman AS, Kniskern DP, eds. *Handbook of Family Therapy*. Brunner/Mazel; 1981:444–482.
3. Gill M, Newman R, Redlich F. *The Initial Interview in Psychiatric Practice*. International Universities Press; 1954.
4. Group for the Advancement of Psychiatry. *The Case History in the Study of Family Process. Report No 76*. Group for the Advancement of Psychiatry; 1970.
5. Bowen M. *Family Therapy in Clinical Practice*. Jason Aronson; 1978.
6. McGoldrick M, Gerson R. *Genograms in Family Assessment*. WW Norton; 1985.

8 Formulating an Understanding of the Family Problem Areas

OBJECTIVES FOR THE READER

- To be able to detail the clinically significant dimensions of family functioning and dysfunction in order to formulate an evaluation of the family
- To examine the process of treatment planning and establishing the treatment contract
- To be able to formulate important problem areas in preparation for planning and choosing the therapeutic approach
- To be able to apply the concepts of treatment planning to a clinical case

For easier reading, we emphasize that the descriptors "couples" or "marital" are used nearly interchangeably in this chapter.

INTRODUCTION

Meeting with the family, the therapist experiences its patterns of interaction and uses the data obtained to begin formulating a concept of the family's problems. These formulations come from historical material and from direct observations made during contact with the family. The data gathered should permit the therapist to pinpoint dimensions or aspects of the family functioning, and its individual members, that may require special attention. As data are gathered, the therapist notes areas of health and dysfunction and creates a priority list for addressing problems. Prioritizing a family's problems allows the therapist to focus on the relative severity of the problems, establishing the order in which they should be addressed. The data also enable the therapist to have greater clarity about therapeutic strategies and the tactics indicated for the particular phases and goals of treatment.

RATING IMPORTANT DIMENSIONS OF FAMILY FUNCTIONING
Communication
Problem-Solving
Roles and Coalitions
Affective Responsiveness and Involvement
Behavior Control
Operative Family Beliefs and Stories
Recent Family Events and Stresses
FAMILY CLASSIFICATION AND DIAGNOSIS

PLANNING THE THERAPEUTIC APPROACH AND ESTABLISHING THE TREATMENT CONTRACT
CASE EXAMPLE ILLUSTRATING EVALUATION AND CASE FORMULATION

RATING IMPORTANT DIMENSIONS OF FAMILY FUNCTIONING

Using the explicit interview data (see Chapter 7), and drawing heavily from observation of the family in interaction during the evaluation sessions, the therapist is in a position to formally or informally summarize and rate the important dimensions of family functioning. (We discussed these dimensions in greater detail in Chapter 7, and in Section IV "Family Treatment" and Section 5 "Couples Therapy" we examine them from the point of view of treatment strategies.)

Communication

> *"Listening is a magnetic and strange thing, a creative force. The friends who listen to us are the ones we move toward, and we want to sit in their radius. When we are listened to, it creates us, makes us unfold and expand."*
>
> —*Karl Menninger*

With regard to communication, the major focus is on the quality and quantity of information exchanged among the family members. Can they state information clearly and accurately? Is that information listened to and perceived accurately by the other family members? Can some family members do this, whereas others cannot? Is the tone of the communication (i.e., the command aspect) respectful? Affirming? Demanding? Insulting?

Problem-Solving

Every family faces problems. One difference between nondistressed and distressed families is that the latter does not come to an effective agreement and action on problems, which then accumulate. The family has come for evaluation with at least one problem, and by asking about current and prior attempts to solve this problem, the interviewer gets a sense of where and how the family has started to deal with it. Many authors (e.g., Jacobson, 1981[1]) have delineated the steps of effective problem-solving, and some have made teaching of these problem-solving steps a major ingredient in family intervention. For example, Falloon et al.[2] have used this model with the families of schizophrenic patients, and many authors have used these steps for less ill populations, including dysfunctional couples[3–5] and couples seeking marital enrichment.[6] In the assessment, the interviewer should note whether the family is capable of each of the following steps in the problem-solving sequence: (1) stating the problem clearly and in behavioral terms, (2) formulating possible solutions, (3) evaluating the solutions, (4) deciding on one solution to try, and (5) assessing the effectiveness of that solution.

Roles and Coalitions

As we detailed in Chapters 3 and 4, the family unit must manage certain tasks: (1) to provide for basic needs, (2) to develop a working marital coalition, and (3) to rear and socialize the offspring. The notion of roles refers to the recurrent patterns of behavior by various individuals in the family through which these family tasks are carried out.

Furthermore, as the individuals in the family carry out their functions, how do they coordinate and mesh with others in the family? How rigidly are roles assigned by age or gender rather than by ability? Who assumes the leadership role, especially regarding decision-making? To what extent does the family seem fragmented and disjointed, as though made up of isolated individuals?

Or do its members appear to be undifferentiated? How are boundaries maintained with respect to family of origin, extended family, neighbors, and community? To what extent is the marital coalition functional and successful? To what extent are cross-generational coalitions stronger than the marital dyad? How successfully are power and leadership issues resolved?

Affective Responsiveness and Involvement

With regard to affective responsiveness and involvement, the clinician assesses the family's ability to generate and express an appropriate range of feelings.

To what extent does the family appear to be emotionally dead rather than expressive, empathic, and spontaneous? What is the family's level of enjoyment, energy, and humor? To what extent does there appear to be an emotional divorce between the marital partners? To what extent does the predominant family mood pattern seem to be one of depression, suspicion, envy, jealousy, withdrawal, anger, irritation, or frustration? To what extent is the family system skewed around the particular mood state or reaction pattern of one of its members? Are the expressed emotions consonant with the behaviors and context?

Affective involvement refers to the degree of emotional interest and investment the family members show toward one another. This could range from absence of involvement to involvement that is devoid of positive feelings to narcissistic involvement, warmth and closeness, angry intrusiveness, or symbiosis (Wynne LC, personal communication, 1987).

Behavior Control

Behavior control is the pattern of behavior the family uses to handle physically dangerous situations (e.g., when a child runs into the road, or when a family member drives recklessly), to express psychobiological needs and drives (e.g., eating, sleeping, sex, aggression), and to engage in interpersonal socializing behavior. Control in these areas can range from rigid to flexible to laissez-faire to chaotic.

> The single most important initial assessment and intervention involves the prevention of physical harm to the family members or the therapist. Abused family members are all too common.

Remember, too, that most families are afraid of psychotic individuals, even when there has been no violence or threat of it.

The therapist must also be aware that violence directed toward therapists is not uncommon, particularly with patients who are angry, paranoid, under the influence of a substance, or impulsive. Neither the family nor the therapist can work on other issues when they fear safety. If a family member makes threats, the available community resources must be considered and employed when appropriate. Encouraging family members to call the police when threatened, to seek shelter when abused, and to inform the appropriate authorities of child abuse should be regarded as the beginning of family therapy and as necessary for its success. Little can be accomplished when family members are too frightened to speak openly.

The family, however, may not be willing to take any of these steps until it trusts the therapist. In some circumstances, the therapist is required to call child protection services whether or not the family wants it.

Operative Family Beliefs and Stories

Families and individuals function with a set of conscious and unconscious ideas pertaining to what the family is about, what the family's history tells about the roles of men and women, what values are important (e.g., money, education, work, resilience), and what adults and children should do and be. Some of these beliefs are clearly cultural or class bound, such as whether family loyalty or career advancement is more important, and whether obedience or initiative is valued more in children. Some beliefs are related to issues in the family's history, such as a story of occupational success or failure, or a parent who has been in a war or was exposed to genocide. Some beliefs are about a particular child, in terms of whether the child is considered good, bad, talented, or pretty, labels with which others, outside the family, might disagree. Some beliefs are about therapy itself and whether people should accept help, do it on their own, or deny and endure problems. These beliefs markedly influence how the family functions and copes. Not all family members share each belief. An awareness of these beliefs is essential to finding ways to help the family to develop new behaviors.

Recent Family Events and Stresses

As we discussed in Chapter 7, in answering the question of why a family comes for treatment at a particular time, the therapist carefully reviews any recent changes in family composition (e.g., births, deaths, separations, recent marriages), location (e.g., when a child leaves home), or stress (e.g., severe illnesses) and life cycle transition points.

FAMILY CLASSIFICATION AND DIAGNOSIS

Several generations of family therapists have attempted to find a reliable and agreed-on way to classify family functioning. Such attempts usually focus on problem-centered descriptive diagnoses, as exemplified by the relational problems and problems of abuse and neglect, which we consider relational issues, listed in DSM-5[7] (Fig. 8.1). The conditions described in these systems are serious ones (e.g., family violence with abuse of children). They are called *relational diagnoses* in that they involve interactions of one or several of the participants (remember, though, that not all families have a diagnosis).

Several dimensions of the family are important for the family therapist: the location and type of the problem (e.g., marital conflict, parent–child conflict with violence); the severity of the identified problem and the severity of general family dysfunction; and the description of the problematic system, which includes both the history and the current patterns of communication, role, affect, and so on. As we mentioned in Chapter 7, it is critical to determine whether the problem is heavily weighted toward issues of the individual (e.g., a child with schizophrenia in a reasonably well-functioning family) or toward issues of the family (e.g., a marital relational disorder with violence, in the throes of a divorce).

In order to do effective treatment, the therapist's first task includes making a diagnosis, meaning systemic and dynamic formulations for both the individual and the family, as well as descriptive diagnoses. Table 8.1 offers an algorithm, a schematic way to address the key questions the therapist must answer:

1. How can the problem best be explained (cells A, B, C, D)?
2. What is the level of family functioning, and how does the family function; that is, what are the family problems and processes (cell C)?
3. Has any family member been given a DSM-5 diagnosis (cell D)?
4. If a serious psychiatric disease is present in any family members (cell D), how is the family involved (cell A)?
5. How can systems concepts help clarify the problem (cell A)? What roles do individual biology and individual psychodynamics (cell B) play in the problem?

These conditions can be found at the end of DSM-5 listed in a section called "Other Conditions that may be as Focus of Clinical Attention." These conditions affect mental disorders but they are not considered mental disorders themselves. In the DSM-5 coding system they receive a "V code" designation and in general are non-reimbursable by insurance companies.

PROBLEMS RELATED TO FAMILY UPBRINGING

- **V61.20 Parent–Child Relational Problem**
- **V61.8 Sibling Relational Problem**
- **V61.8 Upbringing Away From Parents**
- **V61.29 Child Affected by Parental Relationship Distress**

OTHER PROBLEMS RELATED TO PRIMARY SUPPORT GROUP

- **V61.10 (Z63.0) Relationship Distress With Spouse or Intimate Partner**
- **V61.03 (Z63.5) Disruption of Family by Separation or Divorce**
- **V61.8 (Z63.8) High Expressed Emotion Level Within Family**
- **V62.82 (Z63.4) Uncomplicated Bereavement**

PROBLEMS RELATED TO ABUSE AND NEGLECT

CHILD MALTREATMENT AND NEGLECT PROBLEMS

- **Child Physical Abuse, Confirmed**
- **Child Physical Abuse, Suspected**
- **Other Circumstances Related to Child Physical Abuse**
- V61.21 (Z69.010) Encounter for Mental Health Services for Victim of Child Abuse by Parent
- V61.21 (Z69.020) Encounter for Mental Health Services for Victim of Nonparental Child Abuse
- V15.41 (Z62.810) Personal History (Past History) of Physical Abuse in Childhood
- V61.22 (Z69.011) Encounter for Mental Health Services for Perpetrator of Parental Child Abuse
- V62.83 (Z69.021) Encounter for Mental Health Services for Perpetrator of Nonparental Child Abuse

CHILD SEXUAL ABUSE

- **Child Sexual Abuse, Confirmed**
- **Child Sexual Abuse, Suspected**
- **Other Circumstances Related to Child Sexual Abuse**
- V61.21 (Z69.010) Encounter for Mental Health Services for Victim of Child Psychological Abuse by Parent
- V61.21 (Z69.020) Encounter for Mental Health Services for Victim of Nonparental Child Sexual Abuse
- V15.42 (Z62.810) Personal History (Past History) of Sexual Abuse in Childhood
- V61.22 (Z69.811) Encounter for Mental Health Services for Perpetrator of Parental Child Sexual Abuse
- V62.83 (Z69.021) Encounter for Mental Health Services for Perpetrator of Nonparental Sexual Abuse

CHILD NEGLECT

- **Child Neglect, Confirmed**
- **Child Neglect, Suspected**
- **Other Circumstances Related to Child Neglect**
- V61.21 (Z69.010) Encounter for Mental Health Services for Victim of Child Psychological Abuse by Parent
- V61.21 (Z69.020) Encounter for Mental Health Services for Victim of Nonparental Child Psychological Abuse
- V15.42 (Z62.810) Personal History (Past History) of Psychological Abuse in Childhood
- V61.22 (Z69.811) Encounter for Mental Health Services for Perpetrator of Parental Child Psychological Abuse
- V62.83 (Z69.021) Encounter for Mental Health Services for Perpetrator of Nonparental Child Abuse

CHILD PSYCHOLOGICAL ABUSE

- **Child Psychological Abuse, Confirmed**
- **Child Psychological Abuse, Suspected**
- **Other Circumstances Related to Child Psychological Abuse**
- V61.21 (Z69.010) Encounter for Mental Health Services for Victim of Child Psychological Abuse by Parent
- V61.21 (Z69.020) Encounter for Mental Health Services for Victim of Nonparental Child Psychological Abuse
- V15.42 (Z62.810) Personal History (Past History) of Psychological Abuse in Childhood
- V61.22 (Z69.811) Encounter for Mental Health Services for Perpetrator of Parental Child Psychological Abuse
- V62.83 (Z69.021) Encounter for Mental Health Services for Perpetrator of Nonparental Child Abuse

ADULT MALTREATMENT AND NEGLECT PROBLEMS

- Spouse or Partner Violence, Physical, Confirmed
- Spouse or Partner Violence, Physical, Suspected
- Spouse or Partner Violence, Sexual, Confirmed
- Spouse or Partner Violence, Sexual, Suspected
- Spouse or Partner Neglect, Confirmed
- Spouse or Partner Neglect, Suspected
- Spouse or Partner Abuse, Psychological, Confirmed
- Spouse or Partner Abuse, Psychological, Suspected
- Adult Physical Abuse by Nonspouse or Nonpartner, Confirmed
- Adult Physical Abuse by Nonspouse or Nonpartner, Suspected
- Adult Sexual Abuse by Nonspouse or Nonpartner, Confirmed
- Adult Sexual Abuse by Nonspouse or Nonpartner, Suspected
- Adult Psychological Abuse by Nonspouse or Nonpartner, Confirmed
- Adult Psychological Abuse by Nonspouse or Nonpartner, Suspected

Figure 8.1 Relational problems and abuse and neglect.

Table 8.1 A comprehensive evaluation schema

	Type of formulation	For the family	For the individual(s)
Diagnosis	Functional	*A* A systemic formulation	*B* Behavioral or individual psychodynamic model and/or biologic model
Diagnosis	Descriptive	*C* DSM-5 conditions not attributable to a mental disorder that are a focus of attention or treatment (e.g., Relational Problems and Abuse and Neglect)	*D* DSM-5 classification for each family member attributable to a mental disorder or general medical condition

Saying it another way, the therapist can

1. Use DSM-5 or the GAP diagnostic scheme for a descriptive diagnosis, if applicable.
2. Describe the functioning of the family, using the dimensions listed earlier in this chapter.
3. Make a judgment as to the salience of individual pathology.
4. Determine the severity of the family problem, using the Global Assessment of Relational Functioning (GARF) Scale. This instrument was also developed by the GAP Committee on the Family.[8,9] It is a dimensional scale that describes features of a relationship along a health-to-dysfunction continuum. For example, communication is one of the dimensions. The GARF Scale permits the clinician to characterize the overall functioning of a family or other ongoing relational unit on a hypothetical continuum: from competent, optimal performance to disorganized, maladaptive functioning.

(Contrast the GARF Scale with the severity of psychosocial stressors scale [Axis IV seen in DSM-IV], which is dimensional. Axis IV is concerned only with the individual's experience; it rates only stressors and dysfunction, not the protective, health-enhancing factors that help individuals cope more effectively.)

The GARF Scale includes only three areas of family functioning: problem-solving, organization, and emotional climate. As a global scale, the GARF Scale cannot characterize all of the features of families and other relationships that might be important to specialists assessing and treating families, but it is still very useful. The key task is to determine how much each of these theories contributes to an understanding of the development and maintenance of the problem and, even more important, what approach is most likely to foster change at the present time. A purely physical symptom such as invalidism after a heart attack can be maintained by the way family members treat the patient, and a problem such as difficulties in shared decision-making can be the result of individual dynamics. If the therapist has decided that the family is involved in the problem, and they believe that intervening with the family may produce change, then they should discuss this with the family and agree on a contract for consultation or therapy.

This method, albeit imprecise, represents our recommendation for how to assess a family, formulate a working diagnosis, and draw implications for goals and treatment. **To reemphasize, just as individual, psychodynamic theories maintain that symptoms are the result of internal forces, dynamics, and fantasies, so family theories maintain that symptoms are the result of, or are maintained by, the properties of an interaction or the functioning of a family system and the characteristics of the individuals involved.**

> The key task is to determine how much each of these theories contributes to an understanding of the development and maintenance of the problem and, even more important, what approach is most likely to foster change at the present time.

PLANNING THE THERAPEUTIC APPROACH AND ESTABLISHING THE TREATMENT CONTRACT

After the evaluation data have been gathered and formulated into diagnostic hypotheses, the therapist and family together can formulate goals regarding important problem areas (Table 8.2 is a continuation of Table 8.1). Note that in Table 8.2, goals are set *after* the diagnostic evaluation. The therapist is then ready to consider the appropriate therapeutic strategies (see Chapter 11). The therapist should make a concise, explicit statement of the family problem using language the family can understand. Such a formulation will be determined by the treatment model the therapist is using. For example, a behavioral therapist might say to the family, "You two have gotten into the habit of criticizing each other so much that you have neglected to comment on the good things the other one does, or to give each other what each of you needs. We will try to help you communicate more clearly and take care of each other in ways that you both want." A therapist using a more dynamic approach might say, "Each of you had a mother who was depressed and a father who was working too hard to be available. So each of you assumes that if the other one doesn't give you what you want, they must be unavailable or unloving. It makes both of you become tense and withdrawn a lot. Perhaps we can find a way to help you separate your past from your present and learn to take care of each other better." A therapist with a problem-solving approach might say, "You seem to be trying to explain to each other what you need in ways that make each of you angry. So your attempts to solve this problem have been making things worse. Perhaps we could find a better way to do it, by focusing on a new solution or on the solutions that have worked at least some of the time."

As we mentioned earlier in this chapter, if it appears from the initial family evaluation that any family members have an individual disorder, as in cell C of Table 8.2, this must be noted and taken into account in the formulation and treatment planning. The most common way a family gets to the family therapist is through an individual. Common situations include those in which one spouse has a diagnosable depression or phobia, a family member appears to have a severe personality disorder, a member has a serious substance abuse problem, schizophrenia is present in one of the young adults living in the parents' home, or childhood or adolescent antisocial behavior is present. The initial suspicion of a diagnosable disorder in one individual may necessitate further evaluation either in the family setting or individually in order to carefully assess the nature and extent of the individual symptoms as enumerated in DSM-5. **Our assumption is**

Table 8.2 Setting goals after evaluation

	Type of formulation	For the family	For the individual(s)
Diagnosis	Functional	***A*** A systemic formulation	***B*** Behavioral or individual psychodynamic model and/or biologic model
Diagnosis	Descriptive	***C*** DSM-5 conditions not attributable to a mental disorder that are a focus of attention or treatment (e.g., Relational Problems and Abuse and Neglect)	***D*** DSM-5 classification for each family member attributable to a mental disorder or general medical condition
Goals	Based on diagnosis	Specify for each problem	Specify for each problem

that important components of both the individual and the biologic models interact with each other and with the family model.

At this point, a beginning contract with regard to goals and treatment should be established.[11] The contract should include who is to be present; the location, times, estimated length, and frequency of meetings; the fee; and contingency planning with respect to absent members and missed appointments. It is usually not possible to determine in the first sessions how long treatment will take. Some therapists contract for 10 sessions and renew; others leave things open ended. For some families, treatment will be very brief and crisis oriented, lasting only one or two sessions, whereas for other families treatment may continue for months or occasionally years when the resources to maintain treatment are available.

Some therapists may want to refer families to the book *Solving Your Problems Together: Family Therapy for the Whole Family*,[12] which was written specifically for the lay market.

This illustrated book for children, adolescents, and adults is designed to answer typical questions and address feelings of reluctance that arise when a family is considering family therapy: Does our family need therapy? What are the sessions going to be like? Will what we talk about be confidential? If our child has a problem, why must the whole family go? How can I find the right family therapist for us? What if a family member refuses to go?

Families are introduced to the idea of family therapy as a safe place in which strengths can be used and skills can be learned to help solve problems, improve communication, and handle stress more effectively. By not advocating any one school of family therapy, the book is helpful to potential clients regardless of the theoretical orientation of the therapist they may choose.

We highly recommend Lloyd Sederer's (2013) text entitled *The Family Guide to Mental Health Care* to patients and their families. This resource provides families with information to navigate the mental health-care system. Please see Suggested Reading.

CASE EXAMPLE ILLUSTRATING EVALUATION AND CASE FORMULATION

The following case example illustrates the use of the family evaluation outline (see Table 8.1).

> *The R family is a working-class, Irish family consisting of a father, a 55-year-old manual laborer; a mother, a 44-year-old housewife; a 17-year-old daughter, who is a senior in high school; a 20-year-old son, who is a part-time college student; and a 22-year-old son, who is working part time. All three children still live at home. Both mothers-in-law are actively involved in the family. They have been referred for family therapy after Mrs. R's hospitalization for paranoid symptoms following benzodiazepine withdrawal.*

1. *Gathering identifying data and establishing current phase of family life cycle*
   The therapist notes that although the identified patient is Mrs. R, the family is also approaching the empty-nest phase, in which the parents will have to face being alone together. The therapist begins to wonder and to ask to what extent the couple has emphasized the parental role rather than the marital relationship, and to what extent they have discouraged the development of the children's ability to move out of the house and complete their maturation and separation from their parents. The older son, a month prior to intake, had indicated that he was moving out of the house and in with his girlfriend.
2. *Gathering explicit interview data*
   A. What is the current family problem?
   The older son said that the family problem was his mother because she had recently stopped using sedatives on the advice of her doctor and subsequently began having

ideas that people in the family were trying to harm her. Mr. R added that his wife had always been the problem. He was joined in these sentiments by the daughter and by the younger son. Mrs. R, however, said that the problem was that nobody would help her around the house and that she could not get any cooperation from the family members. The therapist then asked the family to think in terms of what the current family (not individual) problem was. The younger son said he thought that maybe the problem was not the mother but the fact that nobody in the family was communicating or was happy.

B. Why does the family come for treatment at the present time?
The family reported that about the time the older son announced that he was going to move out, the parents' quarreling, which had been long standing, intensified. Mrs. R went to a family doctor for a tranquilizer. The doctor said that she appeared confused and suggested that she stop taking the benzodiazepine she had also been using, and she stopped taking them all at once. She then became suspicious and had a fight with her husband in which they threw pots at each other. At this point, everybody felt that she should see her family physician, who recommended admission to an inpatient psychiatric unit. She remained there for a week until her symptoms stopped.

C. What is the background of the family problem?
   1. *Composition of household.*
   Mr. R works as a manual laborer in a shipyard. Although he spent a year in college, he has not advanced in his job and is concerned about finances and worried about retirement. Mrs. R is a housewife. She has never worked outside the home. The older son works part time in a record store. The younger son is a part-time student at a local college. The daughter is finishing high school. Mrs. R's father is dead, and her mother is a frequent visitor in the home. Mr. R's parents are alive. He is close to his mother.
   2. *Developmental history and patterns of each family member.*
   Mrs. R's father was manager of a cemetery, and she described her mother as being sick all the time. Her parents' relationship revolved around her father taking care of her mother through much of the marriage because of her sickness. Mrs. R gave a history of being chronically sick, like her mother. She had been born prematurely and developed sinusitis and asthma at an early age. She had one older brother. She felt ignored by her mother and father and was often called on to care for her mother when her father was absent. She often dreamed of someone to take care of her. In adulthood, she and mother became very close.

   Mr. R's father was the foreman in a factory, and Mr. R was close to his father, but he described his mother as "overprotective" and said that his father essentially catered to his mother. Both parents had hoped that their children would exceed them educationally and professionally and had tried the best they could to encourage this.

   Mr. R was the oldest of four children and took care of two younger siblings who were "always sick." He resented this caretaking and tended to stay in his room or work on his car as he grew older. He never quite lived up to his parents' expectations. He attempted college but quit, did not want to move out of the house, and dated very little before he met Mrs. R.
   3. *Developmental history and patterns of the nuclear family unit.*
   Mr. and Mrs. R were introduced by relatives. Most of their courtship involved family social events, and there was little intimacy during their courtship period. Mrs. R described the marriage as somewhat disappointing. She indicated that she had married for stability and someone to take care of her. He had said that he thought she would provide some of the spark that he lacked. He saw her as an independent

person who would not ask too much of him. Both partners stated that they had no knowledge of contraception, and their older son was born in the first year of marriage. They had had very little experience being alone together as husband and wife.

After they had the other two children, Mr. R began spending more and more time at work. Mrs. R found herself becoming sick more frequently with various respiratory and other ailments. They had to turn to their own mothers: his for financial support, hers for help in raising the children and taking care of herself. Mrs. R. felt uncared for by her husband, and Mr. R became increasingly resentful that his wife was sick and angry rather than the "spark plug" he had married. As the children grew up, Mr. R increasingly retreated, neither helping Mrs. R nor supporting her in her attempts to get the children to cooperate with her. Mr. R also experienced his own sense of failure in that he had never moved up in his job and believed his wife was disappointed in him for not earning more money. She became angry, then anxious, at this withdrawal and then began to take barbiturates. In addition, they had many arguments over the children: Mrs. R wanted them to work harder in school, and Mr. R would tell her to leave them alone.

4. *Current interactional patterns.*

The situation had worsened progressively during the 2 years prior to referral as the two boys reached adulthood and Mrs. R reached an increasingly depressed middle age. Mr. and Mrs. R found themselves drifting further apart and spending less time together, barely talking to each other. Mr. R was working much more than before, which made Mrs. R suspicious that he was chasing other women. Mrs. R continued to complain of physical symptoms, to take more medications, and to become less able to perform child-rearing or housekeeping tasks. The more Mrs. R attempted to get Mr. R's attention, the more he retreated. The older son began to experiment with psychedelic drugs, the younger son had difficulty with his grades, and the daughter attended school less frequently and did poorly when in class. The two mothers-in-law fought over who was helping the family more, each placing the blame for the family problems on the other's child.

It appeared that Mr. R had abdicated his role as a parent and a spouse. The marital coalition was almost nonexistent; instead, the daughter and her father were on one side and the younger son and mother on the other. The older son, although a mediator in the family, had in many ways withdrawn from the battle by using drugs.

D. What is the history of past treatment attempts or other attempts at problem-solving in the family?

Mrs. R had been seeing the same internist for the past 15 or 20 years. The doctor had frequently suggested psychiatric treatment, but Mrs. R had refused. Instead, he prescribed benzodiazepines to help her sleep. She went for individual psychotherapy over a 3-month period but quit. She explained, "It didn't make my husband better." Mr. and Mrs. R also consulted their local clergyman on several occasions, and he counseled tolerance and patience. The children had not been involved in treatment.

E. What are the family's goals and expectations of the treatment? What are its strengths, motivations, and resistances?

The family's motivations at first were to help Mrs. R so that she could get better. During the evaluation interview, they hoped she would "stop being sick and take care of us."

The primary resistances apparent during the evaluation interview were the family members' scapegoating of Mrs. R and a reluctance to change themselves, the latter quite evident in Mr. R's saying that he could not get to treatment sessions because of his job, no matter what time the therapist suggested for the meeting. Although it was less apparent than the resistance, each person in the family did seem to recognize that there was something wrong with the overall functioning of the family and with its individual members and that this problem could be worked on.

3. *Formulating the family problem areas*
   A. Rating important dimensions of family functioning
      1. *Communication.*
         There was little or no spontaneous interaction or communication between Mr. and Mrs. R. The children seemed somewhat at odds, but they were united in a struggle to prevent their parents from taking power. Even when the therapist tried to get the parents to talk to each other, it was impossible, as Mrs. R felt that Mr. R never listened to her, and Mr. R felt that Mrs. R was always complaining and could not do anything. There was very little communication follow-up from one to the other, thus leaving them without continuity of communication or closure. The parental communication was mainly nonverbal. It consisted of Mrs. R clutching her stomach, grabbing her chest near her heart, or rolling her head back, as though she were about to have a stroke or a heart attack, at which point Mr. R would move his chair farther away from everyone in the family. Positive feedback has been virtually abandoned in this family for years. Communication was best between Mr. R and the daughter and between Mrs. R and the younger son.
      2. *Problem-solving.*
         The family had difficulty agreeing on anything, even the making of a list of problems. The topic of the list led to various arguments involving many family members. Sometimes they would follow the lead of the older son.
      3. *Roles and coalitions.*
         Mrs. R, who was currently a daughter, wife, and mother, had been unable to move out of her family of origin to her present family. She seemed almost childlike in her presentation and her functioning. She seemed to be overly involved as a daughter and less involved as a wife and mother. Mr. R was likewise very involved with his family of origin. He had essentially given up his role as husband and turned over the role of father to the older son, who had been managing the family finances, bringing in extra money, and making the kinds of family decisions that Mr. R used to make.

         There had been a reversal of generational roles, with the daughter taking over when Mrs. R was ill and doing the housecleaning and cooking. The daughter also fulfilled part of a spouse's role, in that she and Mr. R frequently went to the movies together, whereas Mrs. R stayed home with her headaches. The strongest coalition in the family appeared to be father–daughter instead of the more usual husband–wife.

         The main alignments and communication patterns pitted the father and daughter against the younger son and mother, with the older son being a mediator. In his role as mediator, the son was the center of all communication. All fights seemed to be resolved in his "court." This seemed to be taking a toll on him. He said he was having trouble finding himself and was having great difficulty in making a job decision or career choice. It became clear that this son's leaving home would be a grave crisis for the family.
      4. *Affective responsiveness and involvement.*
         The therapist noted that the general emotional tone of the family was one of anger and frustration. Any sign of positive emotional expression between family members was lacking.
      5. *Behavior control.*
         There seemed to be no difficulty in this area, as there was no inappropriate expression of aggressive or sexual impulses.
      6. *Operative family beliefs and stories.*

In the R family, the theme of illness and caretaking was central. Both spouses had ill parents for whom they had been caretakers. Mrs. R entered the marriage wanting someone to care for her. Mr. R also had been a caretaker but hated it and was hoping his wife would take care of him. Over time Mrs. R's requests for caretaking were rejected, and she became seen as sick or a nag, while Mr. R became helpless and silent. In one way or another, the children then became involved as caretaker (daughter), assistant man of the house (older son), or good boy (the younger son—the only one to attempt college).

The family operated under the cultural myth that a happy marriage is one in which there are no disagreements. Mrs. R lived with the fantasy that everything should be calm and that any flaws or problems were to be avoided and not to be discussed. This meant that the painful realities of both partners could not be addressed directly. In addition, both partners believed it was possible to change the other by nagging enough. Mrs. R wanted her husband to be a charming prince, and Mr. R wanted his wife to be a happy and supportive spouse who would make up for his feeling of inferiority. Mrs. R also felt that both marital partners should be as unselfish as possible and that she had sacrificed her life for her children and husband. In contrast, Mr. R felt that he had worked himself to the bone to bring home the money to keep the family going, sacrificing everything for everyone else. Mr. R could not see that his wife wanted his presence and support more than the money, and Mrs. R could not see that her anger at his withdrawal made it impossible for her to support him or make him feel better about himself or his work. The children, faced with an ill, scapegoated mother and a retreating father who felt like a failure, could neither succeed themselves nor leave home.

Mrs. R was the scapegoat in the family. Whenever anything went wrong, everyone turned on her. If what she had done did not seem to be an adequate explanation of the problem, an explanation was found that took into account her past transgressions. Her position as the bad person, on the one hand, and as responsible for much of the family's functioning, on the other, is a classic gender bind (note that when she did not do the caretaking, her daughter stepped in). The fact that she had been tranquilized to help her avoid her reasonable frustrations is not unusual.

It was clear that what at first looked like an individual medical illness was predominantly a family problem.

B. Family classification and diagnosis

Classification of relational disorders (CORD) classification (Table 8.3): Couple conflictional relational disorder (without violence)

Score on GARF Scale: 50

C. Individual Diagnoses

Mrs. R met criteria on DSM-5 for Sedative Use Disorder. At the time of evaluation, most of Mrs. R's symptoms of benzodiazepine withdrawal had ceased and she was on no medication. She appeared sad but did not meet the criteria for addiction or major depression. Her physician assured the therapist that her other medical symptoms, particularly the respiratory ones, were present but minor and that she needed no special treatment at this time. Mr. and Mrs. R met criteria for personality disorder features on what was previously known as Axis II in DSM-IV (Mr. R, dependent; Mrs. R, histrionic). The older son met criteria for substance use disorder.

4. *Planning the therapeutic approach and establishing the treatment contract*

The therapist's first decision was to approach the R family's problem from a family standpoint rather than by treating Mrs. R, the identified patient, as an individual, isolated from her family. The family seemed to be in a crisis, facing the imminent departure of the older son, the family mediator. The parents seemed unable to handle this separation. Mr. R seemed to

Table 8.3 Proposed classification of relational disorders (CORD)

I. Relational disorders within one generation
  A. Severe relational disorders in couples
    1. Conflictual disorder with and without physical aggression
    2. Sexual dysfunction
    3. Sexual abuse
    4. Divorce dysfunction
    5. Induced psychotic disorder (folie à deux)
  B. Severe relational disorders in siblings
    1. Conflictual disorder
    2. Physical and/or sexual abuse
    3. Induced psychotic disorder (folie à deux)
II. Intergenerational relational disorders
  A. Problems relating to infants, children, and adolescents
    1. With overt physical abuse or neglect
      a. With intrafamily child sexual abuse
      b. Without sexual abuse Overinvolvement
    2. With problems in engagement
      a. Overinvolvement
        i. Intrusive overinvolvement
        ii. Emotional abuse
        iii. Family separation disorder
      a. Preadolescent type
      b. Adolescent type
      b. Underinvolvement
        i. Reactive attachment disorder
        ii. Failure to thrive
    3. With problems in control
      a. Undercontrol
      b. Overcontrol
      c. Inconsistent control
    4. With problems in communication
      a. Communication deviance (e.g., high expressed emotion)
      b With lack of affective or instrumental communication
  B. Problems relating to adult offspring and their parents
    1. With physical abuse or neglect
    2. With problems in engagement
      a. With burden
      b. With overinvolvement
    3. With problems in communication
      a. With cutoffs
      b With severe verbal conflict

Reprinted with permission from A model for the classification and diagnosis of relational disorders. Committee on the Family, Group for the Advancement of Psychiatry. *Psychiatr Serv.* 1995;46(9):926–931. Table 1.

be behaving in an ineffective manner, and both parents still had a dependent relationship with their own families of origin.

The basic strategy was to strengthen the marital coalition by increasing interaction between the marital dyad, by attempting to decrease the intensity of the interaction between these two people and their families of origin, and by attempting to decrease the cross-generational ties between these two people and their children. The therapist encouraged the mother not to take any sedative medication, which she was happy to do when she felt that the family was being attended to. The older son made a treatment contract with the therapist to stop taking drugs.

The therapist treated the family as a unit, and he also met with the marital dyad alone for many of the sessions; for a time, the children also had a few sessions as a sibling group. A decision was made to exclude the parents' in-laws from treatment and to encourage the marital dyad to take over the parental role that they had abrogated not only to the older son but also to their own parents. In the sessions in which just the marital dyad participated, positive attention was given to reinforcing communication patterns between husband and wife. They were taught to pick up emotional cues and to respond to each other, rather than to withdraw or to somatize. Each was encouraged to find ways to take care of and praise the other. Mrs. R was encouraged to reassume executive functions in the house and to consider whether she wanted a part-time job to help out with finances and to give her a focus of interest separate from the house and children. Mr. R was encouraged to share decisions with Mrs. R rather than retreating and then criticizing her. He also spent some time dealing with the question of whether his own life has been the failure he felt it to be. The older son was steered toward his girlfriend and a career choice, letting his father make the decisions the son had once made. The daughter was encouraged to improve her failing schoolwork and to stop doing the housecleaning and cooking. The younger son was supported in his plans for college and began to deal with the question of what would happen if he surpassed his father educationally. He was also encouraged to do his share of chores around the house as long as he lived at home.

SUGGESTED READING

This book can be required reading for every family with a loved one suffering from mental illness.
Sederer LI. *The Family Guide to Mental Health Care*. WW Norton; 2013.

REFERENCES

1. Jacobson NS. Behavioral marital therapy. In: Gurman AS, Kniskern DP, eds. *Handbook of Family Therapy*. Brunner/Mazel; 1981:556–591.
2. Falloon IRH, Hole V, Mulroy L, et al. Behavioral family therapy, In: Clarkin JF, Haas GL, Glick ID, eds. *Affective Disorders and the Family: Assessment and Treatment*. Guilford; 1988:117–133.
3. Gottman J. *Why Marriages Succeed or Fail*. Simon & Schuster; 1994.
4. Jones J, Jacobson N, Christensen A. *Integrative Behavioral Couple Therapy: A Therapist's Guide to Transforming Relationships*. WW Norton; 1996.
5. Markman H, Renick M, Floyd FJ, Stanley SM, Clements M. Preventing marital distress through communication and conflict management training: a four year follow-up. *J Consult Clin Psychol*. 1993;61:70–77.
6. Guerney BG Jr. *Relationship Enhancement: Skill-training programs for therapy, problem prevention, and enrichment*. Jossey-Bass; 1977.
7. American Psychiatric Association. *Diagnostic and Statistical Manual of Mental Disorders*. 5th ed. American Psychiatric Association; 2013.
8. Dausch BM, Miklowitz DJ, Richards JA. Global Assessment of Relational Functioning Scale (GARF), II. Reliability and validity in a sample of families of bipolar patients. *Fam Process*. 1996;35:175–189.
9. Group for the Advancement of Psychiatry Committee on the Family. Global Assessment of Relational Functioning Scale (GARF): I. Background and rationale. *Fam Process*. 1996;35:155–172.
10. American Psychiatric Association. *Diagnostic and Statistical Manual of Mental Disorders*. 4th ed. American Psychiatric Association; 1994:758–759.
11. Shankar R, Menon MS. Development of a framework of interventions with families in the management of schizophrenia. *Psychosoc Rehabil J*. 1993;16:75–91.
12. Annunziata J, Jacobson-Kram P. *Solving Your Problems Together: Family Therapy for the Whole Family*. American Psychological Association; 1994.
13. Guttman HA, Beavers WR, Berman E, et al. A model for the classification and diagnosis of relational disorders. Committee on the Family, Group for the Advancement of Psychiatry. *Psychiatr Serv*. 1995;46:926–932.

Once the therapist achieves an understanding of what is wrong, the next step is to set treatment goals (Chapter 10). For the reader, however, it is necessary first to understand the current competing models of understanding and treating family disorder—each with its unique mediating and final goals. We review and compare each in Chapter 9.

In Chapter 11, we get to the essentials of how to do family treatment, and in Chapter 12, we examine what treatment looks like over time. At the end of Chapter 12, we specifically focus on brief therapy since it is so commonly done in family work. In Chapter 13, we review the resistances that can occur during a course of treatment and highlight the elements that may be most crucial to make it all work—the therapeutic alliance.

In Chapter 14, we cover some of the ground rules, that is, the issues that are of major interest to beginning therapists. Among these issues are determining who to include in the treatment, choosing to work with another therapist or as a member of a team, establishing where and how to see and schedule families, setting fees, keeping a record of treatment, deciding whether to include family therapy in combination with other psychotherapeutic and pharmacologic treatments, and coordinating treatment with helping agencies and other health care professionals.

Section

IV Family Treatment

9 Major Family Therapy Schools and Their Treatment Strategies 121

10 Goals 128

11 Family Treatment: Integrated Strategies and Techniques 136

12 The Course of Family Treatment 151

13 Promoting Change in Family Treatment: Issues of Alliance and Resistance 163

14 Family Therapy: General Considerations 175

9 Major Family Therapy Schools and Their Treatment Strategies

OBJECTIVES FOR THE READER

- To be able to outline in broad strokes the essentials of the major schools of family therapy
- To differentiate the strategies, techniques, stance, goals, and database used in each school

For easier reading, we emphasize that the descriptors "couples" or "marital" are used nearly interchangeably in this chapter.

INTRODUCTION

An observer of the general psychotherapy scene has stated, "In picking up the textbook of the future, we should see in the table of contents not a listing of School A, School B, and so on—perhaps ending with the author's attempt at integration—but an outline of the various agreed-on intervention principles, a specification of varying techniques for implementing each principle, and an indication of the relative effectiveness of each of these techniques, together with their interaction with varying presenting problems and individual differences among patients/clients and therapists."[1] We agree wholeheartedly, as we have emphasized throughout this book, although this seems like an ideal to strive for rather than a full possibility at present. In the spirit of Goldfried's idea, we present in this chapter (and in Chapter 10) the general schools of family intervention by focusing not primarily on their originators but on their mediating and final goals and related strategies of intervention. Much has been written about the diverse schools of family intervention, often formed around the so-called first generation of bold, revolutionary evolutionary thinkers and clinicians such as Salvador Minuchin, Virginia Satir, Jay Haley, Murray Bowen, Carl Whitaker, and Nathan Ackerman. Different classifications of the schools exist, each with its own assumptions about the origin and maintenance of pathology; goals, strategies, and techniques for intervention; and indications for use. Especially for the 21st century, it is necessary for the student of family intervention to have some general conceptual understanding of these schools, their history, and the contemporary personalities involved (Table 9.1).

INSIGHT-AWARENESS MODEL
FAMILY OF ORIGIN MODEL
SYSTEMIC-STRATEGIC MODEL
STRUCTURAL MODEL
COGNITIVE–BEHAVIORAL MODEL
EXPERIENTIAL MODEL

Table 9.1 Models of family treatment

Treatment approach (school)	Representative therapies	Strategies and techniques	Stance	Goals	Database
Insight-awareness (a.k.a. historic, psychodynamic, or psychoanalytic)	Ackerman, Boszormenyi-Nagy, and Spark Paul Nadelson, Bowen	Observe Clarify Interpret	Therapist is listener Therapist keeps "therapeutic distance" Therapist maintains therapeutic stance of technical neutrality	Foster understanding and insight to effect change	History Unconscious derivatives Transference
Systemic–structural (a.k.a. systems, communications, or structural)	Palo Alto group (Jackson, Bateson, Haley, Satir) Sluzki Bowen Minuchin Erickson Palazzoli	Alter family structure and behavior Observe and transform using directives	Therapist observes and moves in and out of process	Change structure, communication pattern, and roles, which change perception and behavior	Sequences Communication Rules History
Cognitive–behavioral	Weiss Jacobson Patterson Falloon	Teach communication skills and problem-solving skills Use contingency contracting	Therapist is collaborator in the development of interpersonal skills	Eliminate dysfunctional behaviors and learn to utilize new and more effective interpersonal behaviors	Observation of overt behaviors Functional analysis of problematic behavioral sequences
Experiential–existential	Whitaker Bowen Boszormenyi-Nagy Satir	Design or participate with family in the emotional experience Empathize	Therapist offers themselves for interaction to minimize distance between family and therapist	Change ways family members experience (and presumably react to) each other Growth and differentiation	Observed verbal and nonverbal behavior Shared feelings (including the therapist's feelings)
Narrative	White Epston	Externalize the problem Map influence of problem over family and influence of family over problem	Therapist collaborates with family on a therapeutic conversation	**1.** Develop an alternative narrative story about the problem **2.** Liberate the family from being controlled by the problem toward authoring their own study	Linguistic behavior

a.k.a., also known as.

NARRATIVE MODEL
PSYCHOEDUCATIONAL MODEL
CLINICAL PRACTICE IMPLICATIONS

INSIGHT-AWARENESS MODEL

The insight-awareness orientation is also known as the psychodynamic, or the psychoanalytic school. In a real sense, this is the oldest school of family therapy because it grew naturally out of the psychoanalytic tradition. One of the earliest family therapists was Nathan Ackerman, a child analyst who used his analytic background to inform and lend substance to his approach and understanding of families.[2] The marriage counseling movement of the 1930s and 1940s also drew from this tradition.[3] The theoretical underpinnings of this model are the familiar ones of psychoanalytic thinking, including especially topographical concepts of conscious, preconscious, and unconscious; constructs of the id, ego, and superego; and concepts that focus on the interaction of individuals, such as secondary gain, transference, countertransference, enactments, and projective identification.

By changing the transference distortions, correcting the projective identifications, and infusing insight and new understanding into the arena of interpersonal turmoil and conflict, this school of family therapy attempts to change the functioning and interrelationships of the members of the family or marital system. The database is derived from historical material of the current and past generations, from transference and countertransference phenomena, unconscious derivatives, and resistances. A basic assumption is that intrapsychic conflict, interpersonal problem foci, and defensive and coping mechanisms are modeled and played out within the family system. Portions of the database that are of paramount interest to the practitioners of this model are dream and fantasy material, fantasies and projections about other family members, and transference distortions about other family members and the therapist. Understanding the history and mutations of these dynamics over time is considered crucial to understanding current dysfunction.

The terms *transference* and *countertransference* are used broadly here.

Such phenomena can be understood in terms of transference in at least five directions: (1) partner to partner, (2) partner to therapist, (3) couple (or family) to therapist, (4) therapist to individual, and (5) therapist to couple (or family). Just as there are multiple transference reactions, there are multiple countertransference responses. It is assumed that understanding of unconscious derivatives and their resistances is usually necessary to effect change.

The major therapeutic techniques of the insight-awareness model include clarification, interpretation, and exploration of intrapsychic and interpersonal dynamics and development of insight and empathy. Using such analytic techniques with an individual in the presence of a spouse or other family member represented a unique development in its time. However, more important is the understanding of mutual distortions and projections in the couple's process.

The goal is to foster understanding and insight in order to effect change in individuals and in the family unit.

FAMILY OF ORIGIN MODEL

Allied with the insight-awareness model is the family of origin model, pioneered by Bowen.[4] As in the insight-awareness model, historical data are important. This group of theorists is most interested in the realities of the three- and four-generation family—its themes, beliefs, and loyalties from past generations and the current functioning of adult patients and their parents rather than patient fantasies about them. In this model, the spouses are encouraged and coached to deal with their issues directly with members of the family of origin so as not to project them onto their spouses. This model encourages understanding of the parents and individuation within the family rather than confrontation.

Bowen[4] developed family systems theory, in which he focused on the role of the family emotional system in the etiology of individual dysfunction. He is credited with having developed the genogram, the method of collecting three-generation historical information that some liken to a family tree. His theory concentrated on the need to differentiate oneself in the family by distinguishing between intellectual process and the feeling the person is experiencing; he focused on family triangles, the family projection process, and multigenerational transmission. Using his approach, the therapist works with the individual, coaching them on how to differentiate while within the family. McGoldrick[5,6] continued to promote the use of Bowen's three-generational genograms as an organizing framework for working with couples and families.

Framo[7] is usually grouped with object relations therapists, and his model starts with the couple, but he also invites each spouse to separately explore their relationships with all family members. Framo also developed a model of working with couples groups. Boszormenyi-Nagy and Krasner[8] developed contextual therapy, which emphasized loyalty, balance, and relational justice. Boszormenyi-Nagy, Williamson,[9] and Framo[7] all advocated working with multigenerational families in the therapy room. In each of these approaches, the therapist considers the persistence of past and present multigenerational patterns that exert an invisible influence on present day functioning.

SYSTEMIC-STRATEGIC MODEL

As systems theory developed, a variety of therapists decided to see how far they could take a therapy in which the only emphasis was on the here-and-now system and current relationships between people. In these models, it is assumed that the individual is governed and regulated by the family system and that changing the repetitive patterns of communication and behavior between them in the present would eliminate symptomatology. Jay Haley[10] proposed that the symptom was needed for the homeostasis of the family system and that the family's efforts to solve the family problem had led to more problems (i.e., the solution had become the problem). The ultimate goal of the therapy is to change the family pattern.[11] Insight or understanding is not a goal of this therapy, although often it occurs as a result of treatment.

In these models, it is considered the job of the therapist to understand the problem and find a solution, as opposed to models that are seen as more collaborative.

Treatment techniques in this model include focusing on, exaggerating, de-emphasizing, or relabeling symptoms; clarifying communication; interrupting repetitive interactional patterns; or prescribing symptoms (i.e., requesting a family member to continue to do what they are already doing so that the behavior is, in effect, controlled by the therapist). For example, the family may come in with the complaint that the daughter does not obey the mother and is becoming impossible to discipline. If the father and daughter look at each other and smile whenever the mother attempts to make a statement, the therapist could ask the mother and daughter to speak directly to each other and ask the father to support the mother. They could also *exaggerate* the problem by telling the father that every time the girl disobeys her mother, he should congratulate her or give her a dime. This exchange would hopefully bring the problem out in the open and force the father to disown his covert support of the girl's behavior.

STRUCTURAL MODEL

The structural model, pioneered by Minuchin,[12,13] is probably the most popular and influential of the systemic theories. It is less focused on the details of communication and more on the family "dance" or structure. These patterns of complementarity, where one family member's behavior is understood as an inevitable consequence of the other's, often result in rigid patterns of interaction. For example, if one member of a couple or family is viewed as frightened, the therapist would then look for who in the family is scary (or one is pushy leading to an exploration of who feels "pushed"). Minuchin is also interested in hierarchy (e.g., parental subsystems should be in charge of child subsystems) and clear boundaries, so that each member has a sense of self and privacy but also a sense of membership in the family system. It is important to understand, however, that boundaries, hierarchies, and coalitions are repetitive behaviors (both verbal and nonverbal) that are determined by the family's operational rules and beliefs. These patterns set constraints on individual behavior.

A notable feature of the structural approach involves the setting up of enactments or in-session interactions (e.g., "Mrs. A, you and Mr. A sit next to each other and decide how to handle this problem with your child") or in which the family is given tasks to continue the structure at home. From the structural perspective, the health of a couple or family system lies in its capacity to flexibly reorganize itself to respond to both normal developmental and extrafamilial challenges.

The models of systems theory in which present-oriented and family-focused techniques are used exclusively have been modified extensively since the 1980s. Most practitioners see the system as composed of subsystems that must be understood, including the biologic system of each individual and the internal myths, stories, and beliefs by which each individual modifies incoming communications. Most therapists today are interested in how a person's, couple's, or family's story of past affects present behavior and how family members use this knowledge in reframing the current situation or in developing directives.[14]

COGNITIVE–BEHAVIORAL MODEL

The behavioral model emerges from the behavioral orientation, which has historically developed both alongside and in response to the psychoanalytic tradition. Data for this orientation are database for this orientation is quantifiable, measurable behaviors, whether internal (thoughts) or external (actions). Explanatory concepts are derived from learning theories, for example, concepts such as stimulus and response, as well as basic cognitive–behavioral concepts looking at actions, behaviors, and consequences. With the behavioral model being applied increasingly to interactional systems such as the family, other concepts have been introduced to expand the model into the interpersonal sphere.

The goal in the cognitive–behavioral approaches—popularized by clinician-researchers Baucom and Epstein[15] as well as Christensen and Jacobson[16]—is to effect change in discrete, observable, measurable behaviors that the individuals seeking assistance consider to be problematic. As opposed to the insight-awareness model, which often seems to have more ambitious goals of character change and insight, this model tends to focus more on discrete problem areas defined by clear behavior patterns. Thus, treatment in this model tends to be briefer and more circumscribed. Emphasis is placed not on pathology but on behavioral deficits and excesses that are to be changed. If undesired behaviors are eliminated, it is not assumed that more social behaviors will necessarily emerge spontaneously but rather that the therapist might be required to teach new and more adaptive behaviors to the spouses or family members. Integrative behavioral couple therapy adds the element of acceptance to the traditional behavioral and cognitive models, encouraging couples to appreciate areas in their relationship that may not change and modifying their attitudes to accept these areas of difficulty.

Techniques in this model include helping family members learn how to elicit the desired behavior in another member. Some of the major techniques used are behavioral contracting based on good faith or *quid pro quo* agreements (e.g., If you do this, I will do that), training in communication skills, training in effective problem solving, and combining positive reinforcement with a decrease in destructive interchanges. The therapist's stance is quite active because they see their job as a means to introduce behavior change into the family members' repertoire.

EXPERIENTIAL MODEL

Experiential therapy involves a search for meaning through *mutually shared experience* on the part of the therapist and family. Whitaker (1978, Napier and Whitaker[17]) and Satir[18] were two of the best-known founders of the field working within this model. Both had as a goal the idea of increasing the family members' capacity to experience their lives more fully by sharing with the therapist the struggle with the here and now. Whitaker's approach, symbolic experiential therapy, worked to strengthen the unconscious symbolic processes that foster maturation. The approach emphasizes the therapist's participation as a whole person rather than as an interpreter or director in the process. In Whitaker's model, the assumption is that if the family takes the courageous step of talking about usually hidden things, it will let go of its logical defensive structures and reorganize in more constructive ways.

Satir's model operates less in the fantasy dimension and more in the here and now. These models remind us that structure and problem solving are not the only possible goals of family therapy but that a warm and connected listener who is listening for deeper structures and meanings has much to offer. Later integrators, such as Johnson's emotionally focused therapy, also blend elements from Satir's original work. Her emotionally focused approach orientation, which also includes elements from structural and narrative models, focuses on the attachment styles of family members and tries to promote a climate of emotional safety in which anxiety is reduced so new connections can be forged.

NARRATIVE MODEL

The narrative approach is based on social constructivist ideas from the social sciences whereby reality is viewed as constructed by the observer rather than as a truth to be discovered. Translated into the field of therapy, the narrative approach pioneered by White and Epston[19] proposes that the family's reality is in its shared *narratives and meaning systems*, that the personal story or self-narrative provides the principal frame of intelligibility for our lived experience, and that the therapist's assumptions about the family are also constructed rather than truth. The job of the therapist, then, is to help the family explore and re-evaluate its own assumptions, beliefs, and meaning systems.

Specifically, narrative therapists work to externalize problems, or reframe them as being outside of the members of the family, so that family members can objectively identify the influences of family patterns on their functioning and unite to reduce these influences. In some ways, the constructivist position has returned us to our roots, by elevating meaning to a position at least equal in importance to behavior patterns and by increasing the attention given to our own social constructions, meaning, and value systems.

PSYCHOEDUCATIONAL MODEL

Family psychoeducation acknowledges the essentially chronic nature of mental illness and aims to engage families in the rehabilitation process by creating a long-term working partnership with them and providing them with the information needed to understand how mental illness affects family functioning. This model, developed by McFarlane,[20] Miklowitz,[21] and others,[22] seeks to assist the patient and family in ways to minimize discord, learn adaptive strategies, and in developing social support systems to deal with the myriad of emotions experienced by family members. Although the primary focus of family psychoeducation interventions is improved patient outcomes, an essential intermediate goal is to promote the wellness of the family. This model has crucial importance for treating psychiatric disorders (please see Chapters 11, 18, 20, and 24). Multifamily Group Therapy brings together many families including the families' identified patient. These groups are led by co-facilitators and merge elements of family therapy and group therapy with a psychoeducational focus, typically with a focus on severe psychiatric disorders.[20]

CLINICAL PRACTICE IMPLICATIONS

Various strategies are available for treating families. Each may emphasize different assumptions and types of interventions. Some therapists prefer to operate with one strategy in most cases, whereas others intermix these strategies, depending on the type of case and the phase of treatment. At times the type of strategy used is made explicit by the therapist, whereas in other instances it remains covert. Regardless of whether a therapist specializes in one or another approach or is integrative/eclectic, some hypotheses will be formed about the nature of the family's difficulty and the preferable approach to adopt.

SUGGESTED READINGS

Family therapy schools are discussed in detail.
Lebow JL, Snyder DK, eds. *Clinical Handbook of Couple Therapy* (6th ed.). Guilford Press; 2024.
Gurman AS, Kniskern DP, eds. *Handbook of Family Therapy*. Routledge; 2014.

REFERENCES

1. Goldfried M. Toward the delineation of therapeutic change principles. *Am Psychol.* 1980;35:991–999.
2. Block D, Simon R, eds. *The Strength of Family Therapy: Selected Papers of Nathan W. Ackerman*. Brunner/Mazel; 1982.
3. Dicks HV. *Marital Tensions: Clinical Studies Towards a Psychological Theory of Interaction*. Routledge & Kegan Paul; 1967.
4. Bowen M. *Family Therapy in Clinical Practice*. Jason Aronson; 1978.
5. McGoldrick M. *You Can Go Home Again: Reconnecting With Your Family*. Norton; 1995.
6. McGoldrick M, Gerson R, Sueli P. *Genograms: Assessment and Intervention*. Norton; 2008.
7. Framo JL. *Family of Origin Therapy: An Intergenerational Approach*. Brunner/Mazel; 1992.
8. Boszormenyi-Nagy I, Krasner B. *Between Give and Take: A Clinical Guide to Contextual Therapy*. Brunner/Mazel; 1986.
9. Williamson D. *The Intimacy Paradox: Personal Authority in the Family System*. Guilford; 1986.
10. Haley J. *Problem-Solving Therapy*. Harper & Row; 1976.
11. DeShazer S. *Clues: Investigating Solutions in Brief Therapy*. WW Norton; 1988.
12. Minuchin S. *Families and Family Therapy*. Harvard; 1974.
13. Minuchin S, Fishman H. *Family Therapy Techniques*. Harvard; 1981.
14. White, M. Systemic task setting in family therapy. *Australian Journal of Family Therapy*; 1980;1(4).
15. Baucom D, Epstein N. *Cognitive-Behavioral Marital Therapy*. Brunner/Mazel; 1990.
16. Christensen A, Jacobson N. *Reconcilable Differences*. Guilford Press; 2000.
17. Napier A, Whitaker C. *The Family Crucible: The Intense Experience of Family Therapy*. Harper & Row; 1978.
18. Satir V. *Conjoint Family Therapy*. Science and Behavior Books; 1967.
19. White M, Epston D. *Narrative Means to Therapeutic Ends*. WW Norton; 1990.
20. McFarlane W. *Multifamily Groups in the Treatment of Severe Psychiatric Disorders*. Guilford; 2002.
21. Miklowitz D. The role of the family in the course and treatment of bipolar disorder. *Curr Dir Psychol Sci.* 2007;16:192–196.
22. McFarlane W, Dixon L, Lukens E, Lucksted A. Family psychoeducation and schizophrenia: a review of the literature. *J Marital Fam Ther*. 2003;29:223–245.

10 Goals

OBJECTIVES FOR THE READER

- To be able to set the mediating and final goals of family treatment
- To be able to individualize treatment goals
- To relate the goals of treatment to strategies and interventions
- To relate the goals of treatment to process and content of treatment issues

For easier reading, we emphasize that the descriptors "couples" or "marital" are used nearly interchangeably in this chapter.

INTRODUCTION

> *If you would hit the mark, you must aim a little above it: Every arrow that flies feels the attraction of the earth.*
>
> —*Henry Wadsworth Longfellow*

In this chapter, we examine the issue of goals from five perspectives:

1. Mediating and final goals as they relate to family therapy schools
2. Individualizing goals with the family
3. Goals and their relation to process and content issues
4. Mediating goals and their related strategies
5. Goals and related strategies common to all family therapy schools

MEDIATING AND FINAL GOALS AS THEY RELATE TO SCHOOLS
The Most Common Mediating Goals
The Most Common Final Goals
INDIVIDUALIZING GOALS WITH THE FAMILY
GOALS AND THEIR RELATION TO PROCESS AND CONTENT ISSUES
MEDIATING GOALS AND THEIR RELATED STRATEGIES
GOALS AND RELATED STRATEGIES
Common to All Family Therapy Schools
CLINICAL PRACTICE IMPLICATIONS

MEDIATING AND FINAL GOALS AS THEY RELATE TO SCHOOLS

A convenient way to conceptualize types of treatment goals is to distinguish the final goals (i.e., the ultimate results desired) from the mediating (or intermediate) goals that must precede the final results. Although one would conceptualize unique and specific goals for each individual family, we present more general mediating and final family therapy goals in this chapter. These goals are relatively broad areas that allow for considerable flexibility according to the specifics of each particular family or marital unit, and they are not mutually exclusive but often are intertwined. These broad areas help clarify the therapist's idea of what is to be achieved, and they suggest potential treatment strategies and timing of interventions.

The Most Common Mediating Goals

1. *Establishment of a working alliance.* Patients and families size up therapists very quickly, and those early attitudes are likely to persist. Thus, the early connection between family therapist and each family member is crucial to the ultimate outcome of the work. Setting up such an alliance in individual therapy seems relatively simple in comparison with setting up an alliance with the multiple members of a family, who themselves often do not get along with one another. The therapist also must find a way to connect with each person rather than favoring certain family members.
2. *Specification of problem(s).* This would include a detailed delineation of family members' feelings and behaviors regarding the symptoms or problems that brought the family to treatment.
3. *Clarification of attempted solutions.* It is very likely that many families have attempted solutions to their problems before coming to the conclusion that they need outside intervention. Because almost by definition these are solutions that failed, the therapist should determine what did not work (as indeed some would say that many problems are simply ordinary situations to which less effective solutions were applied).
4. Clarification and specification of individual desires and needs as they are expressed, mediated, and met in the total family or marital environment and network of relationships. It is the lack of clarity, and conflict (either overt or covert), about such needs and desires that leads to or constitutes family pathology itself.
5. *Modification of individual expectations or needs.* Almost always, families need/want too much change, too soon. The therapist titrates the rate of family change.
6. *Recognition of mutual contribution to the problem(s).* Although therapists differ in how early they think this recognition must come or how explicit it must be, the very acceptance of the family intervention format (i.e., most or all family members coming to most sessions) implies the family has some recognition that more than one family member may contribute to the problem or at least to solutions.
7. *Redefinition of the problem(s).* Redefining a problem completely and redefining it into various parts, some of which are problematic and others not, are steps to possible solutions. By way of an example, the therapist might say, "You are not 'bad' people; you are responding to stress with anxiety or anger." In this example, the problem is redefined as a need to find alternative ways to respond to stress.
8. *Improvement in communication skills.* This includes an improvement in listening and expressive skills, a diminution of coercive and blaming behavior with an increase in reciprocity, and the development of effective problem-solving and conflict-resolution behaviors.
9. *A shift in disturbed, inflexible roles and coalitions.* This may include helping to improve the autonomy and individualization of family members, to facilitate the more flexible assumption of leadership by a particular family member as circumstances require, and to facilitate general task performance by one or more members.

10. *Increased family knowledge about serious psychiatric illness.* In families in which any member has a serious mental illness such as schizophrenia or bipolar disorder, a common mediating goal is to increase family information about the illness, its course, and its responsiveness to environmental, including familial, stresses.
11. *Insight.* The mediating goal of developing and improving insight regarding historical factors related to current problems or about current interaction patterns may be relatively important in psychodynamically oriented family or marital work but be absent in other orientations. However, other orientations may reframe particular stories about the family's history as a way of changing interaction.

The Most Common Final Goals

1. *Reduction or elimination of symptoms, or symptomatic behavior, in one or more family members.* Symptoms may include major or minor symptoms of mood and affect (e.g., anxiety and depression), thought disorder, disruptive behaviors in children and adolescents, marital conflict and fighting, and sexual disorders.
2. *Resolution of the problem(s) as originally presented by the family.*
3. *Increased family or marital intimacy.*
4. *Role flexibility and adaptability within the family matrix.*
5. *Toleration of differentness and differentiation appropriate to age and developmental level.*
6. *Balance of power within the marital dyad, with appropriate sharing of input and autonomy for the children.*
7. *Increased self-esteem.*
8. *Clear, efficient, and satisfying communication.*
9. *Resolution of neurotic conflict, inappropriate projective identification, and marital transference phenomena.*

The problems of families and the goals specific to these problems, both mediating and final, should determine the therapeutic strategies. Table 10.1 follows sequentially Tables 8.2 and 8.3 in making this concept clear, and the assumptions embodied in this table are central to the rest of the text.

INDIVIDUALIZING GOALS WITH THE FAMILY

The therapist forms a concept of the family's difficulties based on the evaluation of the family's history and interaction (see Section III). The treatment often begins with the issues that

Table 10.1 Determining strategies after goals are set

	Type of formulation	For the family	For the individual(s)
Diagnosis	Functional	***A*** A systemic formulation	***B*** Behavioral or individual psychodynamic
Diagnosis	Descriptive	***C*** DSM-5 conditions not attributable to a mental disorder that are a focus of attention or treatment (e.g., Relational Problems and Abuse and Neglect)	***D*** DSM-5 classification for each family member attributable to a mental disorder or general medical condition
Goals	Based on diagnosis	Specify for each problem	Specify for each problem
Strategies	Based on goals	Specify for each goal	Specify for each goal

seem to be most crucial to the family; that is, the treatment at the outset helps the family to deal with an immediate crisis situation. Only after some stability and rapport have been achieved is it possible for the therapist to begin to help the family in other ways that also will be beneficial. The work is sometimes slow and gradual, but often a few sessions are enough to get the family's own adaptive mechanisms operating again. At most family therapy clinics, the average number of visits is 6 to 11. One hallmark of family therapy is the belief that rapid change is possible. Sometimes a family comes in for a brief period for one problem and comes back later to work on deeper issues. Family therapists do not consider this a failure. When one family member is seriously ill, therapy may be long term, intermittent, and supportive.

In setting goals, it is helpful to think not only of the family as a whole and of the various interpersonal dyads and triads but also of the individuals who make up the system. Each individual will have a history, a personality, and a set of coping mechanisms. A thorough knowledge of individual personality theory and psychopathology is essential for knowing what to expect from the individual atoms and from the family molecule. At times it will be necessary to provide specific treatment for, or to direct specific attention to, the needs of an individual family member (e.g., when a family member is floridly psychotic) with individual sessions, somatic treatment, and sometimes hospitalization (see Chapters 18 and 20).

Even under ordinary circumstances, however, a thorough understanding of the strengths and weaknesses of each family member (e.g., basic personality patterns, reactions to stress) will help to determine the goals and techniques of the family therapy. Especially when separation or divorce impends, the assessment of individual issues becomes critical.

In setting goals, it is also important to assess the needs of the larger family system, that is, those who may be deeply involved in the family but not in the room. For example, if the wife's mother hates her son-in-law and wishes her daughter would divorce, this is a critical issue affecting the nuclear family. In addition, the possibilities within the larger social system must be considered. For example, is it possible for a couple to marry if it means losing a significant amount of money from welfare or alimony?

The goals of family treatment must be in some way congruent with what the family members seem to desire and what they are realistically capable of achieving. The therapist's views of the appropriate therapeutic possibilities, however, may differ from those the family members envision initially. For example, the family may wish for a home with no conflict, whereas the therapist may see a need for more effective ways of disagreeing.

Overall goals encompass the entire family system and its individual members. Ideally, the entire family should function more satisfactorily as a result of family therapy, and each family member should derive personal benefit from the experience and results of the therapy. The family therapist, for example, should not be in the position of taking the focus off a scapegoated member (saying, for instance, "It's not Dad's withdrawal that is the problem") only to consistently refocus on one or another family member as the cause of the family's difficulties. Nor should the family as a whole feel blamed for one member's problems.

Families traditionally enter therapy because of symptomatic difficulty. In the family's eyes, this is often related to one family member, who has already been labeled as the identified patient. For example, a marital partner may blame the spouse for causing their distress or may feel guilty because the children are not behaving properly. Similarly, a child may be singled out as the only problem in the family. Sometimes a specific family member has a problem (e.g., alcohol, cancer, intellectual disability) around which a family system organizes.

Less commonly, family members talk about system difficulties as marital troubles or family unhappiness. One family member may have instigated the seeking of help, or much less often, the family as a whole may have discussed the difficulties and agreed to seek professional assistance. Families may come into treatment on their own with varying levels of motivation and expectations, or they may be referred by other agencies or individuals.

Some families today are seeking professional help, not for these more traditional reasons but for clarification of family roles and as a growth-enhancing experience. Of course, this is less common because of managed care, unless the family is able to pay for treatment on its own. In such cases, a problem-solving model seems less appropriate than a growth-development model.

The therapist will relate the goals of treatment to what has been learned during the initial evaluation period and to whatever develops as the therapy progresses. All specific mediating and final goals need not be spelled out clearly at the outset of treatment. In some schools of therapy, goals are left somewhat vague, with details being clarified only later or perhaps never being discussed explicitly. The particular areas to be dealt with, and a determination of the priority in dealing with them, must be considered carefully. Some family therapists are relatively comfortable with allowing goals to develop as the therapy proceeds. Such treatment sometimes appears as a sequence of short-term problem resolutions. Other therapists attempt to delineate major goals early in the course of treatment, including those aimed at helping the family to cope better with problems that cannot be reversed.

GOALS AND THEIR RELATION TO PROCESS AND CONTENT ISSUES

The relative importance of structure and process, as compared with its content, is an issue sometimes raised by family therapists. The more traditional view tends to favor substantive content issues, whereas the newer, holistic view looks more closely at the characteristic patterning in an interpersonal network, with less emphasis on the subject matter. In some ways, this may be an artificial dichotomy. For example, the communication process may become the most important subject matter of the therapy. Any attempt to deal with a specific content issue inevitably brings process issues to the surface (and vice versa).

Mr. and Mrs. A requested help because their 19-year-old son, Ted, who was living at home, was very angry at Mrs. A and was being verbally abusive and refusing to help the household in any way. The problems started when Ted was supposed to go to college but refused. In sessions that included Mr. and Mrs. A, Ted, and his younger brother, Ted would talk angrily and dominate the sessions, and Mrs. A would complain about him whenever he stopped talking. Mr. A and Ted's younger brother watched silently.

An initial goal was to alter the communication pattern to bring the rest of the family into the session and decrease the intensity between Mrs. A and Ted. The content of what Mrs. A and Ted talked about was less relevant than the context and pattern of the communication. The therapeutic interventions were to insist that Ted make room for the other members of the family, to get Mr. A to support Mrs. A, and to connect the sibling subsystem. Only when the communication pattern was altered did it become clear that Ted had stayed at home because of fear of failure (he had always had some trouble at school, and college would be a big step) and because he was afraid his father's diabetes would worsen and he would be needed at home.

Sometimes major emphasis is placed on a particular process technique and goal such as clarifying a family's communication patterns or helping family members deal with their feelings. Family therapists may see such process goals as being primary, either on ideologic grounds or because of the appropriateness to a particular family, with the family being encouraged to deal with content issues as they arise after the family has the general process tools to do so. Other family therapists, perhaps because of differing conceptual bases applicable to different types of family goals, will tend to work in the other direction—that is, from the more specific content issues toward the more general process issues.

Table 10.2 Mediating goals of family therapy and their strategies

Mediating goals	Strategies
Increased knowledge, decreased guilt, redefinition of problems, increased use of adaptive coping mechanisms	Supporting adaptive mechanisms
Appropriate emotional experience and communication	Expanding emotional experience
Use of communication skills, problem-solving skills, parenting skills	Developing interpersonal skills
Clarification of boundaries, setting of appropriate boundaries between familial subsystems and family of origin	Reorganizing the family structure
Insight regarding current transactions and historical factors, decreased conflict	Increasing insight
Work on family-of-origin issues	Constructing an alternative reality or story

Trainees often feel uneasy about setting goals for family therapy because they are afraid of being perceived as too authoritarian by taking away from the family its right to set its own goals. Indeed, families should be encouraged to set their own goals to the greatest extent possible; however, the therapist's ability to reframe a problem may lead to different goals (e.g., "Your kid isn't bad, but he seems to be very reactive to your marital conflict; perhaps we could look at how he responds to the stress and how you might deal with each other better"). With disorganized families, the therapist will need to be more structured and active.

MEDIATING GOALS AND THEIR RELATED STRATEGIES

The intersection of appropriate mediating goals with the most efficient therapeutic strategies and techniques at the most propitious moment and in the right sequence is by definition the art of psychotherapy. Future research will help specify such combinations, but clinical skill and creativity will always play a role. For heuristic and instructional reasons, Table 10.2 presents a general scheme of family intervention that relates mediating goals to strategies. In later chapters, we delineate more fully the specific techniques of family intervention.

GOALS AND RELATED STRATEGIES

Common to All Family Therapy Schools

Although repetitive with material presented in Chapter 9, we think it is heuristically useful to conceptualize the broad strategies of intervention that cut across the various schools of thought because, in practice, strategies are combined in different ways to treat the individual family. We summarize here the various ways to conceptualize overall strategies of family intervention.

1. *Strategies for supporting adaptive mechanisms.* There are a number of ways to assist families in using existing strategies and developing new strategies for coping. For example, the therapist could provide the family with information (i.e., psychoeducation) about illnesses in family members or about parenting skills. Supportive advice and encouragement of existing coping mechanisms are also included here, as is the strategy of bearing witness (i.e., acknowledging and understanding the family's experience or emotional pain or trauma). These strategies are of critical importance.
2. *Strategies for expanding emotional experience.* The basic skills are listening, labeling, and encouraging supportive family responses to feelings. Sharing the therapist's own response or

that of others (e.g., "Many people would feel great pain in that situation") is a common way of validating and encouraging feelings. Therapists may at times use fantasy, humor and irony, direct confrontation, family sculpting, or choreography (prescribing sequences of what a family should do) to open up new areas of immediate emotional experiencing for the family.

3. *Strategies for developing interpersonal skills.* By a multitude of techniques, including modeling of intent listening to others, insisting that only one person speaks at a time, questioning the exact meaning of what others are saying and wishing to communicate, and providing explicit instruction in communication skills, the therapist brings the family to a better communication level. This improvement can be an end in itself, or it can be used to solve specific problems that brought the family to treatment in the first place.
4. *Strategies for reorganizing the family structure.* Reframing of the problems as presented by the family, enacting the family problems with their attendant interactional sequences (step-by-step enactment of a family, behavior; e.g., father over "A," mother over "B," son over "C," and so on), marking boundaries, and restructuring moves (changing the structure of a family; e.g., bringing in another family member, such as grandmother, to help change a problem behavior, such as mother's cocaine abuse) can all be used to change the structured family behaviors judged to be causing or contributing to the family distress. Paradoxical techniques (which are discussed in Chapter 12), although used less frequently than in the past, can be used for families that are resistive or at an impasse.

   Effective family structure is predicated on the idea that parents work together and that appropriate generational hierarchy be maintained. By insisting in the session that parents make joint decisions about the children rather than leaving the mother in charge and the father passive, insisting that parents take charge of children rather than allow them to control the session, and delineating responsibilities of grandparents and other family adults, the therapist allows families to experience new types of structure. Homework assignments that encourage clear boundaries, such as making sure the parents' bedroom door is closed at night, reinforce these messages.
5. *Strategies for increasing insight.* Traditional techniques of psychodynamic psychotherapy, such as clarification, confrontation, and interpretation either in the here and now or of genetic material, can be used in the marital and family treatment formats in order to bring underlying conflicts to the fore and reduce conflict-laden interactions. Insight here must be relational in terms of how the person's past affects the present and the response of the other. Direct questioning of the parents and analysis of current relationships by family-of-origin work are other useful ways of developing insight.
6. *Strategies for helping the family understand and modify its narrative.* These strategies involve helping the family tell its story and find alternative and less problem-saturated narratives that offer novel solutions. The therapist and family members look for redefinitions (e.g., enthusiastic rather than noisy, survivor rather than victim), understandings (e.g., fear of failure rather than laziness), and novel outcomes (e.g., how about the times it does not fail—what happens then?).

CLINICAL PRACTICE IMPLICATIONS

We have emphasized that there are both short-term and long-term goals. Please note—we have also briefly discussed short- and long-term goals for families when one member has a psychiatric disorder in Chapter 18.

The beginning therapist is cautioned against trying to produce instantaneous behavioral change that may prove to be evanescent. As Winston Churchill said, "It is a mistake to look too far ahead. Only one link in the chain of destiny can be handled at a time." The chronicle of unconventional psychotherapies is replete with claims of being able to change behavior in the short term. In contrast, family therapists should aim for a more permanent, long-term change in family structure and function but should do it step by step. Many therapists and families might find it useful to create a brief written contract to define goals and expectations from the treatment.[1]

These differences in outlook and practice can be bewildering to the inexperienced therapist who is not aware of the underlying rationales and guidelines. Given the current state of the field, with no unifying theory of family pathology, nomenclature, or even of treatment, each new situation represents an experiment of sorts, in which the therapist is required to clarify and test hypotheses.

REFERENCE

1. Keitner GI, Heru AM, Glick ID. *Clinical Manual of Couples and Family Therapy*. American Psychiatric Publishing; 2009:182–183.

11 Family Treatment: Integrated Strategies and Techniques

OBJECTIVES FOR THE READER

- To understand the common elements of psychotherapy as they apply to family treatment
- To become familiar with the general strategies of family therapy and their related techniques
- To become familiar with the notion of treatment packages for specific situations and disorders

For easier reading, we emphasize that the descriptors "couples" or "marital" are used nearly interchangeably in this chapter.

INTRODUCTION

Before describing how to treat families, we first examine family therapy in the general context of the strategies and techniques of psychotherapy. In this chapter, we recommend treatment modalities that look beyond the notion that success is merely an unconditional acceptance of life and what it brings. Subjective and objective improvement should occur in behaviors, emotions, and individuals' capacities to live. We conclude the chapter with reference to current treatment packages for various diagnostic or problem situations that families face.

GENERAL ELEMENTS OF PSYCHOTHERAPY AND THEIR RELATIONSHIP TO FAMILY THERAPY
BASIC STRATEGIES OF FAMILY INTERVENTION
Techniques for Supporting Adaptive Mechanisms and Strengths: The Psychoeducational Approach
Techniques for Expanding Emotional Experience
Techniques for Developing Interpersonal Skills
Techniques for Reorganizing the Family Structure
Techniques for Increasing Insight and Conflict Resolution
Techniques for a More Effective Construction of Family Reality
TREATMENT PACKAGES
INDICATIONS FOR DIFFERENTIAL USE OF THE BASIC STRATEGIES
CLINICAL PRACTICE IMPLICATIONS

GENERAL ELEMENTS OF PSYCHOTHERAPY AND THEIR RELATIONSHIP TO FAMILY THERAPY

Most schools of psychotherapy share the following elements:

1. An effective patient–therapist relationship
2. Release of emotional tension or development of emotional expression
3. Cognitive learning
4. Insight into the genesis of one's problems
5. Operant reconditioning of the patient toward more adaptive behavior patterns using techniques such as behavioral desensitization
6. Suggestion and persuasion
7. Identification with the therapist
8. Repeated reality testing or practicing of new adaptive techniques in the context of implicit or explicit emotional therapeutic support
9. Construction of a more positive narrative about oneself and the world
10. Instillation of hope

Family therapy involves all of these elements, but it does so in the context of the whole family, with the goal of improving the entire group's overall functioning. The particular mix of therapeutic elements will vary with the family's specific needs. There are few, if any, specific techniques used in other therapy formats (i.e., individual and group) and orientations (e.g., insight-oriented, cognitive–behavioral, systemic–strategic, experiential–existential) that could not in some way be adapted for use in family intervention.

Somewhat parenthetically, the question is often asked, "Can a 'psychotherapy,' such as family therapy, change the brain?" Gabbard[1] pointed out "that the brain is characterized by considerable plasticity and that genes are not static but responsive to environmental factors which we are only beginning to understand." Kandel[2] suggested that by producing changes in gene expression, psychotherapy may alter the strength of synaptic connections. Biologic and psychosocial factors appear to have equal weight in development. There is a reciprocal effect of gene expression on environment and environment on gene expression in every family system. We can no longer afford reductionism in either a biologic or a psychosocial direction.

BASIC STRATEGIES OF FAMILY INTERVENTION

Because much overlap exists among the schools of family intervention (both in theory and techniques), and because our bias is that the field must advance beyond strict schools to basic principles of change, we present our choice of basic strategies of family intervention. We also describe in this section the techniques used in each strategy:

- Supporting adaptive mechanisms and strengths, including imparting new information, advice, suggestions, and so on—the so-called psychoeducational approach
- Expanding individual and family emotional experience
- Encouraging explicit development of interpersonal skills (e.g., communication skills, parenting skills, problem-solving skills)
- Reorganizing the family structure
- Increasing insight and fostering intrapsychic conflict resolution
- Helping the family find new and more positive ways of understanding its situation (i.e., the narrative approach)

Even these strategies, abstractly stated in terms of their aim or goal in treatment, are not mutually exclusive. To some extent, they represent different frames of reference for understanding and dealing with the same family phenomena. Nevertheless, each strategy seems to offer something unique in its conceptualization and execution. The choice of strategy depends on the goals (see Table 10.2). In general, however, all families can profit from review and support of their strengths.

In a clinical situation, the therapist will be hard-pressed to remain a purist. For example, a therapist's efforts to clarify communication may produce shifts in family coalitions or may initiate an exploration of family myths that may lead to a considerable outpouring of previously concealed emotion.

Although we list specific therapeutic strategies here, there is no one magical technique that will "cure" the family. Interventions are instead a series of repetitive maneuvers designed to change feelings, attitudes, and behaviors. If the overall goals and strategy are kept in mind, specific interventions will suggest themselves and be modified by the family's circumstances and the therapist's own style.

> What is unique in family therapy is not so much the specific techniques used but rather that these techniques are used not with an isolated individual but within a relationship and that the overall focus and strategy aims to evaluate and produce a beneficial change in the entire family system.

Techniques for Supporting Adaptive Mechanisms and Strengths: The Psychoeducational Approach

First and foremost, the therapist uses many techniques to support the active or latent positive coping mechanisms the family has at its disposal. **Every family has some degree of health, and that should be acknowledged and actively encouraged.** Empathic listening and concern, positive feedback about the use of adaptive defenses (such as healthy denial in the face of terminal illness), education about poorly adaptive defenses, and well-timed advice are helpful to the family in distress.

The therapist is constantly in the role of a teacher, either directly or indirectly. Without saying a word, they are modeling mood, tempo, and interpersonal acceptance. The therapist also teaches values, often implicitly. For example, in structuring the treatment so that only one person in the family speaks at a time, the therapist is modeling good communication but is also indicating implicitly the value of respecting the thoughts of every person in the family.

More recently there has been a growing emphasis on providing explicit information that might be helpful to families in their coping. This approach has been most obvious in the psychoeducational strategies used with families in which a member has been given the diagnosis of a disorder such as schizophrenia or mood disorder. Information can be communicated through written material, in lectures and discussions in family groups, and in workshop format. Anderson et al. have described a day-long survival skills workshop, which the family attends without the patient.

During this workshop, information is provided on the nature of schizophrenia (e.g., the history and epidemiology of the disorder, its biologic basis, and personal experiences of patients and family members), the available treatments (e.g., medication and psychosocial treatment), and the role of the family (e.g., family reactions to the patient and the illness, methods for coping with the condition).

Consider the following case example:

Ms. A, a 20-year-old single, female college student, had long-standing major depressive disorder and persistent depressive disorder since her teens. She was in the midst of an 8-month episode of acute depression characterized by psychomotor retardation, cognitive slowing, lability, and overeating. She was being treated with a combination of individual therapy, family therapy, and antidepressants. Although she had been ill for 3 or 4 years, she had never understood her illness. Her physician spent time explaining in detail the multiple roots of her depression. She reported that before receiving the psychoeducation, when she thought about her illness it was "like a huge something I didn't understand." After psychoeducation, she said, "I could pick apart pieces of the illness, ask questions about it, and understand it, and I felt better immediately after the session." When asked why she felt better, she said her thoughts were now more cohesive and thus she could better cope with her illness.

In Ms. A's case, a second nuance of psychoeducation involved the family therapist's focus on her parents' perception that she was lazy because she spent so much time on the couch watching television. The intervention directed to Ms. A and her family was partly psychoeducational (i.e., it was explained that leaden paralysis is a cardinal symptom of atypical depression and that weight gain is a side effect of antidepressants) and partly dynamic and systemic.

The psychoeducational approach need not be limited to situations in which there is a clear diagnosis of a condition that has biologic components in its etiology. Communication skills and problem-solving skills are taught in many forms of marital therapy. For example, Patterson[3] provides information to parents with antisocial children so that they can improve their family management skills (described later in this chapter). In some situations, therapists give advice to families that function relatively well. This may include discussing parenting alternatives such as discipline styles or helping the family to make difficult decisions (e.g., determining whether a child should go away to school or stay at home).

The use of psychoeducation should not lead to an exclusive focus on either biology or behavior. As Hunter et al.[4] have pointed out, "Family therapists should not abandon a concern with the inner lives of severely ill patients and their families 'after they are educated about an illness.'" Families that have been asked about their experience in therapy repeatedly cite as helpful the therapist's ability to listen respectfully, to notice their strengths, and to be active—that is, to offer suggestions and advice but in a way that is respectful and not commanding. Families need to have the sense that their therapist has ideas they can try but that the therapist will not be hurt or angry if they don't agree with the plan.

Families that have been asked about their experience in therapy repeatedly cite as helpful the therapist's ability to listen respectfully, to notice their strengths, and to be active—that is, to offer suggestions and advice but in a way that is respectful and not commanding.

Techniques for Expanding Emotional Experience

Techniques used to help individuals and family units expand their experience repertoire tend to focus on the here-and-now experience in the sessions themselves. These techniques are designed to help the individual family members to quell anxiety, slow their reaction process, and maximize the emotional and cognitive experience of the moment, experiences that may have been denied, defended against, and missed in the past. In many families, feelings are either avoided or detoured. For example, some members of the family, or the entire family, may not admit to feelings because they are afraid of hurting other family members. Alternatively, certain feelings may be avoided or denied, so that, for example, anger instead of sadness may be expressed. Rebellious or inappropriate behavior may be used as a nonverbal protest (e.g., forgetting, daydreaming, or bowel control problems may occur as a way of demonstrating helpless rage or anxiety).

In some families, the affect, especially rage or anxiety, may appear all too obvious and overwhelming, but invariably there are also hidden feelings and silent family members. Some families may appear too full of affect, and some families may seem to have none. The therapist's job is to slow down or speed up the family's process and allow the variety of feelings to surface in a safe environment, allowing everyone to feel heard and to see how hidden or detoured feelings, or long-standing rage or anxiety, have affected the family's functioning. Often the most important thing for an individual family member is to know that other family members understand how they feel, even when they cannot fix it. For a child especially, the most difficult thing, even worse than disagreement or punishment, is to be disconfirmed—that is, to have a feeling of being completely ignored.

Often the most important thing for an individual family member is to know that other family members understand how they feel, even when they cannot fix it.

The therapist's main role is to look for the family's underlying feelings and, using empathy and clarification, to help family members to express them. Simple examples of such expression include "That really must have hurt," "How did you feel then?" or "I hear you were angry, but you also look sad; why is that?" The therapist may also use disclosure, by saying, for example, "That story makes me feel sad." This approach is especially helpful in younger patients who are less experienced in expressing emotions, especially strong emotions that are often feared by children to be overwhelming. The therapist then asks how other family members felt or reacted because the issue in families is not only the feeling but the reaction or anticipated reaction of other family members. For example, the therapist could use the following series of questions: "Did you tell your mom or your dad how you felt? What did they say? How did you feel, Mom? Dad? What happened next? Were there other people in the family who felt differently? Why? If you didn't tell them then, how do you think they feel when you tell them now?" The therapist acts as witness and support, making sure that everyone is heard and protected.

The therapist examines which feelings are acceptable in the family and which are not, and whether only certain family members express feelings for other family members (e.g., only the mother expresses anxiety, and she is told she is crazy). This is a particularly important technique in marital therapy, in which the spouses' feelings about each other form much of the basis of the therapy. The sense that one partner is not heard or respected by the other is a common underlying reason for divorce in a society in which the fulfillment of emotional needs is the center of marriage. The use of this technique is critical when violence, acting out, or mourning is present. When the feelings are of great grief, or there is great anger and a need to forgive, rituals are often designed to support or accentuate the process. For example, families that have been unable to mourn may be asked to prepare a new memorial service, to share stories and perhaps pictures of the deceased with the therapist, or to design a new holiday celebration that would include memories of the person who died but allow for new activities.

A number of techniques adapted from other therapies are powerful emotional catalysts. Such techniques include psychodrama and the techniques adapted from it (e.g., role-play, gestalt, family sculpting), family marathons, and guided fantasy. Although these techniques are all interesting and often extremely powerful, they are best left to those with special training. In the long run, there are few techniques as powerful as a therapist who can sit with a family, hour after hour in the face of its pain, and bear the pain with the family and help it find ways to heal.

Techniques for Developing Interpersonal Skills

Many families and marital units do not use basic skills of communication, parenting, or general problem solving, either because they never learned such skills as a result of poor or absent parental modeling or because of interpersonal conflicts that interfere with the use of such skills.

The therapist is, by training, an expert in communication and thus can help family members express their thoughts and feelings more clearly to one another. These are not skills traditionally learned in residency, and beginning therapists do not always have these skills. The therapist should be certain that they are familiar with these techniques, and they should have attempted to use them at a personal level before teaching them to others. The therapist tries to promote open and clear communication, emotional empathy, a positive rapport between family members, and good problem-solving skills. Good problem solving requires an additional set of skills beyond the clear communication of feeling. Problem solving is different from sharing feelings in that the emphasis is on cognitively finding solutions to problems rather than simply expressing feelings about them. Although expressing feelings may involve great positive or negative affect, problem solving needs calm affect. Communication requires both a speaker and a listener (or a communicator and a receiver, in the case of nonverbal communication) and consists of not only the message sent but also the message intended and the message received. The therapist's goal is to help the family look at intended messages, the way the messages are sent and their content, and what the receivers think about them. Although it is impossible not to communicate in a family (even silence plus nonverbal signals present a powerful message), many troubled family members spend very little time talking meaningfully with one another. Both thoughts and feelings can be distorted, hidden, negated, or blurred. The person sending the message may or may not be aware that their intention and the message do not match. Unless the person sending the message asks, they will never know what the other person understood.

> Although expressing feelings may involve great positive or negative affect, problem solving needs calm.

The therapist supplies an arena for family discussion, being cognizant of the different levels of meaning in messages and how these levels of meaning influence and sometimes contradict one another. The therapist does not allow anyone to monopolize a session or to speak for someone else. The therapist helps the family look at how messages are sent, what messages are hidden, and why it is often hard to hear them. A common technique to slow down a conversation so that it is clearer is to insist that before someone can reply to a communication, they have to repeat it, first verbatim and then in paraphrase. The therapist attempts to encourage interpersonal sensitivity and empathy and tries to help each person become more aware of their own thoughts and feelings. Consider the following examples:

Example of a problem.

Husband: I was really upset that you didn't do the dishes last night.
Wife: You think I'm a bad wife and mother! Well, you didn't do the breakfast dishes either!

Example of communications practice.

Husband: I was really upset that you didn't do the dishes last night.
Wife: You were really upset that I didn't do the dishes?
Husband: Yes, that's what I said.
Wife: That makes me angry, and I think you think I'm a sloppy person.
Husband: I don't think you are sloppy, but you promised to do them. I am upset because you broke your promise to me, and that makes me feel as if you don't care about me.

The therapist encourages family members to be specific, to state who did what to whom (e.g., "Dad hit me with a stick," rather than "He did it"). The therapist encourages more productive and supportive communication. They emphasize finding both positive and negative ways of saying things and noticing nonverbal messages. They help parents speak to their children in ways appropriate to each child's age. The therapist looks for family members who speak for others (e.g., a mother who always answers for her daughter) and for family members who don't speak to one another (e.g., a son who speaks only to his father, not to his mother). They work to get family members to speak for themselves (i.e., using "I" statements) and to get family members who have issues with another family member to speak directly to that member rather than through a third person. The therapist stresses that individuals are held accountable for their actions. They fill in gaps in communication, points out discrepancies, and deals with nonverbal communication. The therapist points out nonproductive verbal and nonverbal family communication patterns and tries to identify the implicit, unstated patterns or attitudes that may be causing trouble. Through these efforts the covert is made overt, the implicit made explicit. Blocked channels of communication and feelings can be opened. The therapist counsels that good communication includes listening. Often three or four family members are heard talking at exactly the same time during a session, presumably to avoid hearing thoughts and feelings other than their own. In such a situation the therapist may function as a communication traffic cop or referee.

Marital and family life is filled with problems, large and small. In many cases, distressed families have no more problems than do nondistressed families, but nondistressed families use effective problem-solving techniques so that problems are handled and do not multiply. Distressed families can be taught problem-solving methods. The steps of problem solving are (1) defining a problem, (2) brainstorming, (3) negotiating, and (4) making clear the behavioral contract.

In general, distressed families have trouble with problem solving not only because of skill deficits but also because of hidden agendas, many of which involve power issues. For example, if a wife wants her husband to share the work around the house more and he doesn't want to, a behavioral contract about how many nights he is to wash dishes isn't of much help. He is likely to forget, do the job badly, and be angry, even if she agrees to do something for him in return. The problem must be defined as a larger issue about equality in family life, and if the husband is strongly against doing any more than he is already doing, it is difficult to solve this problem. It will have to be clear to him that he will get something of equal value that will not injure his sense of self-esteem or manliness (the cognitive issue behind the behavioral problem). A couple or family that comes up with seemingly reasonable solutions that are not put into practice needs to spend time with the therapist redefining the problem and looking for the issues behind the issues.

> Distressed families have trouble with problem solving not only because of skill deficits but also because of hidden agendas.

In addition to the communication and problem-solving skills needed by a marital dyad, other skills are needed to raise children effectively. Patterson[3] referred to these skills as family management skills and devised techniques for teaching these skills to families with an antisocial child. The family management skills that can be taught include rule setting, parental monitoring (detection and labeling), and parental sanctions, including the appropriate use of positive reinforcement and punishment. Each of these skills must be carefully taught, role-played, and supervised.

In the social learning theory tradition, Stuart[5] has outlined a behaviorally oriented marital therapy approach that begins with assessment and proceeds through so-called caring days (i.e., each partner offering specific requested caring behaviors). Techniques are organized to increase (1) small, high-frequency, conflict-free behaviors; (2) communication skills; (3) contracting procedures; (4) training in problem-solving skills; (5) training in conflict containment; and (6) strategies for maintaining the changed interaction.

Stuart gives as a clinical example a holistic agreement in which several behaviors by one spouse are exchanged for several by the other, with no requirements that the offerings by one exactly match those of the other.

This model is workable only if the therapist has evaluated carefully the power, intimacy, and justice issues underlying the problematic behaviors. Most behaviorally oriented marital therapies stress cognitive issues (e.g., How does this fit with my picture of myself? Is this an acceptable behavior in my culture?) and the careful and gradual increase of positive and caring behaviors.

Techniques for Reorganizing the Family Structure

In many ways, the unique contribution of the family orientation is the recognition of structured (i.e., repetitive and predictable) behavioral sequences in family groups that cause or maintain symptomatic behaviors. Figure 11.1 provides a graphic representation of common family coalitions. In the figure, a typical four-member family is taken as the unit, with the squares representing the males and the circles the females. The larger symbols stand for spouse/parent, and the smaller symbols represent the offspring/siblings. The solid straight lines joining these symbols are intended to represent positive communication, emotional, and activity bonds between the individuals involved, in a semiquantitative fashion, according to the number of straight lines used. Dotted lines are used to represent the relative absence or negative quality of the interactions.

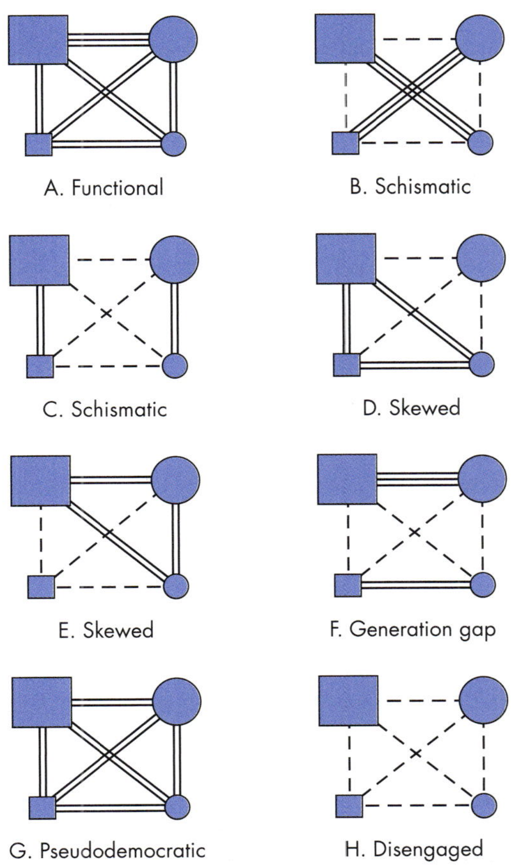

Figure 11.1 Types of family coalitions.

In example A, the functional family, the marital coalition is the strongest dyad in the family, the generational boundary is intact, and all other channels are open and about equal to one another in importance. In contrast to this example are various types of dysfunctional families (see Chapter 3).

In example B, the marital coalition is relatively weak or absent, and instead there are strong alliances across the generations and sexes—between father and daughter and between mother and son—with a relative absence of other effective channels. In example C, cross-generational alliances exist between same-sex parent and child. Examples B and C can be thought of as representing types of the schismatic family.

Examples D and E depict skewed families in which one family member is relatively isolated from the other three, who form a fairly cohesive unit. Example F represents the generation-gap family, in which the marital unit and the offspring both form a fairly cohesive duo, with little or no interaction across the generational lines. Example G represents the pseudodemocratic family, in which all channels seem to be of about equal importance, with the marital coalition and the parental role not being particularly well differentiated. Example H, the disengaged family, represents an extreme case in which each family member is pretty much cut off from every other member, and in which one would expect very little sense of positive interaction, feeling, or belonging to a family unit.

Clearly these representations are highly oversimplified and are pictured only for a two-generation, four-member family. Infinite variations could be added. Such representations enable the therapist to conceptualize more clearly the nature of the coalitions in a particular family and to begin planning a strategy to bring those coalitions into a better functional alignment, presumably more closely approximating example A. In example B, for instance, the therapist might focus on activating the marital coalition, the coalitions between parent and offspring of the same sex, and those between the offspring themselves. Also, the therapist might attempt to attenuate the force of the existing cross-generational, cross-sexed interactions.

The tactics and strategies of family therapy, viewed in this light, might include changes in the marital coalition (very commonly the case) and in the parent–child dyads. Although triads are not considered to any great extent in this model, an isolated family member might be brought into interaction with the rest of the family unit. In some of the families depicted in Figure 11.1, the problem is an overly connected triad, in which case decreasing less functional coalitions will automatically make space for the isolated family member. Looking outside of the nuclear family for a moment, it is critical to consider coalitions and cutoffs with the extended family (e.g., parents and siblings of the adults and other significant family members) and to examine relationships with other significant systems (e.g., peers of children, therapists, other helping professionals in the system, secret relationships such as affair partners). Remarried families in particular will have immensely complicated structures, and it is critical that the therapist uses a genogram to include all members of the family (see Chapter 7). When outside interactions, especially those with in-laws, seem problematic, modifications should be considered. Sometimes outside interactions may need to be encouraged, especially if no one has contacts outside the family.

Temporary triads, for example, incorporating the therapist, are often purposely formed in order to produce structural change. In example D, the father is connected primarily with his son, and both men are disrespectful to mother and daughter. If the daughter enters therapy with depression, rather than treat the daughter's depression in isolation, the therapist looks at how the father's disrespect and mother's passivity have made her feel hopeless. The therapist encourages the husband to insist on his son being respectful (i.e., fathers teach their sons respect) and works with the parents to encourage the mother to speak up for herself and the father to look at why he is treating his wife badly. (Perhaps he is really angry because she is paying attention to her own mother and not to him.) The parents are encouraged to support their daughter and to deal with their own issues. The daughter's depression lifts because she no longer has to be her mother's support.

Techniques that enable the family therapist to interrupt and change such structured family behaviors are central to reorganizing the family structure.[6,7] The techniques include the following:

- *Reframing.* Each individual frames reality from their own unique perspective. When the therapist perceives and understands the patient's or family's frame and then counters this frame with another, competing view, this is called a *reframe.* Such a therapeutic move can be sudden, dramatic, or humorous and often models a more relaxed, less conflicted, or more positive view of the world and the basic details of family life. The goal of a reframe is to allow the family to find different ways of behaving. For example, if the parents of a misbehaving child label the child as being sick or creative, they may not discipline them, but if they label them as being spoiled, then they may find more creative but firm ways of getting them to behave.
- *Enactment.* It is one thing for a family to describe what has happened, and it is another thing for the family to enact what happened in front of the therapist. *Enactment* is the technique of eliciting during the therapeutic hour the playing out of interpersonal problems of which the family complains. Enactment enables the perceptive therapist to observe the interpersonal behaviors in the problem sequence, rather than hearing the typical censored versions of what goes on, as offered by each participant.
- *Focusing.* The individual therapist is flooded with a multitude of data from the patient. With the recent developments in the brief therapy field, literature has accumulated on patient ability and therapist factors in focusing the sessions. This multiplicity of data is compounded in family therapy by the number of individuals involved. For there to be organization, highlighting, and progression in the treatment, someone must focus the group's attention. From multiple inputs, the therapist must select a focus and develop a theme for the family therapy work.[7] According to Minuchin and Fishman,[7] there are three major techniques to challenge the structure of the family: (1) boundary making, (2) unbalancing, and (3) creation of a systemic reality.
- *Boundary making.* Boundary-making techniques are ways of focusing on and changing the psychological distance between two or more family members. A common example is when the therapist moves the mother away from the daughter and insists that the daughter speak. In triadic interactions, a typical situation is one in which the unresolved conflicts between the parents are acted out by the misbehavior of a child, who then either sides with the mother or the father or becomes a judge or go-between for the two parents. The therapist can intervene in the session by distancing the child verbally or physically from the mother–father dyad. The therapist can make boundaries through verbal reconstructions (e.g., they could say, "Mom and Dad, you are the bosses of your children; now act like it"), the giving of tasks, special rearrangements of seating in the sessions, or nonverbal gestures and eye contact.[7]
- *Unbalancing.* The family therapist uses unbalancing techniques in order to change the hierarchical relationship of members of a family system or subsystem. There are three basic ways of unbalancing the existing family hierarchy and power distribution: (1) affiliating with certain family members, (2) ignoring family members, or (3) entering into a coalition with some family members against others. A therapist unbalances the family's existing power system by, for example, allying with a family member low in the power hierarchy. Unbalancing is a technique that is somewhat controversial because many therapists prefer either a more neutral stance or one that supports all family members equally. Unbalancing may have unintended consequences and needs to be done with a clear sense of its use and an awareness of whether the intervention is working.
- *Creation of a systemic reality.* By using mainly cognitive interventions, the family therapist attempts to help the family members perceive and understand the workings of their mutual interdependence and membership in an entity (i.e., the family) larger than themselves. Family members generally perceive themselves as acting and reacting to one another, rather than seeing the larger picture of the family dance (or family script) over time.

The family therapist commonly challenges the family's usual rhetoric (i.e., formulation) in three areas: (1) the family notion that there is only one identified patient, (2) the family notion that one person is controlling the family system, or (3) the family's time-limited vision of its interactions. First, even if one person is obviously symptomatic, the therapist introduces the notion that family interactions are probably helping to maintain the problem. Second, the therapist counters the idea that one person controls the system with the conception that each person provides the context for the other. That is, symptoms in one person are maintained by the interpersonal context. Finally, the therapist helps the family achieve an understanding of its interactions over a large time frame so that it (the family) can perceive (i.e., bring into their awareness) the family rules that transcend (i.e., govern) the individual family members.

- *Paradoxical techniques.* These techniques are called paradoxical because they appear to be opposite to common sense. They are based on the fact that although people are often aware of the reasons they want to change, hidden reasons for not changing keep the symptom going. Faced with a symptom that does not respond to support, insight, logic, and so on, the therapist may suggest that the person keep the symptom to study its effects, make a list of all the reasons the symptom is useful or cannot be changed, or increase the symptom frequency in order to make sure it is working (thereby proving that it is also under the person's control). For example, a couple that has been unable to either make a commitment or split up may be told that their current arrangement of indecision is the best process, giving reasons that are believable and yet slightly off base (e.g., each needs the sense of distance and remoteness, the tension is good for their work, they are not yet ready to give up their mothers). They are given the task of planning how to remain in this ambiguous state for a long time. The therapist must give this intervention with seriousness, which means they must believe in its inherent truth. This injunction to hold on to the symptom usually jars the continuing process and helps the couple focus more clearly on what is going on; it may also unite the couple against the therapist and cause them to rebel, which would also break the logjam. (Because it seems manipulative, many family therapists have argued against this type of intervention.) Although it is possible to conduct a whole therapy in this manner, most therapists reserve this type of intervention for more resistant couples.[8]

A common intervention is to request that the family members (or individuals) intensify the occurrence of the symptoms. When the family does this, the symptoms begin to lose their autonomy, mystery, and power. Whereas the symptoms previously seemed to have been out of control, they now appear to come under the therapist's and the family's control. The participants, in increasing the behavior, become more conscious of it, and often the disruptive behavior begins to lessen or disappear. Consider the following example:

Mr. and Mrs. C, a married couple that have engaged in nonproductive arguing, now find that the therapist has asked them to continue fighting and even to increase it. They tell the couple to fight about the menu before dinner, so that they can enjoy the food. After the first few fights Mr. and Mrs. C decide that this ruins dinner. They refuse to fight. The therapist expresses doubt that this is a good idea, that is, remaining in the no-change position relative to their own suggested intervention. The couple now insists that they can and will stop fighting—taking the change position relative to the intervention. The resistance to change is now coming from the therapist, leaving Mr. and Mrs. C free to experiment with change.

If the therapist gives directives or homework, they are obligated to follow through to make sure that the directions have been followed in the way that was intended. The therapist does so by seeing the family in their office on an ongoing basis and by asking more than one family member what changes have taken place. In some situations, the therapist may choose to make a home visit, but this must be done with considerable care and preparation.

Techniques for Increasing Insight and Conflict Resolution

Although the experiential–existential and insight awareness schools of psychotherapy have different goals, they both use techniques to further the emotional–cognitive horizons of the patient(s), with the assumption that such expansion will lead to behavior or character change. In family therapy with dynamic and expressive undertones, the therapist uses the context of relative therapeutic neutrality (and empathic support) to use techniques such as clarification, confrontation, and interpretation, either with the individual or with the marital dyad or family unit. In family therapy, insight is always given in a family context. In general, family therapists are clearer than other types of therapists that insight is more constructed than revealed. The goal is to link past with present reality of the family in such a way that family members can stop trying to solve the past with the present.

- *Clarification.* In using the technique of clarification, the therapist asks the family members to elucidate their understanding or emotional reaction to present and past events.
- *Confrontation.* Confrontation is the pointing out of contradictory aspects of the patient's behavior, often between verbal and nonverbal behavior.
- *Interpretation.* Interpretation is the elucidation by the therapist of links between present contradictory behavior and present or past distortions that are out of the patient's awareness. In making interpretations, often immediately preceded by clarification and confrontations, the therapist is providing a conceptual link for the patient and the family. The interpretation should connect current behavior (as distorted or guided by internal templates) and past experiences (distorted by anxiety and defense mechanisms) timed so as to maximize cognitive and emotional affect. Interpretations can be made in the here-and-now interaction between family members or between therapist and family member(s), or interpretations can link current behavior to past experiences. Probably the former are of more use in family intervention. Ackerman[9] was a pioneer in using dynamic techniques (along with a multitude of others) in a family therapy format in order to interrupt intrapsychic conflicts being played out in the interpersonal sphere (e.g., if you are mad at a parent, you take it out on your spouse). Dicks[10] has more than any other author spelled out the use of dynamic techniques in interventions with married couples.

Mr. and Mrs. D, a couple in their thirties who are married and have three children, came into therapy complaining that Mrs. D was not interested in sex. Although she was honestly very busy with three young children, that did not seem to be the central issue. It was noted that Mr. D was very depressed and critical and had serious depressive symptoms for years. He was treated with fluoxetine with excellent results. As Mr. D's irritability lessened, Mrs. D realized that she responded to his annoyance with fear and anxiety far beyond the usual response. At that point she began to discuss her abusive father and how if she made him angry, he would hit her, or go into a total rage, and how desperately she had tried to be good. She was projecting onto her husband her fears about her father. Mr. D's mother had been intrusive and anxious, and when his mother became anxious, his father would retreat, as he was doing with his wife. As each saw their projections, they began to learn to reassure the other, and Mrs. D was able to relax and have satisfactory sex.

In the preceding case the issue was not oedipal (i.e., resulting from repressed sexual feelings toward the father) but rather was the projection of an old family interaction into the present. Similarly, Dicks[10] describes the brief marital therapy case of H, a 45-year-old man, married for 20 years to W (the names Mr. E and Mrs. E are used here):

Mr. E and Mrs. E had three adolescent children. The presenting complaint was Mr. E's sexual impotence of 10 years' duration and his depressive moods and irritability, especially at his wife and children, all of which threatened his marriage.

In the initial diagnostic interview with Mr. E alone, he was asked about his early sexual attitudes. His associations shifted to his parental home and its atmosphere, noting that his sulking did not work as it did for his father, as he knows it is wrong. This was followed by an interpretation by the therapist: There seemed to be a similarity between general sulking and sexual withdrawal.

The patient's next association was to his wife, whom he saw as having her own way as to times for intercourse. He then described the many talents of his wife in contrast to himself. Another interpretation was offered: Mr. E feels inadequate in comparison to Mrs. E, as if she has all the potency, much as it was in Mr. E's parents' case.

In the diagnostic interview with Mrs. E, she described a strong bond to an idealized father, who died when she was 17, and a scarcely concealed hostility toward a weak mother.

In the first conjoint marital session, it appeared that the couple had a stereotyped and unvarying pattern of simultaneously attempting intercourse and anticipating failure, followed by some symptomatic behavior on the wife's part. In the second conjoint session, Mrs. E suggested that they discontinue sleeping together, as the strain left her without sleep and constantly tired. An interpretation was made: Her symptoms showed her emotional frustration, which might reflect her disappointment that Mr. E was not the strong, potent man she expected. She had tried to improve him, and Mr. E had met this attempt with anxiety and resistance. Mr. E conceded that he left his office cheerful, but when he entered the home, he felt depressed, nagged, and belittled. Mrs. E responded by saying that it was not she but the children who received the brunt of his moods. She described her husband's belittling and sarcasm toward the children. Another dyadic interpretation was given: There is a vicious circle around power and control. Mr. E feels Mrs. E is trying to control him, whereas he is feeling a great need to control the family through the children. Mrs. E becomes anxious and resentful because she would like to run things her way. This battle has invaded their relationship, and the struggle to contain the urges to dominate has produced mutual strain and pushed out affection. Mrs. E responded to this interpretation by conceding that she is driven to control and that she sees how Mr. E responds by becoming controlling with the children.

At this point the therapist suggested that this pattern may relate to earlier experiences in their families of origin. Mrs. E recalled that she felt a lack of support from her mother and a devotion to her prematurely deceased father, a need to support and control the weak mother, and a desire that in marrying Mr. E he would make up for it all. An interpretation was made that she must feel very complicated about Mr. E's sexual difficulty and his feelings as the weak one. She now saw him not as the interested, inspiring father for her children in whom she saw her own needs mirrored. This interpretation was followed by a show of great feeling on the part of Mrs. E, in which she recalled that her father was not only loving but had also been very demanding and sarcastic, the latter so intolerable to her in Mr. E's behavior toward their children. Another interpretation: Perhaps Mrs. E had not seen the similarity before between her feelings for Mr. E and for her father, with great disappointment that like her father Mr. E had weaknesses that she must control because she could not bear them.

Mr. E responded with some emotion about how as a child he had been very strong willed and strove to compel his mother to give in to him. This was followed by a final dyadic interpretation: It was the strong-willed part of Mr. E that Mrs. E liked. Because of his fear of weakness, the failure in sex, which could have happened to anyone under the circumstances, was quite disproportionately seen by Mr. E as an utter failure, with a compensatory need to be in control in the home. Mrs. E, attaching her aspirations for strength and success to Mr. E, felt disproportionately disappointed in him because it destroyed her fantasy that he was like her father. Her reaction to disappointment, both in the past and now, was to take control.

By the third session, the couple reported that their general relationship was much improved and that Mr. E had been completely potent on a number of occasions.

Techniques for a More Effective Construction of Family Reality

The critical issue for understanding the family's story is a respectful conversation in which the family members are asked to consider their beliefs and ideas about the problem. The therapist must have on hand a number of alternatives that can be offered to the family to see if a consideration of these ideas would offer new possibilities. To the extent possible, the family should participate in the creation of a new story. Consider the following case example:

Mrs. F is distressed by her husband's unwillingness to talk about problems, and Mr. F is distressed by his wife's constant talking. They both assume the worst—Mrs. F sees Mr. F as withholding, and Mr. F sees Mrs. F as demanding. After discovering that Mr. F is from the mid-western United States and that Mrs. F is an Italian woman from New York, the therapist points out that these are ethnic and regional differences that must be understood, rather than hated, and reminds the couple that Mr. F had originally liked Mrs. F's energy and Mrs. F had liked Mr. F's calm. The couple was then engaged in a discussion of how they could turn their differences to their advantage.

TREATMENT PACKAGES

Clinical work and research suggest that so-called treatment packages, which contain a combination of techniques delivered in a specified sequence, are effective with targeted patient populations. These packages include the prescribed use of various techniques from the major strategies outlined in this chapter. Many of these packages have manuals that add to an abstract listing of strategies and techniques by indicating the overall goals (mediating and final) of the treatment for the targeted families, with a rationale for the timing and sequencing of the intervention techniques. Much psychotherapy research is focused on investigating treatment packages as they are applied to specified disorders. We discuss these packages in more detail in Chapter 24 and in other parts of the text.

INDICATIONS FOR DIFFERENTIAL USE OF THE BASIC STRATEGIES

Family therapy trainees are often uncertain about the circumstances in which various strategies and techniques are to be used. As we discuss in Chapters 22 and 23, this is an unresolved area, not only in family therapy but in all psychotherapy. Clinical writers often do not specify the situations in which their proposed strategies and techniques are indicated. Clinical research that compares one therapy technique with another indicates that by and large no one technique is clearly superior. It remains for future research to clarify the differential application and effectiveness of the techniques. In the interim, clinical decisions about the thrust of strategies in family intervention must be made on every case and in every session.

In order to choose a strategy, the therapist must consider both motivation and family style. Families that enjoy talking and analyzing, for example, may prefer a dynamic model, whereas action-oriented families may want specific homework and a behavioral model. Many, if not most, families want some educational interventions—families want and need information. The therapist also must consider speed. For example, low-motivation families need intervention more quickly, so that brief therapy techniques are often the first ones to try. Many apparently low-motivation families increase their motivation when they see results and begin to trust the therapist. The therapist should always remember the following basic rule: try the simplest thing first.

The simplest thing is usually an explanation of the problem and some suggestion for making it better. Before the therapist offers an elaborate discussion of why a couple has become more distant, it is helpful to prescribe 15 minutes of talking to each other every night and see what happens. Sometimes it's all that's needed. If not, the therapist will gather a lot of information from observing how the couple avoided or sabotaged the task. We will look at this topic in more detail in Section VII, in which we discuss guidelines for therapy. Patient diagnostic issues are beginning to factor into recommendations for the type of family therapy techniques to be used. For example, patients with serious mental illness, such as schizophrenia or bipolar disorder, and their families should receive psychoeducation about the illness and how to cope with it.

What the family wants is an important consideration. Most critical, however, is the family members' sense that they are heard, understood, and respected and that the therapist believes the problem is solvable or at least can be made more tolerable.

Some family therapy strategies have received research support for their effectiveness, whereas others have been the focus of very little if any research. Because most therapy research has found little differential effect for the various treatment strategies and techniques, we believe that elements common to the various strategies are most important. These elements include careful assessment, focus as negotiated by the therapist, a reasonable rationale for proceeding, the generation of hope that intervention will help, and orientation to a goal. From this point of view, the organized approach of the family therapist is more important than the specific strategies and techniques. One clinical application of this notion is that the family therapist should not be eclectic in strategies to the point of shifting constantly from one set of strategies to another. A clear focus on the central family problems with a combination of a limited set of strategies is probably more efficient, less confusing to the family, and more effective than is a less-focused approach. This is congruent with the fact that negative outcomes in family therapy are associated with a lack of therapist structuring and guiding of early sessions and with the use of frontal confrontations of highly affective material early in treatment.[11]

CLINICAL PRACTICE IMPLICATIONS

It has been wisely noted that a therapist, not unlike an artist, spends years of hard practice acquiring and honing techniques. Once acquired, these techniques become relatively invisible. During the last three decades, family therapy has seen a great deal of outcome research, from which many manuals have been written. "The manuals attempt to carefully describe treatments, and therapists are taught to perform as the manuals describe. And, yet, with this careful attention to scientific rigor, researchers have noted that the same technique in the hands of a 'pro' and a 'neophyte' (despite years of practice) can have quite different effects on the patients" (M. Weissman, personal communication).

REFERENCES

1. Gabbard GO. The impact of psychotherapy on the brain. *Psychiatric Times*. 1998;15:26.
2. Kandel ER. A new intellectual framework for psychiatry. *Am J Psychiatry*. 1998;155:457–469.
3. Patterson GR. *Coercive Family Process*. Castalia; 1982.
4. Hunter DE, Hoffnung RJ, Ferholt BF. Family therapy and trouble: psychoeducation as solution and as problem. *Fam Process*. 1988;27:327–338.
5. Stuart RB. *Helping Couples Change: A Social Learning Approach to Marital Therapy*. Guilford; 1980.
6. Minuchin S. *Families and Family Therapy*. Harvard University Press; 1974.
7. Minuchin S, Fishman HC. *Family Therapy Techniques*. Harvard University Press; 1981.
8. Weeks G, L'Abate L. *Paradoxical Psychotherapy: Theory and Technique*. Brunner/Mazel; 1982.
9. Ackerman N. *The Psychodynamics of Family Life*. Basic Books; 1958.
10. Dicks HV. *Marital Tensions: Clinical Studies Towards a Psychological Theory of Interaction*. Routledge & Kegan Paul; 1967.
11. Gurman AS, Kniskern DP. Deterioration in marital and family therapy: empirical, clinical and conceptual issues. *Fam Process*. 1978;17:3–20.

12 The Course of Family Treatment

OBJECTIVES FOR THE READER

- To acquire techniques for gathering history
- To become familiar with some of the processes of each phase of family treatment
- To identify various opportunities and interventions appropriate to each phase of family treatment
- To be aware of and understand the indications for brief family therapy
- To be able to describe the course and techniques of brief intervention

For easier reading, we emphasize that the descriptors "couples" or "marital" are used nearly interchangeably in this chapter.

INTRODUCTION

In this chapter, we review the phases of a typical course of treatment—somewhat arbitrarily dividing them into an early phase, a middle phase, and a termination phase. By necessity, some material in this chapter overlaps material in earlier chapters—here it is presented in relation to the course of family treatment. Readers may also wish to refer to the R family case example in Chapter 8.

EARLY PHASE
- Identifying Objectives of the Early Phase
- Choosing Strategies to Get Started
- Distributing the Available Time
- Gathering History and Simultaneously Building a Treatment Alliance with the Family
- Distinguishing Evaluation from Treatment

MIDDLE PHASE

TERMINATION PHASE

CONDUCTING BRIEF FAMILY THERAPY: TREATMENT AS IT IS INFLUENCED BY TIME CONSTRAINTS
- Indications for Brief Family or Couples Intervention
- Course of Brief Therapy
- Techniques
- Setting Limited Goals and a Definite End Point
- Active Focus: Reinforcement of Family Strengths, Reconceptualization

Active Exploration of Alternatives: Behavioral and Emotional Rehearsal
Homework and Family Tasks
The Problem-Oriented School of Brief Therapy
Crisis Intervention
CLINICAL PRACTICE IMPLICATIONS

EARLY PHASE

The early phase is the most difficult of the phases, especially for trainees. Before the early phase of treatment begins, the therapist needs to consider the following issues:

- Identifying objectives of the early phase
- Choosing strategies to get started
- Distributing the available time
- Gathering history and simultaneously building a treatment alliance with the family

We discuss each of these issues in the sections that follow.

Identifying Objectives of the Early Phase

The primary objectives of the early phase include the following:

- Detailing the primary problems and nonproductive family patterns
- Clarifying the goals for treatment
- Solidifying the therapeutic contract
- Strengthening the therapeutic relationship
- Shifting the focus from the identified patient to the entire family system
- Decreasing guilt and blame
- Increasing the ability of family members to empathize with one another
- Assessing the family's strengths
- Assessing the family's preferred style of thinking and working
- Defining who is in the family
- Getting a clear idea of the ethnic and cultural issues that are part of the family's functioning
- Determining the life cycle phase for each individual and for the family

Choosing Strategies to Get Started

1. Before describing in detail the techniques that enable the therapist to achieve the final goals of family intervention, it is important to note the general strategies used in beginning work with the family. These skills are basic, assumed by all orientations, and crucial for the new therapist to master. Without such skills, a therapist is likely to find families dropping out of treatment, which precludes the possibility of change. **Accommodating to and joining the family**. The family is a biologic–psychological unit that over time has evolved rules (overt and covert), procedures, and customary interactional patterns. The therapist must join this group by letting the family members know that they understand them and want to work with them for their better good. Every family therapist will use their own unique personality, combined with sensitivity and warmth, to join with the family in distress.
2. **Interviewing subgroups, extended family members, and other networks**. Family therapy is by definition a therapeutic approach that emphasizes the tremendous power and influence of the individual's social environment. This social environment includes immediate family, family of origin, extended family, neighborhood, school, and community. A crucial decision that often takes place early in treatment is which parts of the social environment to

include directly in the treatment. Various groups of individuals can be included for assessment only or can be more involved in the ongoing treatment. We discuss this topic further in Chapter 14.

3. **Negotiating the goals of treatment.** The family or couple usually comes to treatment with their own goals in mind. Unlike individual therapy, however, in which one individual comes with their own goals, the family comes with a few individuals having specific goals, often for other people (not themselves) to change, and with some individuals not wanting to be there at all.

Distributing the Available Time

If the therapist is engaged in short-term crisis intervention, 30 minutes may be all the time that is available for evaluation. The therapist must join the family group quickly and will evaluate the family only for the presenting problem, with further evaluation occurring during the intervention. In a training or practice setting, with no fixed time limit for treatment, the therapist may be able to allot more time for thorough evaluation (e.g., to complete a quick genogram). Some clinicians take the time at an initial phone contact to gather detailed biographical and historical information. This may save time initially, but is not a substitute for a complete interview with the entire family.

Gathering History and Simultaneously Building a Treatment Alliance with the Family

Styles and techniques of gathering history are very much related to the crucial task of building a treatment alliance with the family. These techniques vary depending on the phase of treatment. Although we covered some of this material in earlier chapters, we repeat it here in the context of the course of family treatment.

We recommend that most therapists obtain a fairly extensive history, perhaps mainly in the opening sessions. Some family therapy models, such as those that are solution focused, place less emphasis on an extensive history diagnosis and more emphasis on the here-and-now, working more with what happens in the session and gathering longitudinal data only as needed during the course of the meetings.

The therapist may decide to hear from each family member in turn on certain important issues or may let the verbal interaction take its own course. The therapist should allow for at least a few minutes of unguided conversation among family members in order to see their patterns of interaction. However, to allow fighting among family members to go on for too long, once the therapist has seen the pattern of the fight, is demoralizing to the family. A decision may be made to call on one parent first, then the other, and then the children in order of descending age. Or it may appear more advantageous to call on the more easily intimidated, weaker, or passive parent (or spouse) first, or to allow the family to decide who speaks first. The therapist may decide to use first names for all family members to help put everyone on an equal footing, or they may prefer to be more formal in addressing the parents in order to strengthen relatively weak generational boundaries and parental functioning. Some therapists may encourage the family members to talk with one another, whereas others may focus family members' conversation largely through the therapist, at least during the first sessions or at times of stress or chaos.

The assumption is made that the family's behavior in the office and at home is similar. This is not always true: the family's behavior is usually modified in some ways in the office by the therapist's presence. In the beginning, the therapist is somewhat the outsider, whose main function may be to allow everyone, including the weakest members of the family, to be heard. Some family members will often be on the attack, whereas others will be defensive at first. An identified patient who is an adolescent will often demand changes at home because those in this age group are often the ones most interested in change. An angry, frustrated spouse will demand that the marital partner change. Some therapists may point out that they will not be decision-makers for the family but will help the family members clarify their problems and help them with their decision-making processes. Such therapists may act as communication referees or traffic cops when necessary, making sure that one person speaks at a time, that no one person is overwhelmed by attacks during the sessions, and that nonconstructive family patterns are not allowed to continue unchallenged during the therapy sessions. They create an atmosphere that encourages the verbal expression of feelings toward constructive ends.

The therapist should indicate to the family that, in an unhappy family, everyone hurts and therefore everyone wants to get something positive out of the sessions. The therapist should convey the feeling that all the family members are doing the best they can and that each family member needs to understand their motives and the motives of others. The therapist also should explain that well-intentioned attitudes and actions sometimes have less than completely positive outcomes.

Families vary considerably in their readiness to move from a discussion of the current crisis situation to an exploration of their patterns and histories. The therapist will follow the family's lead in this respect. For example, a couple may refuse to discuss issues related to themselves as a couple, focusing only on the children. Or a therapist may be willing to start the sessions even though the father is absent and may sense that the family members need some time to talk about the "badness" of one of the children. The therapist must get an idea of the family's mode of operations in order to convey a sense of respect for and understanding of the family's initial point of view. At the same time, the therapist will need to guard against being so passive and accepting that nothing new will be added to the equation. The family's experience in the therapy hour should not be merely a repetition of the nongratifying interactional patterns for which it originally sought help. It may be helpful to indicate to the family members that individual problems are often related to family problems and that they all need to find out more about the family as a whole, in order to enable each member, and the family as an entity, to benefit from the treatment.

As we discussed in Chapter 6 (in the context of choice points), it may be desirable to move on to a longitudinal, chronologic narrative of the family's history (perhaps through three generations) or alternatively to begin with a cross-sectional inventory of how the family currently functions. Which of these areas will be discussed first depends on the therapist's predilections, the family's distress, and the nature of the difficulty. The major longitudinal data to be gathered will refer to the parents' courtship, engagement, wedding, honeymoon, and early years of marriage prior to the arrival of children as well as changes in the family as a result of the first child and each subsequent child and so on through the family cycle.

The therapist may start with the courtship period (which is, in part, predictive of marital patterns), move on to the marriage, and then work backward, with each partner going back to their original family. The therapist can discuss the life history prior to the marriage of each partner, including any previous marriages. In going back to the couple's families of origin, the therapist gets a picture of the functioning of those previous families. This picture serves as a foundation for understanding the present family and its problems. Careful attention must be given not only to recollections of the past and to expressions regarding attitudes and values but also to overt behavior. Difficulties in sexual adjustment should be delineated carefully by taking a complete sexual history. It is our experience that such a history is rarely taken in the field of family therapy, as though sexual problems are regarded as only secondary to other interpersonal difficulties. The timing of the sexual history is critical, even with presenting sexual problems. Consider the following two rules of thumb: (1) The history of sexual problems should be taken after other history is known, and (2) it is best not to begin taking a sexual history in the last half hour of the session. The sexual history should not be taken with children present.

Distinguishing Evaluation from Treatment

For clarity's sake, we have separated the discussions of family evaluations and family treatment. In practice this rarely happens and is not particularly desirable. A process of continual evaluation and hypothesis testing takes place throughout the course of therapy, with the therapist constantly checking their perceptions. At the same time, every session should have some beneficial outcome. The more skillful and experienced the therapist is, the less rigid the approach, the more total the blend of evaluative and therapeutic aspects, and the more extensive the use of improvised variations, condensations, and extensions on some of the themes.

MIDDLE PHASE

The middle phase of treatment is often considered to be the one in which the major work of change takes place. Because Section IV is devoted to treatment, we will say less here regarding this phase. What the therapist does during the middle stage will vary, depending on the goals that have been identified. During this phase the therapist may repeatedly discuss common examples of persistent, nongratifying interpersonal patterns and attitudes, preferably drawn from recent or here-and-now interactions. They challenge old, nonfunctional coalitions, rules, myths, and role models and present the possibility of alternative modes. New habits of thinking, feeling, and interacting take time to develop, and much repetition is often required. At the same time resistance to change comes to the fore and must be dealt with accordingly (see Chapter 13).

The initial focus may be on the identified patient, but the focus then moves to the family. Often the identified patient may improve before the family does. A crisis often develops when the problems that have been hidden away or have been too painful to face are brought to the conscious awareness of the family members.

In the middle phase of treatment, symptomatology may accelerate, new symptoms may arise, and families may talk about quitting treatment. This upheaval usually is related to the family's barely perceived awareness that for things to get better, some family member will have to change. Rather than change, a family member may accentuate or exaggerate symptoms. Family therapy changes have to be made sequentially. As for the process of doing therapy, at the start of therapy the therapist must meet the family where it is coming from and gradually draw it toward the therapeutic scenario. Figure 12.1 illustrates this process.

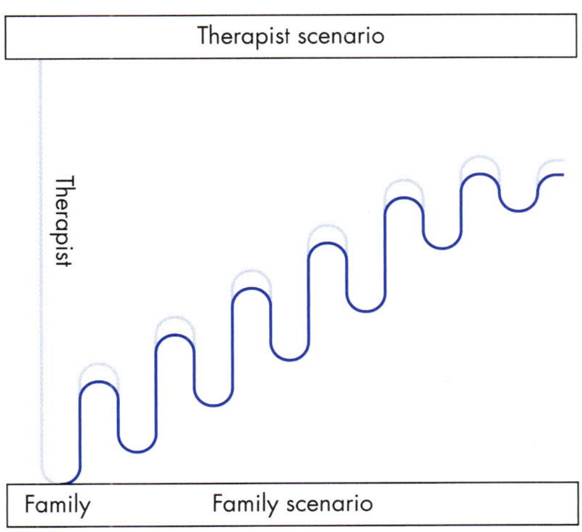

Figure 12.1 Schematic of the joining of therapist and family scenarios. (*Source:* Forgatch MS, DeGarmo DS. Adult problem solving: Contributor to parenting and child outcomes in divorced families. *Social Development.* 1997;6(2): 237–253. https://doi.org/10.1111/j.1467-9507.1997.tb00104.x. Reproduced with permission of Oregon Social Learning Center.)

In this figure, the family (bottom of the figure) has its own scenario of what it thinks the problem is. Similarly, the therapist (top of the figure) has their own scenario of what they think the problem is. If the family is left to its own devices, its patterns are scripted, repetitive, and unchanging. The same can hold true for the therapist. That is, without interaction with the family, the therapist's scenario does not vary. The essence of the therapy is to bring together the two scenarios, beginning at the top left of the diagram as the therapist and the family interact. Presumably, the family's behavior changes as the family interacts with the therapist's strategies. The figure also points out that therapy is never a smooth line. As it continues, frequent oscillations occur. The point is that therapy should be moving forward to achieve the goals that were established earlier in the process (see Chapter 10).

TERMINATION PHASE

In the termination phase, the therapist reviews with the family the goals that have been achieved and those that have not. It is often useful to review the entire course of therapy, including the original problems and goals. A useful technique is to ask each family member to say what they would have to do in order to make the situation the same as it was at the outset of treatment. For example, the father would have to yell at the mother, who would have to yell at the daughter, who would have to stop going to school. In essence, the family reconstructs the sequences leading to the pathology. Videotape playback may be helpful at this time, so that the family can see what it looked like at the start of treatment, compared with its present state. It is important to acknowledge that some behaviors cannot be altered and that life will continue to change, that is, unexpected and periodic problems will occur. The family should be provided with the skills for solving future conflicts and challenges.

What are the criteria for suggesting termination of therapy? If the original goals have been achieved, the therapist may consider stopping the treatment. When the treatment has been successful, new coping patterns and an enhanced empathy by family members for one another will have been established. There will be recognition that the family itself seems capable of dealing satisfactorily with new situations as they arise. There may be little to talk about during the sessions and little sense of urgency. Nonproductive quarreling and conflict will have been reduced; the family will be freer to disagree openly and will have methods of living with and working out its differences and separateness. The family will seem less inflexible in its rules and organization and appear more able to grow and develop. Individual family members will be less symptomatic, and positive channels of interaction will be available between all family members. There will be improved agreement about family roles and functions. Even if the goals have not been achieved but have been worked out to the best capabilities of therapist and family, therapy can stop. If the therapist feels stuck but believes more change is possible, it is helpful to consult with another therapist before ending therapy. Families often cannot or do not recognize changes that have occurred during therapy. A therapist should check carefully for any change and amplify it, giving positive reinforcement. If a family can produce a small change, then bigger changes may be possible. With some families, no change may occur until the therapy is completed.

After a successful therapy, when termination issues have been resolved, the family may experience a recurrence of presenting symptoms. These eruptions are usually short-lived and may represent a temporary response to the anxiety of terminating treatment, rather than being a sign of treatment failure or a new problem. Such anxiety is part of the separation process, which is a key issue to be worked on in termination and which, in some theoretical orientations, may represent the major theme of the entire therapy. One way to deal with this is as follows: the family is encouraged to experience the recurring symptoms to see if it wants to keep any of them. If the family says no, it is encouraged to examine how symptoms occur and to review what happens on the days when symptoms do not occur. The family is encouraged to see this as a review or final examination.

CONDUCTING BRIEF FAMILY THERAPY: TREATMENT AS IT IS INFLUENCED BY TIME CONSTRAINTS

The current focus on time-limited therapies has resulted from a multitude of factors. Economic limitations of patients and clinics helped press for an intervention package that was time-limited and cost-effective. The existence of long waiting lists of clinic patients expecting assignment to therapists also pressured clinicians to consider and experiment with shorter forms of intervention. Another reason for the increased use of brief therapy was the need for research on psychotherapy, coupled with the realization that to research 10 sessions of therapy was much more practical than observing and recording a therapy that spanned some years. Most important, some clinicians began to formulate the theoretical advantages of a short, preplanned intervention and linked it to the historical roots of the beginning of psychotherapy, pointing out that Freud's initial work, for example, was brief.[1]

Gurman[2] suggested some interesting hypotheses as to why marital therapy tends to be brief. Because marital therapy is not based just on the insight awareness model, the therapist focuses on the current problem rather than examining the antecedent of the problem. Many of the patients who enter marital therapy have shown themselves as capable of having at least one (more or less) meaningful relationship judged by the fact that they are married; thus, these individuals are likely to constitute a selected good-prognosis population. In addition, the interpersonal or transferential aspects of the problem are not only talked about but also exhibited in the therapy sessions themselves because both parties are present. Finally, the loss of the therapist at the end of the treatment is not as threatening as the termination of an individual treatment, because the primary affect is always toward the partner rather than the therapist.

Indications for Brief Family or Couples Intervention

Indications for the use of planned, brief family, or marital intervention would include the following:

1. When there is a current, relatively focused family or marital conflict. Examples include the need to separate from the family of origin[3]; to establish marital commitment; to resolve mixed feelings about intimacy and dependency; to establish modes of conflict resolution, decision-making, and negotiation in the marital dyad; to clarify role expectations; to develop channels for expression of positive and negative feelings; to explore the decision to divorce or gain assistance in negotiating a separation or divorce that is least harmful to spouses and children involved.
2. When evidence indicates that family members are contributing to an identified patient's focused symptom or problem complex.
3. When family cooperation must be mobilized as an induction to another mode of therapy.
4. When the family situation is baffling, and brief therapy is chosen partly as an extended evaluation and partly as therapy.

Not only is the specific problem area important in indicating time-limited family intervention, but also the family members' specific capabilities for focused brief work factor into the decision to use this treatment mode. These capabilities include the family's ability to meet together without uncontrollable fighting, the presence of family agreement and the family's ability to focus on specific problems, and the motivation of significant family members to participate. For the most part, these capabilities are not as crucial in lengthier family work.

Many current practitioners believe that the issue is not the presenting problem but defining the problem in such a way that it is amenable to solution (as we discussed earlier in the chapter on strategies) by highly systemic formulations. In the hands of experienced practitioners, brief therapy models have been applied with success to all family issues.

Course of Brief Therapy

The initial referral contact and evaluation interview can be used to set the stage for the brief family treatment. The therapist in collaboration with a family can focus on specific issues, clarify the goals and expectations, and channel the interactions in ways suited to short-term, focused work. For example, if the family situation fits one of the indications listed earlier in this chapter, then the evaluation data gathering will focus on material and processes relevant to that category and its goals, and other types of data will be given less attention.

Before the end of the first session, the therapist will have made a contract with the family outlining the goals and duration of treatment. An agreement may also be made about the goals that will not be pursued. Anything else that is made explicit to the family about the process of treatment may vary, but the therapist should have a blueprint in mind.

As the therapy proceeds, the therapist will actively keep the family on track and discourage derailments of various sorts. Depending on the type of treatment involved, the family will be rewarded for continuing in the necessary stepwise sequence or for gaining mastery in a more adaptive way of dealing with an old pattern. The therapist will be conductor, traffic cop, referee, mentor, and model, using their knowledge of individual and group dynamics, as well as family processes.

The therapist will remind the family of the limited nature of the treatment. They will be aware that termination anxiety may occur, with distress reemerging as the end of the treatment approaches, even if positive gains have been made during the earlier phase of treatment. The therapist will resist attempts to prolong therapy beyond the agreed-on time. They will deal with the family's desire for dependence on the therapist and the family's fear of being unable to cope. The family members will be helped to summarize the gains they have made during treatment and to rehearse their future problem-solving efforts.

Techniques

In this section, we discuss specific techniques established as especially useful in brief, focused family evaluation and treatment. Although these techniques are by no means the only ones available, readers should gain from their descriptions an adequate understanding of the variety of therapeutic options available.[4] There is no necessary and absolute connection between any one technique and the five general strategies we outlined in Chapter 11, although some techniques obviously lend themselves more easily to one strategy than to another.

Experienced therapists are most likely to be flexible in what they do, from case to case and from minute to minute. The techniques we describe, then, should be thought of as freeing the therapeutic imagination rather than as restricting it with a straitjacket.

Setting Limited Goals and a Definite End Point

When brevity is not part of the agreed-on contract, the reasons for therapy often remain vague and ambiguous. Sessions are likely to continue with no fixed termination agreed on in advance and with goals and directions changing as treatment proceeds. Symptomatic and behavioral progress is not taken as a sign that treatment can end but rather as confirmation of the positive effects of the treatment and the desirability of continuing it.

It is essential in brief therapy that the therapist be clear as to the focused and limited goals of treatment. In every session, the therapist must keep clearly in mind that the amount of contact with the family will be limited and will have a definite end point, in terms of either the number of hours or the achievement of a specific goal. The therapist's concept may be centered on the least that needs to be done to help the family to continue on its own rather than on more ambitious, if not grandiose, notions of the family's potential.

During the first few sessions, the therapist should state and discuss with the family the focused goals of the treatment in concrete and specific detail. The family can be asked to specify in concrete terms how family life would be 6 or 10 weeks from then if interactions in the problem area were better. This approach can flush out individual family members' grandiose or unrealistic goals, vagueness, or resistance to visualizing change. Stated in concrete and observable terms, the goals can then stand as barometers to be observed during the course of treatment and can be used to assess progress at termination, thus reinforcing the efforts of successful families and challenging the more resistant families.

The content of the goals will, of course, vary according to the situation. If the evaluation indicates that the family has been functioning satisfactorily until a recent crisis, efforts will be made to restore the preexisting equilibrium as quickly as possible. For example, crisis intervention techniques may be used in a family in which the 22-year-old son, who is living with his parents, has had an exacerbation of positive symptoms of chronic schizophrenia. The parents may panic, demanding hospitalization of their son and his permanent removal from the home. With ventilation, attention to what triggered the upset, support, symptomatic relief for all concerned, and a setting that allows for daily visits to the therapist, brief but intensive therapy may avoid hospitalization and quickly restore the family's ability to cope. If the family's distress seems more related to long-lasting patterns of interaction, some attempt can be made to set goals in one or two crucial areas in a way that will open up new possibilities for the family to grow and develop on its own, without further reliance on the therapist. For example, when a wife's suicide attempt seems related to chronic unspoken doubts about the viability of the marriage, the therapist will work toward the goal of getting the husband and wife to express more openly to each other the extent of their current needs, disappointments, and frustrations and make at least one thing better. As soon as the couple is able to engage satisfactorily in these transactions, they may be ready to carry on without the therapist's presence. But there is always the danger of making things worse temporarily, in which case the therapy may need to be longer. Because problem avoidance was at the root of the suicide attempt, a no-treatment option is not indicated.

Setting a fixed number of sessions with the family at the beginning of treatment is often desirable, as it makes explicit and concrete the limited time in which the goals are to be achieved. It is essential that this commitment to terminate be adhered to, despite various attempts the family may make to undermine it. The essence of such treatment may be to help families begin to understand how they do not keep agreements and how they sabotage attempts at changing dysfunctional patterns.

Active Focus: Reinforcement of Family Strengths, Reconceptualization

The therapist will be alert to the need to stay on target during the course of the treatment and will continually help the family to stick to the one or two primary goals that have been agreed on. Other issues that emerge can be conceptualized as relating to the core issues in some important ways or as resistances to dealing with those issues. Alternatively, extraneous matters can be noted as important but not germane to the current focus, and perhaps they can be left for the family to deal with later, on its own. Whatever treatment focus has been selected will benefit from underlying and positive reinforcement from the therapist whenever possible.

Family therapy requires the active contribution of the therapist, possibly more so than in some other formats of therapy. In brief family therapy, even more therapist participation is usually needed. Passivity and indecisiveness tend to activate the family's dysfunctional repetitive patterns.

Existing and emerging family strengths should be reinforced and supported, as should the concept that all family members are doing the best they can. Especially in brief therapy, in which there is little opportunity for the gradual development of rapport, the therapist must be active and encouraging and must indicate that an attempt is being made to understand the situation from each member's, as well as the whole family's, vantage point. For effective brief therapy, each family member needs to feel that the therapist understands and accepts them. Informal moments before, during, and after sessions are invaluable for the therapist to add a personal touch of contact with each family member.

The therapist should reward successes in substituting more functional patterns during the course of the therapy. They should highlight indications that the family can change and should emphasize the important idea that the therapist is there to catalyze the changes and help the family learn how to carry on this process alone. The therapist may temporarily be extremely active and directive but always with the goal in mind that the family needs to learn how to monitor and direct itself. The therapist should discourage any long-term reliance on outside experts and should challenge and educate the family to take charge of itself in more gratifying ways.

Active Exploration of Alternatives: Behavioral and Emotional Rehearsal

Sometimes families need to be given permission and encouragement to consider alternative patterns to those they have been living with or feel they will be facing in the future. The mere raising of such an issue can be a liberating experience. For example, a middle-aged couple, facing the oncoming empty-nest syndrome in which their parental role will be curtailed sharply, may find it exhilarating to consider rethinking their marital contract and marital roles. Once the therapist has opened such a door, the couple may find quickly that they are able to proceed on their own.

Couples who have secretly thought about separating but have never dared to express such a thought may at first feel threatened by a therapist who openly wonders whether they have considered it. With a skillful therapist, such a couple can face ideas and feelings they have been too afraid or guilty to express before, allowing for intensity and change.

During the therapy sessions, family members should be given the strength to express themselves more openly to one another than before. The therapist should make it safe for them to do so but should also explore with the family the consequences of such openness. Repeated rehearsals of possible consequences may be required before more open communication can be established as being safe.

When a child is considered to be the problem, rehearsals aimed at strengthening the parental coalition may be essential. The parents may be undermining each other's authority, which is often related to weaknesses in their marital relationship.

Homework and Family Tasks

For therapy to be effective, changes must be noted outside the treatment sessions. To speed up this process, and to maximize the effect of the limited number of sessions, family members can be asked to carry out homework assignments. These should be relatively simple and achievable and should bear on those crucial problems that are the focus of treatment. They may involve, for example, various types of marital or family communication exercises. The husband and wife may be asked to practice negotiating differences at home. They can be told to make explicit to each other their position on a given issue, with the expectation that they will repeat to each other their understanding of the other's position.

Interaction and behavioral exercises are often helpful. For example, two estranged family members can be asked to jointly plan and carry out a dyadic activity that they would enjoy and to report about it at the next treatment session. The therapist can make negative injunctions, such as prohibiting family members from bringing up recriminations from the past.

Sometimes the therapist can help a family member clarify or modify an important outside relationship, such as with that member's family of origin. For example, a wife who has felt squeezed between her love for her husband and her mother's disapproval of him can be asked to start talking to her mother about this situation in an attempt to resolve it.

To encourage rapid transactional changes, the therapist can negotiate explicit contracts between family members. For example, a mother may be asked to agree to let her teenage daughter stay out until midnight on weekends in return for the daughter having all her homework completed by then. Such contracts can bring a temporary halt to bickering, offer a model for mutually satisfying negotiations, and allow the family sessions to move on to other issues.

The Problem-Oriented School of Brief Therapy

One school of brief therapy is based on the notion that change can be accomplished by identifying the problem and changing the family's solution to it.[5] The model ignores all historical material except as it pertains to why the clients have chosen a particular solution to the problem and what other solutions they have attempted. The rationale is that the family's attempted solution maintains and compounds the problem. The therapeutic intervention then is to intercept and redirect the family's solution. Other therapists may search with the family for exceptions—that is, times when the problem did not occur—and emphasize what went right at those times.

In the A family, the presenting problem was that the adolescent son got into fights with his single-parent mother and refused to help with basic household maintenance. The mother's solution had been to reason with her son as to why she couldn't fulfill his demands. Her solution escalated the problem. Taking as an example the son's demands for her always to prepare meals despite her busy work schedule, she was instructed to tell her son that she wouldn't be able to get supper every night because she was not a good enough mother. This intervention pushed the mother to decide whether she was good enough. After she made a list of all that she was doing, she concluded that she was carrying 90% of the workload in the house. She could then deliver the line with a smile and a shrug. After eight sessions, mostly with the mother, the son began to be more helpful, and his fighting in the home stopped completely (as determined over a 1-year follow-up period).

Crisis Intervention

In one sense, an extreme form of brief intervention is the crisis intervention needed when a family is in acute distress that threatens the very life of an individual, the family unit, or family adjustment. This would be analogous to a serious medical emergency in which primary efforts would be directed at maintaining vital body functions, stopping any loss of blood, and providing for supportive conditions until the system stabilizes. At such a time, no definitive reconstructive or elective procedures can be undertaken.

For family emergencies, attention must be given to the carrying out of necessary family tasks, including the basic provision of food, clothing, and shelter. Physiologic needs, such as sleep, may require professional intervention, and outside sources of help (e.g., relatives, friends, agencies) may need to be called on. Behavioral controls and at least a modicum of emotional stability should be sought while the therapist evaluates the specific situation that resulted in the acute family disequilibrium. Every effort should be made to eliminate, contain, buffer, understand, or conceptualize this situation so that the family can return quickly to its former level of adjustment. After the acute crisis has passed, further intervention may not be needed or desired. Often, however, a new contract (or referral) can be made for ongoing treatment with new goals.

CLINICAL PRACTICE IMPLICATIONS

We have gone to considerable lengths to describe the processes involved in an entire course of family therapy. This is because during training, therapists rarely see a case from beginning to end (primarily because of the dropout problem). The point is that treatment (like anything else) has a certain natural course (i.e., rate of change), and therapists must be aware of these changes in order to do effective therapy.

SUGGESTED READINGS

An exploration of the therapeutic alliance in brief couples and family therapy.

Rait D. Perspectives on the therapeutic alliance in brief couples and family therapy. In: Safran J, Muran JC, eds. *The Therapeutic Alliance in Brief Psychotherapy*. American Psychological Association Press; 1998:171–191.

REFERENCES

1. Malan DH. *A Study of Brief Psychotherapy*. Tavistock; 1963.
2. Gurman AS. Integrative marital therapy: toward the development of an interpersonal approach. In: Budman SH, ed. *Forms of Brief Therapy*. Guilford; 1981:415–457.
3. Haley J. *Leaving Home: The Therapy of Disturbed Young People*. McGraw-Hill; 1980.
4. Cade B, O'Hanlon WH. *A Brief Guide to Brief Therapy*. WW Norton; 1993.
5. Watzlawick P, Weakland J, Fisch R. *Change: Principles of Problem Formation and Problem Resolution*. WW Norton; 1974.

13 Promoting Change in Family Treatment: Issues of Alliance and Resistance

OBJECTIVES FOR THE READER

- To understand how the connection between the therapist and the family facilitates change
- To understand how to build an alliance with a family and to know those factors that make it more difficult
- To be aware of and understand family resistances to treatment and change
- To understand therapist reactions to the family that interfere with progress in treatment
- To identify strategies for countering resistances

For easier reading, we emphasize that the descriptors "couples" or "marital" are used nearly interchangeably in this chapter.

INTRODUCTION

In this chapter, we discuss two issues that at first glance may not seem related: the therapeutic alliance and resistance. By *therapeutic alliance*, we mean the collaborative relationship between therapist and family aimed at promoting change. By *resistance*, we mean, broadly speaking, the processes in the patient or family that impede change. Both issues are central to the process of therapy, and without the therapeutic alliance, it is almost impossible to deal with resistance.

THE THERAPEUTIC ALLIANCE
MODELS FOR DEALING WITH FAMILIES THAT HAVE TROUBLE FORMING AN ALLIANCE
- Medical Model
- Coaching Model
- Conflict Model
- Strategic Systems Model

PROBLEMS IN CREATING CHANGE: RESISTANCE AND DISCONNECTION
- Problems in Creating Change: Emanating from the Family
- Problems in Creating Change: Emanating from the Therapist
- Problems in Creating Change: From the Therapist–Family System
- Problems in Creating Change: Stages of Treatment: At Evaluation and Early in Treatment

Problems in Creating Change: In Ongoing Treatment
Problems in Creating Change: At the Termination Phase of Therapy
Problems in Creating Change: Family Secrets
TECHNIQUES TO DEAL WITH RESISTANCES OR STALLED THERAPY
Assume Nothing
Collaboration
Emphasizing Family Responsibility
Focus on the Present
CLINICAL PRACTICE IMPLICATIONS

THE THERAPEUTIC ALLIANCE

The family unit is often portrayed as sanctified. Certainly, popular politics touts it thus, celebrating the importance of family values as a means to alleviate a variety of societal ills. Much like in religion, those within the intimate sect of the family use the utmost caution in questioning the rules governing its functioning. The therapist is an outsider, initially unaware of the family's complex (and often dysfunctional) rules. As has been proven throughout history, religious convictions are remarkably resistant to change, especially if suggested by someone outside the church.

To alter the system, one must first be accepted by the system. This is also true in marital and family therapy. The success of any therapeutic endeavor depends on the participants establishing and maintaining an open, trusting, and collaborative relationship or alliance. In marital and family therapy, the therapeutic alliance offers the opportunity for corrective experience and is a necessary condition for therapeutic change. A growing body of empirical evidence demonstrates that the therapeutic alliance is the best predictor of psychotherapy outcome in individual therapy, and a similar line of clinical research in relation to marital and family therapy has begun to emerge. The functions of a therapeutic alliance include instilling hope in the family and creating an environment safe enough for the family to engage in new behaviors that take it past its comfort zone. The family members must believe that the therapist not only has the skills to help them through the problem but also respects and appreciates them as people.

- The family therapist faces the following issues in establishing an alliance:
- The therapist must form at one time an alliance with several people, who often have quite different feelings and agendas.
- The therapist must keep in mind the need to adopt a conceptual framework to account for interactions within triangles or systems of three (or more) people.
- The system will operate in powerful ways to induct the therapist into it.
- Because multiple participants are present, people with different motivations, goals, and beliefs about how to change must all be attended to. If the participant has come involuntarily, as with many adolescents and most court-ordered patients, the situation is even more complicated.

Sessions with any family tend to be more complex and more openly conflicted than most individual sessions. The therapist must work to develop a connection with each person, with the various subsystems, and with the family as a whole. In this process, the therapist must be constantly aware of the presence of triangles among family members and among themself and family members. No dyadic relationship in therapy can exist outside a series of interlocking triangles. This means that, for example, if the therapist develops a strong relationship with one spouse, the other may feel left out or angry. Any move the therapist makes may be seen from a variety of different angles.

No dyadic relationship in therapy can exist outside a series of interlocking triangles.

The therapist joining the system experiences the pull of the system—that is, the request to operate within the system's rules and beliefs—to help the family members change the problem without changing the system. This process is subtle and very strong. If the therapist, for example, buys into the family's definition of the problem as "We have a bad child," they may not pay attention to the marital problems or to the problems of the child who is labeled as being good. The therapist must see the constraints on behavior (e.g., this cannot be talked about, this cannot be changed) as information to use in understanding the system, and they must remain separate enough not to be bound by these constraints.

Alliance formation for the therapist is complicated by multiple countertransference reactions. The therapist may be drawn to, or prefer, some family members. Family dynamics may replicate the therapist's family in some way, producing wishes to save, or punish, certain family members. In addition, the therapist can see how badly one person is treating another, in a way that does not happen in individual therapy. Watching a parent verbally abuse a child in session, the therapist may find it difficult to ally with the parent and the child, but unless the therapist can connect with all family members in some way, the family will exclude them.

Different family theorists use forms of connection and joining that are related to their overall model. For example, Satir and Baldwin[1] modeled warmth, support, and respect for give-and-take and emphasized that therapists and patients are equals in learning. Bowen's[2] model took the position that the therapist is a coach, or researcher, and should stay more distant to avoid being affected by the family's emotional process. In Bowen's work, most of the session is focused on one individual. The therapist seldom sees the whole family together. Haley and Hoffman[3] and many solution-focused models use the therapist's position as expert. These models differ in their beliefs about the use of the therapist's power and the level of appropriate closeness. At one end are therapists who see themselves as defining the problem and having the job of fixing it. At the other end are (with the family) coconstructors of a new reality for the family—who hope to change the family's perception of their family life. This second group of therapists are quite humble about their suggestions. The position that a particular therapist chooses will relate both to the therapist's model of therapy and to their specific personality and situation. The therapist's ability to form an alliance with a particular family is partly skill and partly a matter of style and tolerance for certain kinds of interaction. Beginning therapists will find certain families dramatically harder to ally with than others. Different therapists, by virtue of their position with certain patients, will be able to take some positions more easily than others.

MODELS FOR DEALING WITH FAMILIES THAT HAVE TROUBLE FORMING AN ALLIANCE

In the family therapy field, there are at least four different models for dealing with families who present difficulties in forming a therapeutic alliance.

Medical Model

In the medical model, it is assumed that the identified patient has an illness, such as schizophrenia or a major depressive disorder, and that the family is not the only, nor necessarily the principal, factor in the etiology of the illness. With this assumption, the major strategy in reducing family resistance to treatment is psychoeducation for the family members, in which they are taught about the symptoms, etiology, and course of the illness. In this model, it is emphasized that the family did not cause the illness, thus reducing the family guilt and resistance to meeting with the therapist. The family therapist takes on the role of a teacher who instructs the family about the illness and what the family can do to ensure optimal coping.

Coaching Model

Therapists who work in individual and family formats that use behavioral techniques tended until recently to ignore the concept of resistance in their writings. Instead, they emphasized that individuals in families must learn certain basic social, communication, and negotiating skills for harmonious interactions and that individuals lacked these skills because of deficiencies in prior learning. In this model, it was assumed that the therapist was a coach and rational collaborator who elicited the cooperation of the patient and family in learning skills that were missing. More recently, behavioral therapists have become interested in what prevents learning of these skills and have developed cognitive-behavioral models that consider the role of the cognitive meaning of behaviors, so that resistance is also examined as a series of cognitive distortions and beliefs that impede learning (e.g., "If I'm nice to her and give in, I won't be a real man," or "He is really a bad person, so why should I give him anything?").

In a coaching model, it is assumed that the therapist helps the couple locate problem areas and address them in a rational and focused way. Resistances in learning skills, such as failure to do homework or diverting attention from practice during the session, may be met first with rational argument (e.g., "You need these skills in order to function well"), encouragement, and positive reinforcement. Therapists also work with the couple or family to uncover distortions and replace dysfunctional cognitions with more functional ones.

Conflict Model

In a continuation of the psychodynamic tradition, the conflict model assumes that particular individuals in the couple or family system may exhibit resistance to intervention and change based on their own internal conflicts and defense mechanisms. In this model, the family therapist, like the individual dynamic therapist, uses techniques of confrontation and interpretation of the here-and-now interaction, especially negative interactions that might destroy the therapeutic relationship and the very survival of the therapy itself.

Strategic Systems Model

A unique contribution of the family therapy field is its theoretical position regarding the strength of a pattern of family interactions that shape and mold the behavior and psychopathology of an individual member of that group. In this orientation, it is assumed that family systems in homeostasis, even when the homeostasis involves severe problems, will resist change. When faced with resistance of a whole system, the therapist may use strategic interventions to change not individual behaviors but a pattern of systems behaviors.

Consider the following case example:

The A family sought treatment after the younger son, aged 25 years, refused to leave home or get a job. The son was not psychotic or suffering from a serious mental illness, and he had worked previously. Mr. A was subtly encouraging his son to stay. The therapist suggested that the son should not leave because, after all, he was a good companion for his father, and the family had plenty of money. The therapist began to discuss building an addition onto the house so that the son would be more comfortable, implying that this would certainly be a permanent plan. He talked about how pleasant it would be that the son would keep his parents company into their old age and that even though it meant the son could not marry, it would be a small sacrifice. At this point, Mrs. A, who had remained quiet, said that she would begin house hunting because one of them was leaving, either she or her son. Within a week the son was looking at graduate school catalogs, and within a month he had left home.

The concept of prescribing the symptom, or encouraging the no-change position, is a helpful alternative to the therapist being the voice for change. If the therapist pushes too hard for change, the family will become the keepers of the no-change position. Once the therapist backs off, the family's demand for change can be activated. For example, the family can be asked to list all the negatives that would occur if the supposedly desired change occurred (e.g., "If we gave up arguing, we might get too close, and I would feel vulnerable," or "If we gave up arguing, we might not have anything to say," or "If we gave up arguing, I wouldn't feel angry and I might feel depressed").

PROBLEMS IN CREATING CHANGE: RESISTANCE AND DISCONNECTION

Resistance in family therapy is usually defined as those forces within the patient or family that impede apparently wished-for change. Although resistance is usually seen as negative, it is also clear that because personal and family stability depend on certain consistencies of thought and behavior, psychological mechanisms and family rules are not designed for instant change. In general, families are likely to have an idea of what changes they want to make and are confused about why they cannot make these changes. The task of the therapist and family then becomes understanding the specific ideas and fears that stand in the way of change. Some families are not open to change at any level at a particular point in time. However, lack of change in therapy is often attributed to family mechanisms when the real problem is a disconnect between the therapist and the family, meaning that the therapist is not correctly assessing the system or has lost the family's trust. Problems in creating change during therapy can come from the family, from the therapist (e.g., as a result of inexperience, mistakes in judgment), or from disconnects in the therapist–family system.

> Resistance in family therapy is usually defined as those forces within the patient or family that impede apparently wished-for change.

We strongly emphasize to residents that when a family discontinues treatment, the clinician must be active in trying to bring the family back into treatment. This means actively contacting the family member most aligned with the clinician to get the family reengaged in treatment. The clinician should not be passive when one or more members of the family discontinue therapy. We discuss a very difficult case where a family member continually discontinues treatment in Chapter 23.

Problems in Creating Change: Emanating from the Family

Families fear change for many reasons. Most problem behaviors were originally adaptive mechanisms that are now failing but are frightening to let go of unless something can replace them. For example, if an overly close relationship between a mother and her daughter made up for the mother's poor marital relationship with the father, the mother will need to believe she can change the relationship with her husband, or feel better herself, before she can wholeheartedly let her daughter go. Similarly, if a father believes that his son will be a sissy unless he yells at and bullies him, the father will have to change that belief before he can change his behavior.

Sometimes the family has a toxic secret that it is afraid to reveal. For example, no one may be willing to speak about the father's sexual abuse of his daughter because they are afraid he will retaliate with violence, so they are unable to mobilize themselves to change any of the resulting problems. Certain conditions in individuals make change far more complex. For example, alcoholism or drug addiction sometimes responds to family interventions, but if these conditions do not, only limited change is possible. Similarly, with severe mental illness in a parent, family therapy must be accompanied by appropriate psychiatric medical management, or the situation will be difficult to change.

Problems in Creating Change: Emanating from the Therapist

Therapists face many challenges, including their own powerful countertransference feelings, as they begin to deal with a family. Therapists who become angry at or too connected to some members of the family will be unable to form the necessary alliance with the whole system. Therapists may blame the family for the symptoms of one member, as did many early practitioners who treated schizophrenia, making their hostility so apparent that the family members were unable to take anything useful from them.

Basic therapist mistakes will make it appear as though the family is resisting. For example, failing to diagnose attention deficit hyperactivity disorder in a child, the therapist may insist that the problem is an overprotective mother and spend time working to get her less involved, when the child actually needs both medication and more structure. Similarly, if a couple presents for treatment of wife abuse, and the therapist concentrates on communication and does not directly interdict the husband's violence, it is unlikely that much will change. Even if the therapist correctly understands the family system, problems ranging from the therapist's failure to be clear about goals and directions, or to explain their theory to the family, to the therapist's failure to give tasks small enough and clear enough for learning to occur, to the therapist's inability to control the session will result in inability to move the family forward. In summary, in the spirit of our integrated model, let us quote from William Vogel,[4] (p. 972).

The issue of countertransference is, arguably, even more important in couples therapy than in individual treatment. The patient couple is ever alert to the danger that the therapist might favor (or disfavor), or be more identified with, one of the two partners; the wise therapist will ever be alert to the same possibility. The therapist's differential response may be a function of any combination of almost an infinite number of factors and will, of necessity, determine their response to the couple, as well as to the outcome of the treatment.

To give one obvious example, a therapist who, all unaware, tends to behave seductively with the same-sex (or opposite-sex) member of the patient couple, or who, conversely, disfavors the same-sex (or opposite-sex) member of the couple is a therapist who will always be in serious difficulty. The fact that the therapist is simultaneously dealing with two patients immeasurably complicates all of the problems that are associated with countertransference.

Problems in Creating Change: From the Therapist–Family System

1. **Mismatch between therapist and family.** Although most therapists learn to work with a variety of patients over time, some therapist–patient systems are too difficult to manage, especially for beginning therapists. For example, a very young female therapist, who was newly married, was assigned to work with a midlife couple in sex therapy. The wife, who was depressed, angry, and feeling unlovable because of years of sexual disinterest on the part of her husband, could not stand being treated by a woman she saw as a rival and who did not have the life experience necessary to understand midlife issues. The couple did well when transferred to an older therapist who could connect more directly with the couple's life experience and circumstances. Sometimes the therapist's style of functioning is too far from the needs of the patient system (e.g., too aggressive, too passive, too distant).
2. **Disagreement as to treatment goals.** Problems can occur if the therapist believes that one goal is central and the family wants to focus on another goal. For example, the therapist may see couple issues as critical, whereas the family wants to talk only about the child. If the therapist moves too fast or does not wait to see if the family has accepted the new goal, treatment will stall.
3. **Inclusion in the system of others besides the nuclear family and the therapist not taking this into account.** Common systems to be considered include family elders (e.g.,

grandparents or other relatives), who may have very definite ideas about what should be done, the school system, the legal system, and the medical system (e.g., if a family member is physically ill). Families with multiple problems are often involved with several caregivers who may have very different ideas about the problem's definition and solution—this may involve child welfare, the school, a social worker, legal services, or other therapists seeing family members. If the therapist is working in an agency, another set of systems is involved. For example, the family may be suspicious of therapists working in social welfare or probation agencies, seeing them as agents of social control rather than support. In addition, the treatment that the family or the therapist desires may be in conflict with agency rules or with the therapist's supervisor.

Problems in Creating Change: Stages of Treatment: At Evaluation and Early in Treatment

The therapist's first task is to set the structure within which the family intervention can occur. Many resistances can surface during this process of negotiating the structure with the family. In contrast to individual therapy, family or marital therapy necessitates the attendance of a number of people, most of whom do not have overt symptoms. The therapist must first decide whether to insist on seeing the whole family. Napier and Whitaker[5] describe their approach in doing family therapy (with a mother, father, and three adolescents) in which all family members were required to attend. In an initial session, when the adolescent son did not appear, the therapists refused to begin therapy even though the parents were concerned that the adolescent daughter was suicidal. The therapists assessed the situation, felt that the suicide potential was not significant, and told the parents to return with the whole family. In this case, it was felt that to let the family dictate the terms of the therapy would result in a loss of what the authors called the battle for structure. However, some families would not return after such an experience.

At times it is best to begin work with whoever comes to treatment first and to support the family member(s) in getting the rest of the family to come. In general, it is best to insist on seeing the whole family as close to the beginning of therapy as possible. Getting fathers into and involved in family therapy has classically been seen as the most difficult task, especially for inexperienced therapists. In the past, many fathers did not see their role in the emotional life of the family as significant and often were afraid of their own vulnerability in a setting in which words and feelings were paramount.

Strategies for getting fathers (and other important family members) to sessions include the following: reassuring the missing member of their importance, pointing out that changes depend on their presence, noting that their absence can sabotage therapy, providing flexibility in scheduling, and spacing appointments. If it seems appropriate, the therapist can refuse to continue without the family member. Stanton and Todd[6] generated a number of principles to ensure attendance in starting family intervention with substance abusers and their families (these principles are probably appropriate for other symptom groups):

- The therapist, not the family, should decide which family members will be included in the treatment.
- Whenever possible, family members should be encouraged to attend the evaluation interview.
- The identified patient alone should not be given the task of bringing in the other members of the family.
- The therapist should obtain permission from the identified patient and personally contact the family members.
- The therapist should contact the family with a rationale for family intervention that is nonpejorative and nonjudgmental and that in no way blames the family for the symptoms and problems of the identified patient.

Often the critical issue is in supporting the overtly symptomatic patient to ask for help from the family. Consider the following case example:

> *In the B family, the identified patient was Mr. B, who had a long history of major depression. After his depressive episodes had been regulated with medication, he told the therapist that his wife was unhappy with their relationship. The therapist suggested marital therapy. Mr. B said that this was his cross to bear because Mrs. B would not come in for therapy. The therapist suggested that he again try talking to her about this. Surprisingly, Mrs. B appeared for the next session and said that she was unhappy with the relationship but had never been asked to come in for therapy. Mr. B said that he had asked her but admitted he might have "mumbled the invitation."*

Families in which one member exhibits current self-destructive behaviors (e.g., suicidal threats, gestures, and attempts; anorexia or bulimia; drug abuse; physical violence) present special challenges in the initial structuring of the therapy. Clinicians vary in how they address these behaviors in the early structuring of the treatment. Although there is little research evidence as to the most efficacious approaches, it is our clinical opinion that from the beginning, even in the very first session, the family therapist must address their responsibilities and the family's responsibilities if and when these destructive behaviors occur. The therapist must often spell out in great detail what they will and will not do when these behaviors occur. The therapist can also help the family members plan how they will behave. If this is not done, the first resistance will come in the form of destructive behaviors that derail the possibility of change.

As we mentioned earlier in this chapter, disagreement about treatment goals is an area of potential resistance and deadlock in the early phase of treatment. We also addressed this issue in Chapter 12 in our discussion of the process of bringing together the family's and the therapist's views of the problem (see Fig. 12.1). The family members themselves may disagree about the problem and the goals of treatment. For example, the family of an identified adolescent patient may see the adolescent as the only problem, whereas the adolescent sees no problem in themselves and sees the parents as authoritarian, narrow, and hostile. Similarly, covert disagreement about the problem and especially the goals of intervention occur in marital therapy when one spouse wants the marriage improved and the other secretly wants out and is intending to leave the spouse, using the therapist for assistance in the breakup.

Strategies to overcome family differences about the problem include searching for a new definition of the problem with which all family members agree, labeling the disagreement as part of the problem, and asking the family to give up idiosyncratic notions about its version of truth and reality. Covert goals can be approached by encouraging family members to say what has remained unsaid.

Disagreement about goals of intervention can also occur between the therapist and the family. This seems most prominent when the therapist sees the problems of the identified patient as related to the interactions of the family, whereas the family sees no contribution of its own and wants the identified patient changed or cured. The therapist can approach this problem by initially accepting the family's view of the problem, or at least not challenging this view, or by broadening the family's definition to include other aspects of interaction.

In families in which a member has been hospitalized for the first time with the emergence of psychotic symptomatology subsequently diagnosed as either schizophrenia or mood disorder, a common resistance of the family is to deny either the presence of the illness or its severity. If such denial persists, the family is in danger of avoiding follow-up care for the patient and family and furthering expectations for the identified patient that are unrealistic and thus cause stress for the vulnerable individual.

A particularly troublesome resistance for the beginning family therapist, especially if they are a psychiatric resident, psychology intern, or social work student, is the family's attack on the therapist's competence or personal characteristics (e.g., age, sex, race, socioeconomic level). These resistances can come in subtle barrages (e.g., "You're so good for a youngster, but you probably don't know much about older people") and not so subtle barrages (e.g., "This is probably your first case, and we are not making any progress. Have you talked to your supervisor about this?"). Contact with an experienced supervisor is most helpful in these situations. The therapist, if able to see the remarks in the context of resistance, can explore the meaning of the questions about competence by empathizing with the family's concern. With equilibrium and, at times, humor, the therapist can admit differences and limitations (e.g., youth, relative inexperience), appeal to the family for its assistance and help, and ask for a period in which to give the therapy a chance to succeed.

If it is clear that the family cannot tolerate the situation, a transfer to a therapist it has requested (e.g., older, younger, different race or gender) is indicated. Either when the family was correct in its assessment that it needed something different or once the family has proved it has some control in a situation, the family may feel it is safe to begin work.

Problems in Creating Change: In Ongoing Treatment

It is extremely common for a therapy to move rapidly in the early weeks and then stall. This is the point at which old habits reassert themselves, the natural homeostasis of the family takes over, and small failures begin to seem insurmountable. The process of working through change is difficult. The therapist needs to review the treatment and decide whether to change direction or to simply support the idea that change is sometimes difficult and continue in the same direction.

Anderson and Stewart[7] have listed several situations that threaten treatment.

- A family member who is consistently too talkative and dominant
- A family member who refuses to speak
- Chaotic and disruptive children
- Use of defenses such as intellectualization, rationalization, and denial
- Constant focus by one or more family members placing blame on others
- Unwillingness to do assigned tasks or homework that is necessary for change

The therapist can limit overly talkative family members or can encourage other family members to do so. Parents of chaotic children can be educated by words and by the therapist's modeling of limit setting in the sessions. Most important is the therapist's understanding of why the behavior is occurring. If the behavior serves a purpose, it will be less amenable to requests to stop it, unless the underlying meaning is addressed. However, if the therapist can create a different experience in the session, such as getting a quiet husband to talk while his wife listens, the family may be able to repeat the experience at home without needing to have specific insight into why things have changed.

When couples argue as a regular pattern, usually they are not trying to understand what each other is saying. More likely feeling defensive and out of control, the partners listen for weaknesses in logic to leap on or selectively mishear what each other says. Such couples misread each other's intent, feel defensive, and believe if they don't attack first, they will be injured. Behind this behavior is a deep sense of hurt. The truth is more likely to be found in the complex middle than in the simplified extremes. Therefore, the therapist must discuss the process of the argument and its underlying meanings.

If tasks are not being completed, then the therapist can challenge the couple or redesign the task. Refusal to do homework should always be discussed because the discussion will contain cues about what is really going on. Several techniques are available for handling defenses, not unlike those one might use in individual or group therapy. For example, to counteract intellectualization and rationalization, the therapist can go with the theme by emphasizing the intellectual aspects of the therapy or by giving intellectual explanations. Relabeling of feelings as facts may help. A family in denial can be slowed down so as to emphasize aspects of the interactions before they are glossed over. Nonverbal and experiential techniques can also be used to get to denied material. As a last resort, the therapist can focus on and support a no-change position as a way to eventually get change.

Problems in Creating Change: At the Termination Phase of Therapy

Often after a successful therapy, the family experiences a resurgence of symptoms when termination begins. This usually indicates anxiety over ending rather than a new problem. The family can use this time to review its progress and understand its issues further. The family may be encouraged to have the symptoms to see if it would like to keep any of them. It may use the situation to understand how the symptoms occur and when they are avoided, so as to lock in new behaviors. The therapist should be alert to the idea that the family is asking for more support and should plan appropriate follow-up care.

Problems in Creating Change: Family Secrets

Individual family members often have secrets that in most cases are known but not acknowledged by other family members. They may involve overt behaviors that one couple partner feels they have been able to conceal from the other (e.g., couple infidelity), or they may involve thoughts, feelings, and attitudes that family members believe others are not aware of. For example, parents may not realize (or may deny) that their children pick up the general emotional tone existing between parents.

They may act as if marital discord is hidden from their children and may want to keep that discord secret. The family can also keep secrets from the therapist, as in the following case example:

> *The C family consisted of a hospitalized adolescent, the parents, and two older siblings. For 10 weeks, the family therapy seemed to be bogged down. The family stopped treatment. Two months later, the family therapist discovered a secret that the entire family already knew—the identified patient had been having sexual relations with a ward nurse. The patient had told his siblings, who told the parents, who then signed the patient out of the hospital. The secret served the purpose of denigrating the hospital staff (including the family therapist) and effectively halting the family therapy.*

Helping the family bring these secrets into the open usually results in a clearing of the air and eventually leads to a sense of relief and greater mutual understanding. Interestingly, it is commonly the children who talk openly in the family sessions about what was thought by others to be a secret. The therapist should be prepared to deal with acute shock waves at the time the secret emerges. When a family member requests an individual session for the purpose of revealing a secret, the therapist may listen and try to explore the consequences of discussing the issue within the family setting. If, for example, one of the spouses has an incurable illness and the other spouse does not know about it, the reasons for the secrecy would be examined and the spouse would be encouraged to share the information with the whole family.

If the secret does not seem critical to the relationship, the therapist might take a more neutral stance. Imber-Black[8] provides a good discussion of secrets and the distinction between secrets and power. The therapist must guard against becoming a repository of secrets. They have the right to tell the patient the therapy will end unless the secret is told. It is not recommended that therapists themselves reveal a family secret unless a no-confidentiality agreement has been made in advance.

At times a family member may insist on total honesty, either because of emotional insensitivity or as an active way of hurting another family member. For example, a parent might report to a child every negative feeling that crosses their mind in the guise of honesty. Needless to say, the therapist must be alert to these kinds of resistances (i.e., "honesty") in the service of stopping the treatment. Usually, the therapist will reframe the behavior and place it in context so that the family can work with the issue.

TECHNIQUES TO DEAL WITH RESISTANCES OR STALLED THERAPY

Regardless of the type of resistance or when it occurs, a therapist can do several helpful things:

1. **Announce to the family that the therapist feels stuck and ask if the family does.** Sometimes the family is doing fine and only the therapist is anxious. If everyone feels stuck, then everyone can work on the problem together.
2. **Retake a history.** The most common reason for problems in therapy is that the therapist does not have all the facts and so has not formulated the problem or the solution properly. Sometimes information is not shared with therapists until late in therapy when the patients are more trusting. Sometimes if a family came in crisis, the original history was too sketchy. The best way to regroup is to start over, preferably with a more complete genogram related to the problem (see Chapter 7).
3. **Go up or down a system level.** Often the problem is that too many or too few people are involved. If the therapist is seeing a couple, they can go up a level by involving more people (e.g., the couple's children or parents). Likewise, the therapist can go down a level by doing some individual work.
4. **Do the opposite of what has been done so far.** With therapy, as with life, sometimes the solution becomes the problem. If pushing hard doesn't work, the therapist can prescribe the symptom. If the therapist has been gentle and nonconfrontational, they can try pushing harder.
5. **Request a consultation.** A consultation serves notice to everyone that there is a problem and opens up the system for new ways of thinking. Consultants can often see a problem or blind spot because they are less connected to the family system and can visualize the therapist–family system as a whole. In the same vein, Alves,[9] (p. 8) suggested that therapists often refer to their families as being "stuck" when movement in the therapy process breaks down. Often, when this occurs, it is the therapist who has gotten off track and contributed to, if not directly reinforced, the lack of progress.

Therapists have a major responsibility in getting the therapy process back on track. A return to a few basic, fundamental principles often dislodges even the most stubborn roadblocks to progress. Here are a few trusty techniques, that is, standbys on which we rely.

Assume Nothing

A thorough assessment of a family's presenting problems and overall functioning is key to the therapy process. Problems in therapy presented in supervision can often be traced back to a hurried, haphazard assessment. Therapists either don't ask all the questions or jump to conclusions based on limited information. Assumptions by therapists on family treatment goals will typically create blocks to progress if the family has not agreed to such goals. A quick check of this area often reveals that what the therapists once labeled "family resistance" is in fact a lack of clarity on the part of the therapist.

Collaboration

Without collaboration between family members as well as between the family and the therapist, there is no therapy. Collaboration is an active process, with each step in the treatment needing to be negotiated and agreed upon. It can happen that family members will change their minds in the midst of treatment. If not addressed, this can result in a breakdown in progress.

Emphasizing Family Responsibility

Therapists will describe a sense of "working too hard" with some families. In such cases, shifting the balance of responsibility evenly between the therapist and family is necessary. Ultimately, it is the family who must do the work necessary to reach their desired goals. It is the therapist's responsibility to facilitate an environment in which change can take place.

Focus on the Present

There are times when the family continues to discuss the same issues incessantly with no signs toward resolving to change destructive patterns. Allowing families to continuously wallow in the unfortunate water that has gone under the bridge is not only unproductive but can be dangerous. Inadvertently, the therapist may be facilitating a sense of hopelessness in the family. It can be helpful for the therapist to focus the family to the present moment and encourage them to consider how the past affects today's functioning.

CLINICAL PRACTICE IMPLICATIONS

Doing family therapy is very different from doing individual treatment. Therapists are usually apprehensive at first, but as they gain experience, they are excited by the challenge and fascination of working with family units. Many therapists find themselves uncomfortable doing family work and should not force themselves to undertake it. In some ways, the experience for the therapist is like sitting in between the couple in the play *Who's Afraid of Virginia Woolf?* or in the middle of the family in the play *Long Day's Journey Into Night*, or it can be like watching a three-ring circus. The therapist has to pay attention not only to the feelings of individuals in the family system but also to the tone in the family unit and at the same time must be aware of their own feelings toward the family. The task is to stay focused on the objectives to be achieved with each family.

SUGGESTED READINGS

These texts go into great depth on the psychotherapy of family therapy.

Lambert MJ, ed. *Bergin and Garfield's Handbook of Psychotherapy and Behavior Change*. 6th ed. John Wiley & Sons, Inc.; 2013.

Norcross JC, ed. *Psychotherapy Relationships That Work: Evidence-Based Responsiveness*. 2nd ed. Oxford University Press; 2011.

REFERENCES

1. Satir VM, Baldwin M. *Satir Step by Step: A Guide to Creating Change in Families*. Science and Behavior Books; 1983.
2. Bowen M. *Family Therapy in Clinical Practice*. Jason Aronson; 1978.
3. Haley J, Hoffman L. *Techniques of Family Therapy*. Basic Books; 1967.
4. Vogel W. Enriching therapy for couples and families. *Psychiatr Serv*. 1998;49:972–973.
5. Napier A, Whitaker C. *The Family Crucible*. Harper & Row; 1978.
6. Stanton MD, Todd TC. Engaging resistant families in treatment. *Fam Process*. 1981;20:261–293.
7. Anderson C, Stewart S. *Mastering Resistance: A Practical Guide to Family Therapy*. Guilford; 1983.
8. Imber-Black E. *Secrets in Families and Family Therapy*. WW Norton; 1993.
9. Alves JW. *Back to Basics Is Good Move When "Stuck" in Family Therapy*. The Brown University Family Therapy Letter; 1992.

14 Family Therapy: General Considerations

OBJECTIVES FOR THE READER

- To be able to decide which family participants to include in treatment and to be aware of the guidelines for including children, adolescents, grandparents, and others
- To know the advantages and disadvantages of various therapist combinations
- To be aware of the variety of settings in which family therapy has been used
- To be able to manage the complexities of combining family treatment with medication or with other psychotherapies
- To know the similarities and differences between family therapy versus individual or group therapy

For easier reading, we emphasize that the descriptors "couples" or "marital" are used nearly interchangeably in this chapter.

In a family, you live close to people that you otherwise may not even want to talk to. Over time, you learn their most miniscule, most private habits and characteristics. Today, professionals are preoccupied with the dysfunctional family. But to some extent, all families are dysfunctional, with most having serious problems. A family is a microcosm reflecting the nature of the world; a place that runs on both virtue and evil. You cannot change this, you can only learn to live in it.

—Thomas Moore, *Care of the Soul*

INTRODUCTION

By now, the reader should have some understanding of how families function and how their difficulties may be conceptualized. In addition, we have presented material relevant to the evaluation of troubled families and to the setting up of appropriate treatment goals. In this chapter, we consider more general features of marital and family therapy, namely, the participants, the setting, the scheduling of treatment, and the use of family therapy in combination with other treatment methods and helping agencies. Finally, we compare family therapy with other therapy formats.

FAMILY PARTICIPANTS
Extended Family and Significant Others
Caregivers

INCLUDING CHILDREN AND ADOLESCENTS IN FAMILY THERAPY
Diagnostic Family Evaluation
Treatment
THERAPIST COMBINATIONS
Co-Therapy
Working as a Team
SETTING
TIME, SCHEDULING, AND FEES
KEEPING A RECORD OF TREATMENT
FAMILY THERAPY IN COMBINATION WITH OTHER PSYCHOSOCIAL THERAPIES
Practical Guidelines
Effective Family Intervention
Comparison of Therapy Formats and Strategies
CLINICAL PRACTICE IMPLICATIONS

FAMILY PARTICIPANTS

In practice, it is often preferable to begin treatment by seeing the entire family together. The family can be defined broadly to include all persons living under the same roof; all those persons closely related to one another, even though they do not live together; or even more broadly, all persons significant to the family, even though not related to them—including friends, caregivers, or the family's social network.

Sometimes family therapy is carried out with the same therapist meeting with the whole family and with *each* family member individually. This approach, termed *concurrent family therapy*, is uncommon today. At other times, two therapists who maintain some contact with each other, but who do not work jointly, may both see separately one or more members of a family in what is known as *collaborative family therapy*, which is also rare. *Conjoint family therapy* has been defined as family therapy in which the participants include at least two generations of a family, such as parents and children, plus the therapist, all meeting together. *Conjoint couples therapy* is limited to the two spouses plus the therapist meeting together.

The preferred model for family therapists is to see the whole family together for most of the sessions, occasionally having sessions with one of the subsystems (e.g., parents alone, siblings alone, father–son) as needed. Therapists who are interested in family-of-origin work will also have some sessions with one of the spouses and the spouse's parents. Opinion is divided over whether individual therapy with one or more family members should be done while family therapy is in progress and whether the individual therapist should also be the family therapist. Concurrent individual therapy is sometimes done by a different therapist, who it is hoped has some communication with the family therapist. Frequently a child's or spouse's therapist will suggest family therapy and then continue to treat their patient while family therapy is ongoing.

The preferred model for family therapists is to see the whole family together for most of the sessions, occasionally having sessions with one of the subsystems (e.g., parents alone, siblings alone, father–son) as needed.

Although it often seems desirable to meet with all family members present, in practice this may be impossible or even contraindicated. For example, children should not be present when their parents' sexual adjustment is being discussed. (We discuss the issue of taking a couple's sexual history more fully later in this chapter and in Chapter 20.) Often, too, the therapist will be unable to include certain family members because of illness, divorce, or death, or because one or more family members temporarily or permanently refuse to participate. In the latter case, a decision will have to be made, either at the outset of treatment or after the evaluation, as to whether it is worthwhile and possible to continue working with the incomplete family. Hard-and-fast rules as to when such therapy is worthwhile are not easy to give, but our bias is that if the pros and cons are about equal, it is better to give treatment a try even if the family is incomplete.

Sometimes individuals will feel uncomfortable talking about certain topics in front of other family members. The family therapist will then have to decide whether individual interviewing might be indicated. Such an approach might be taken, for example, with the goal of eventually bringing the material from the individual session to the entire family group. However, there may be family secrets that cannot be productively shared with other family members and that should be kept private between an individual family member and the therapist. For example, one of the most complex current issues is whether children should be told they are products of artificial insemination or assisted pregnancy (e.g., surrogate mothers). Current thinking is that the emotional problems for the family caused by not knowing or by having a secret are worse than the emotional problems associated with dealing with the secret, but there is no real proof for this conclusion. (We discuss more fully the issue of secrets in Chapters 12 and 25.) On the issue of secrets, too, no rigid guidelines can be established. Consider the following example of an unshared family secret:

Ms. A, the identified patient, was a 20-year-old woman with schizophrenia. After Ms. A's birth, her mother experienced a postpartum psychosis, during which she jumped in front of a train, resulting in bilateral amputation below the knees. Ms. A's grandmother had also experienced a postpartum psychosis after the birth of her daughter, Ms. A's mother. Ms. A had not known about these secrets. Her father revealed the story in a family session that did not involve Ms. A. She was not informed of her mother's psychosis, based on the judgment of all concerned that she was not psychologically capable of dealing with this material at that time. However, because this information surely affected Ms. A deeply, the therapist might choose to share it with her when she is in a more compensated state.

The family concept can be extended to cover nonrelated people who have an effect on the individuals in treatment. These might be friends, neighbors, professional helpers, or legal guardians. Such people often do not have the same kind of emotional impact and influence that the natural family unit has, but at any one particular time, these significant others may be quite important. Many experienced family therapists believe that the probability of improvement increases as the number of nuclear family members involved in treatment increases. We tend to agree.

Extended Family and Significant Others

Family therapists include grandparents or in-laws as participants when these individuals seem to influence significantly the family's difficulties. Grandparents and other extended family members play vital roles in many families. In some families, they may provide important help financially and functionally in carrying out the family's tasks. They may be a repository of emotional support and warmth, available in times of crisis and need. Their contributions and participation may at times be viewed as interference or infantilization. They may create or demand obligations in return for their involvement.

The grandparents may provide money with strings attached, which may be in the form of rules and regulations concerning the rearing of their grandchildren; such aid may also imply an obligation that the family visit the grandparents on a prescribed schedule. The 1976 film *Lies My Father Told Me* provides an excellent example of a family in which a child may feel much closer to a grandparent than to his father or mother. In this film, a 7-year-old boy is being raised by a mother who is totally devoted to a rather insensitive and inadequate spouse. The boy spends most of his time with his grandfather, who acts as a father substitute.

The question of whether a friend, fiance(e), boyfriend, or girlfriend should participate in a therapy session is raised occasionally. Sometimes the inclusion is vital, and such individuals should be included if their involvement is judged to be important to the progress of the therapy. However, there are potential drawbacks of including such outsiders. For example, they may be less motivated to change than are family members, thus hampering the usefulness of the family therapy; they are more likely to drop out of family therapy; and they may learn more intimate knowledge than is appropriate in a noncommitted relationship.

Caregivers

Caregivers (e.g., babysitters or housekeepers) are playing an increasingly important role in the function of families, especially in families in which both parents work. They are sometimes usefully included in treatment. Consider the following case example:

In the B family, Mr. and Mrs. B were separated. Mrs. B had great difficulty functioning as a mother and in general, secondary to her depression. Mr. B, therefore, had custody of the children. Care of the children, aged 14, 12, and 10 years, was left to a babysitter, who was the 21-year-old sister of Mr. B's current girlfriend. Feeling despondent, Mrs. B attempted suicide. It was at this point that attempts at family therapy were initiated, but Mr. B refused to attend because he was angry with his wife. At the outset of family therapy, Mrs. B complained that she was unable to get the children to attend. They were on Mr. B's side. The children refused to attend when the therapist called them, saying the babysitter would not let them travel to the sessions. The babysitter was, of course, on the father's side. Furthermore, once the children began to attend therapy, the babysitter would, after each session, belittle the mother to the children. They would then berate their mother, who would again become suicidal. Only after the husband, the babysitter, and the husband's girlfriend were included in family therapy could this sequence of interactions be understood and modified.

INCLUDING CHILDREN AND ADOLESCENTS IN FAMILY THERAPY

It would seem obvious that family therapy would be a useful modality in the treatment of the problems and disorders of children. Children are usually brought by their parents to mental health professionals for help. The child's family is often involved with and affected by the problem. Family members are concerned, usually motivated, and may have their own theories about the causes expressed in terms of some family dysfunction. It is common for parents to blame themselves for their child's problem.

Historically, child psychology and psychiatry have been shaped principally by theories of the individual, the development cycle, and the psychoanalytic model. These theories might have a similar point of view, as does family systems theory, with regard to the family's role in causing the problem, but when it comes to therapeutic intervention, the theories lead to very different approaches. Family systems thinkers believe that family treatment involving the child and various family members is the optimal way to produce change. Psychoanalytic thinking has taken a less central role in psychiatry training. Increased emphasis on family and systems issues is a more common component of child psychiatric training programs.[1] Nonetheless, studies confirm that although instruction in family therapy is required in child psychiatry training programs, most training does not include it.[2] A new concern has arisen, with the advent of managed health care, that an emphasis on medications as the only approach may undermine the gains family therapy has made within child psychiatry.

Working with families that have children compels the family therapist to first think developmentally. Some theorists have looked at families as the laboratories in which children are socialized and first learn about order, discipline, respect, cooperation, conflict resolution, and enjoyment. At the same time, every clinician has working models of the tasks that families with children of varying ages encounter and must master. For example, parents of young children must make room for their children, learn new parenting roles, and guide their children's behavior through rules and words. As children enter school and progress through adolescence, the parent–child relationship is based less on parental authority and more on parent–child collaboration.

For the family therapist, it is important to understand that the stable family and/or marital partner is a good buffer (possible healer) of childhood psychiatric disorder.[3]

Diagnostic Family Evaluation

All children require careful medical, neurologic, and developmental evaluations by professionals qualified to do them. To assume that a symptom has an interactional basis or that it is acting as a metaphor for the systems problem is premature and unprofessional. In addition to these evaluations, any evaluation of a child must include a family assessment. But family assessment means different things to different people. A family therapist would interview all family members and significant others at the same time. They would believe that such a procedure would give the most information about the child's and family's problems and that a child psychiatrist, who interviewed the parents and child separately and excluded siblings, was getting less information and not doing a family evaluation. Many good mental health professionals who work with children intuitively work with families. For example, individual psychotherapy for a 15-year-old adolescent who exhibits school avoidance won't produce change if the child psychiatrist missed the family evaluation and didn't pick up that the adolescent's 6-year-old sister is being abused by the parent. Conversely, child psychiatry has a lot to offer the family therapy field. For example, family therapy for that same adolescent won't help if the family therapist misses the adolescent's severe learning disability. Child psychiatrists, who in addition to being trained to evaluate and treat individual children are competent in family therapy, become fine generalists capable of working in both modalities of treatment.

Most family therapists assume that assessment of the family environment is crucial when a child presents with emotional–behavioral symptoms. By looking at the problem in its natural context, such as the home, the therapist can determine how family members' responses to the child's behavior may be contributing to the problem's persistence. For example, a child with oppositional behavior may elicit contradictory reactions from their parents. The father may react by punishing the child, whereas the mother tries to modify what she views as her husband's extreme reaction. The astute family therapist will choose to see the problem in action, asking the family to show the problem rather than simply describe it. The therapist, guided by a developmental framework, may then identify the problematic pattern that maintains the child's difficulties, clarify the parents' conflict over discipline, help the parents to define a common strategy with which they both feel comfortable, and coach them in applying their plan with their child.

Many therapists prefer to involve everyone in the household, including infants (and perhaps even pets), during the evaluation period in order to observe how family members relate to one another. Helpful observations may be gathered, such as differences in how parents relate to each other with and without the infant present, how one parent holds an infant, and what the other parent's role is. After the initial evaluation is completed, the therapist must decide whether the continued inclusion of an infant or relatively nonverbal child aids or disrupts the work of therapy. An increased appreciation of the family variables involved in taking care of infants has developed in recent years and attachment theory and research has served as the foundation for therapeutic work.

Most family therapists would agree that infants and children should be included at least once for diagnostic purposes. Certainly much can be gained from having children present for many of the sessions, if for no other reason than that they are often more open and direct than adults and will say what they think.

Many family therapists can get confused and distracted by young children in a session, commonly maintaining that children don't sit still, that they just play. Because children's play and drawings can add much information to a family session, the therapist should keep some toys in the office. At different stages of family therapy, excluding younger children may be appropriate, just as seeing the sibling subsystem or the parental subsystem may be. Children and adolescents have delicately balanced internal psychological forces, which are in constant interaction with the external forces of the family. Where and how to intervene should come out of a careful evaluation of these factors.

As we have emphasized throughout this book, other individuals such as teachers, pediatricians, clergy, and neighbors may be important to the problem and should be consulted if they are part of the system.

Treatment

Family therapists not only assess but also treat the problems of children and adolescents within the context of the family. Therapists must ally with the family, invite the family members to enact the problem, recognize the developmental tasks that need to be accomplished, and devise therapeutic interventions that assist family members in continuing through the course of normal development. In addition, therapists who work with children and families need to appreciate the important socializing roles that schools and friendships play in contributing to the positive social development of children and adolescents.

When young children are present, the parents are expected to exert appropriate behavioral control over them. If not, the therapist helps the parents to accomplish the task. The therapist explains the house rules, including behavioral limits and freedom of communication. The therapist must decide who should handle requests to go to the toilet or the water fountain. The therapist may wish to provide materials for play, such as toys, papers, and crayons.

Adolescents will be crucially involved in the family unit's concerns and interactions and often are the identified patients. They should be included in the sessions so that intergenerational conflicts and inadequate communications can be addressed. One of the primary tasks of the late adolescent, however, is to achieve increasing psychosocial autonomy from their family of origin. If such adolescents are consistently included in all family sessions, their involvement in all of the family's interactions is structurally reinforced. In addition, there may be little recognition of those specific interactions of the husband–wife pair that do not, and should not, involve their children. Thus, it may be useful to have some sessions with only the husband and wife. Other sessions may be devoted to seeing an adolescent alone for the special purpose of reinforcing or increasing autonomy. Conjoint sessions may also be used successfully to explore issues of differentness and separation. Occasionally a marital relationship has ruptured to the extent that treatment is stalemated. For example, two spouses may sit in the room and not speak to each other. A last-resort technique is to use adolescent children, on a temporary basis, as buffers, neutralizers, or reality testers, until such time as the couple is able to resume functioning as a dyad.

Careful recognition must be given to the readiness and ability of the adolescent and their family to separate. Although individual autonomous functioning is seen as a desirable goal, in some situations the therapist must be realistic with respect to the family's ability to tolerate an abrupt separation. They should also consider the possibility that the adolescent may have brain damage, chronic schizophrenia, or severe characterologic difficulties. Child psychiatrists may face other issues, including the child's need for medication and the effect of this situation on families.

THERAPIST COMBINATIONS

Co-Therapy

Most family therapists work alone; however, some therapists still prefer to work with a co-therapist to help monitor the complexity of the transactions and to use as a system of checks and balances with the other therapist. Co-therapy is seldom used except in teaching sessions, and it poses a problem in such a setting because of the unequal balance of power involved when a student and a teacher do therapy together. One-way mirrors and video have supplanted this method as a learning technique. Some collaborative modules use one therapist for each spouse and involve periodic four-person sessions.

For training purposes, a student therapist can work with either a more seasoned veteran or a student of another discipline. Co-therapists can present an experiential model of a two-person interaction that is similar to a marital dyad by dealing openly with their own differences and by providing models for healthy communication. If, in contrast, the co-therapists feel that they need to present a united front or that they need to be identical in their attitudes and interactions with the family members they are treating jointly, the family will then be provided with a very unrealistic model.

Co-therapists may come to be seen as parents or as husband and wife by the family and may therefore be the recipients of the typical patterns, feelings, and attitudes that the family has toward people in these roles. The co-therapists may find themselves in danger of being split and having to take sides, in a manner very similar to that which takes place in family treatment. The co-therapy team must avoid falling into this trap. A solution is for one co-therapist to be sensitive to a family member who is in distress and who may need support, while the other therapist focuses on someone else. A co-therapist may in style or in behavior either complement (i.e., be different from) or be synergistic with (i.e., be similar to) the other therapist.

It is necessary to consider whether a therapist can work effectively with a co-therapist and if co-therapy is the best use of each therapist's time. An older study suggests that therapist satisfaction with co-therapy decreases as experience in family therapy increases.[4] Furthermore, some authors have found that co-therapy causes problems that can impede family progress. For example, if a male co-therapist has had significant problems with his mother and is in the process of treating a family that has a difficult mother, he might have difficulty working effectively with a female therapist. Another obvious reason for the more common use of a single therapist is that it costs less.

In order to make co-therapy a successful experience, the co-therapists should know and like each other. They should have worked together, so that they are able to appreciate each other's therapy style and attitude. They should have time to discuss together what has been going on in their therapy sessions and to work out their mutual roles with respect to the family and each other. Ideally, co-therapists should get together before each session in order to review their objectives and ideas. Co-therapists should meet after each session to review what went on and to plan for the next session.

An innovative approach is the use of co-therapists from different disciplines, a desirable approach for beginning therapists. This technique has the advantage that each therapist may complement the other because each discipline has different training and may bring its own areas of expertise. This method requires the use of extra staff time, however, and to justify it, one would have to prove its differential effectiveness over family therapy as it is usually practiced.

Working as a Team

Several groups have experimented with the use of a treatment team (i.e., three or four therapists) to work with the family[5], although this practice is less common now than in the past.

Typically, one or two therapists are in the treatment room with the family, while the rest of the treatment team is behind a one-way mirror. The team communicates with the therapist in the room by telephone or by having a conference (without the family) during or toward the end of the therapy hour. The team assists the therapist by providing directives to the therapist trainee or by helping to formulate messages and tasks, including paradoxical tasks that the therapist will convey to the family.

In some settings, team members may join the therapist in the room or may send in contradictory messages (e.g., the team can insist that the couple shouldn't change so that the therapist can defend the change position). Although some families are put off by the one-way mirror and the idea of several people watching, most become comfortable with the setting and the idea that many people are involved in their care.

A treatment team is an extraordinary advantage to a trainee or even a seasoned therapist, particularly those working on the cutting edge of innovation. Having several people focus on a case at one time gives a sense of the broad possibilities for intervention and offers an opportunity to try things out, get immediate feedback, and correct course if needed. For the trainees behind the mirror, it offers a chance to see many cases in process and to work on formulating intervention. These sessions are usually taped so that work on the case can continue between sessions.

Problems can occur when no one is monitoring and supporting the team's dynamics. Sometimes the treating therapist freezes at the thought of several people watching behind the mirror or becomes so dependent on the team's interventions that they stop feeling as if they are running the session. Of course, this is also a very expensive way to do therapy, because although the patient is charged for only one therapist, many people may be involved.

Although expensive in terms of therapist resources, the team approach has the advantages of many heads being better than one and of using outside observers who are not enmeshed in the family interaction. It seems clear that with a number of team members, the team must generate its own smooth systems functioning, including clear leadership, cooperation, and so on.

SETTING

Family therapy has been carried out in virtually all mental health settings, including child guidance clinics, psychiatric hospitals, emergency rooms (walk-in or crisis clinics), outpatient clinics, juvenile probation offices, domestic relations courts, private offices, schools, social welfare services, and so on. In the past, there have been cases in which entire families have been hospitalized for treatment or for research purposes. Other therapists have carried out treatment in the family's own home.

The issue of effectiveness in relation to location of treatment (e.g., in the hospital/clinic or in the home) has been raised. Some researchers feel that there is no carryover from the office to the home and have described the situation using the metaphor of training in the zoo (i.e., office) versus in the jungle (i.e., home). Although there may be a modicum of truth in this argument, in most countries, practical problems associated with home visits (e.g., time and money) may make this approach a nonissue in the current treatment climate.

TIME, SCHEDULING, AND FEES

Most family therapists will see a family once a week for 45 to 90 minutes. In outpatient settings, a minority of therapists will see a family more than once a week. In inpatient settings, family sessions may be scheduled more frequently. There is nothing sacred about once-a-week scheduling. Because the frequency of sessions is somewhat arbitrary (once a week is the most common), meeting less frequently may be strategically better for some families. In multiple-impact therapy, families are seen on an intensive basis and in different combinations—marital couple, mother and son, whole family, individuals, and so on—over a 2- or 3-day period by various members of a therapy team, consisting of a psychiatrist, a psychologist, a social worker, and a vocational counselor. Techniques focus on bringing about rapid change in the family during this time because its members have come for therapy from distant locations.

The overall duration of treatment depends in part on the treatment goals. On average, family therapy is a short-term method compared with individual or group psychotherapy or psychoanalysis. Other ground rules include the following:

1. Missed appointments should be rescheduled that week, if possible.
2. When one member of the family comes late, the therapist may start the clock at the arranged time and proceed with whoever is present. The therapist can present the position of the absent member. In contrast, many therapists don't start therapy until everyone arrives, in order to put pressure on everyone to come on time.
3. What can be done if one member of the family will not come to treatment? Often the resistance is not only from the member who will not come but also from the other family members who encourage the absence (either covertly or overtly). They may be unaware of their collusion, however, and often ask for help to get the reluctant member to participate. One possibility is for the therapist to contact the absent member.
4. Fees are usually set by time (i.e., the length of the session), not by number of family members present.

KEEPING A RECORD OF TREATMENT

Opinions differ as to the value of keeping written notes on the course of family treatment. Such a record may be useful in monitoring goals and in recording changes. The problem-oriented record modified for families provides a concise overall picture of the identified patient and the family and outlines problems, goals, and strategies. Ongoing progress notes record significant family developments, enable goal achievement to be measured, and provide a record of treatment and modalities used for achieving these goals. Referrals to other agencies are also noted. Such a system has a definite advantage over the traditional practice of keeping a separate record for each family member.

Many therapists focus on the process rather than the content of the sessions and therefore believe that there is no need to write down the details of what goes on. Others prefer not to keep any records of treatment to protect themselves against possible subpoenas. We disagree. Our bias is to keep succinct and relevant records in all cases. We believe, too, that records are very helpful for legal and training purposes.

The American Psychiatric Association has set forth the following guidelines:

> *In family therapy, although it may be preferable to keep records on a family basis, it is usually more practical to keep them in one of the participant's individual charts, as most facilities maintain records in this manner. Since authorization from the patient named in the chart is generally sufficient for the release of information, care must be taken about information included about other family members. Whether or not the record is kept on an individual or a family basis, it may be wise to have all of the involved family members sign a statement at the beginning of therapy acknowledging that it will contain information about all of them and specifying which signatures or combination thereof will be required to authorize access to the chart or release information from it. In the event of substantial family change, such as divorce or a child's reaching majority, particular care should be exercised not to release information inappropriately.*[6]

FAMILY THERAPY IN COMBINATION WITH OTHER PSYCHOSOCIAL THERAPIES

It is becoming more common for the same therapist to use individual psychotherapy sessions combined with family therapy. In this case, the therapist has the advantage of knowing both the individual and the family. This combination, however, changes the nature of the therapy as follows: (1) The patient in individual therapy feels that what they reveal in the one-to-one situation may in some way (either overtly or covertly) be communicated to the family by the therapist; (2) family members may be reluctant to deal with sensitive issues in the conjoint sessions, preferring to reveal them in individual sessions; and (3) transference in individual sessions does not develop as fully because the patient can directly express their feelings about their family in the family therapy. The first two items must be dealt with directly; the last item is not a major problem because in these situations the therapy is usually not transference based. Inexperienced therapists may tend to identify with the individual patient, thus seeing the family from the patient's point of view. For example, the therapist may see all problems as resulting from a cold, passive, authoritarian father and a smoldering, double binding, rejecting mother, and from what the parents have done to the poor patient. This attitude may make it extremely difficult to work conjointly with the whole family.

In addition to conjoint family treatment, individual therapy has been carried out simultaneously in separate sessions with one or both parents. In this case, individual therapy is often carried out by a colleague of the family therapist. It cannot be stressed too strongly that communication between therapists is necessary for effective collaborative treatment.

In the E family, the son, who had chronic schizophrenia, was the identified patient.

He was aged 20 years when he was brought for treatment because he had not left his room for a year. Mr. and Mrs. E were bringing him his meals in bed, and he had stopped attending school. The patient history revealed that there were two older sisters who were functioning well. Mr. and Mrs. E had met 25 years earlier. Mr. E was shy and withdrawn. Mrs. E was handling most of the burden and brought in most of the money. She worked as a cashier. Life for them had been good until the birth of the youngest child—the identified patient—at which point Mr. and Mrs. E stopped having sexual relations (the previous frequency had been about two times per week). Mrs. E said that she was uninformed about contraceptive methods and that because she did not want any more children, the only way she could think of was to stop having sex. Because Mr. E was a noncommunicative person, this issue had not been discussed for 19 years, until their son returned to the hospital.

Treatment intervention was initiated with an individual therapist who prescribed medication for the symptoms of the son's schizophrenia. Once the son's symptoms (negativism and autistic thinking) began to clear, treatment was directed toward his rehabilitation. To this end, and to place the patient in a work setting, the parents had to let him out of the nest. Family meetings were held with the mother, father, sisters, and the identified patient. Mr. and Mrs. E were also seen as a couple to help them rebuild their marital relationship. A series of progressive behavioral exercises markedly improved their sexual relations, which resumed with a satisfactory frequency. After this had occurred, Mr. and Mrs. E helped to find a halfway house for their son.

A major shift in the 1990s was the notion of using different formats over different stages of therapy and periods of time. A common sequence of treatment starts with the couple presenting with a sexual problem. Sexual therapy solves the problem. At this point, marital problems often come to the fore. Marital therapy is then used, and the marital relationship improves. Then one or both members of the couple may decide they want to explore different aspects of their own growth and development; therefore, individual sessions or therapy is scheduled. Numerous variations on this concept are possible, and this kind of sequencing represents an increasing trend. Sugarman[7] described some rules of thumb to follow in making decisions about combined therapy, which are still useful:

> *(1) It is useful if it appears that different modalities would help significantly in different dimensions, such as the biologic, social, and psychological; (2) if it appears that a given modality is either not helpful or of limited usefulness without an additional modality; (3) if there is significant motivation on the part of the individual or family to combine modalities; and (4) if the modalities are synergistic and enhance one another. On the other hand, the following reasons would be contraindications to combining modalities: (1) The epistemologic foundations of the various modalities are often based on contradictory assumptions. Since the goal of clinical work is to provide a coherent cognitive ordering of the world, combining modalities can at times be unproductively confusing for the patient system. (2) The additional time and money involved may be unnecessary.*

A single modality is often powerful enough to accomplish what is therapeutically necessary. (3) Different modalities can dilute the potential catharsis available for each separate therapeutic involvement. To the extent that there is meaning to the concept of psychic energy, it could be divided between the various modalities with not enough available in any one for the "critical mass" necessary to accomplish therapeutic work. This is similar to the concept of "diluting the transference" in psychoanalytic thought.

Practical Guidelines

1. **Diagnosis.** The therapist must be sure to make a DSM-5 diagnosis, a family systems diagnosis, and an individual formulation of dynamics. Without a diagnostic map, the appropriate drug will not be prescribed. Similarly, without a map of the family system dynamics, the clinician will be lost in the complexity of family issues.
2. **Goals.** The therapist must set target symptoms for all modalities. The issue here is to determine which symptoms are responsive to drugs and which are responsive to individual or family interventions. Without this delineation of target symptoms, it is impossible to know which treatment (or combination) is effective.
3. **Untoward effects.** The therapist must be aware of the side effects of drug therapy, family and individual psychotherapy, and their interaction. For example, increasing medications may enable the identified patient to discuss issues that were previously too emotionally charged for careful family discussion. Untoward effects must be monitored at each session. For example, antipsychotic medication may create side effects (e.g., sedation, dysphoria) that not only are unpleasant to the patient but also may decrease the patient's ability to socialize inside and outside the family. In some situations, a patient, with or without the family, may use the improvement that results from medication to avoid exploring relevant family issues. In such cases, the family therapist should continue prescribing medications as necessary rather than discontinuing a treatment that is efficacious.
4. **Contraindications.** The therapist should be aware of situations in which combined family or individual treatment plus medication is contraindicated. Obviously, this combination is not for everyone. We believe in the principle of therapeutic parsimony. If one modality is effective, a second should not be added. To be explicit, for some clinical situations we start with family therapy; for others we start with medication. In still others we start both approaches simultaneously and may withdraw one (or both) modalities over time. Given the shift in the field of psychiatry to psychopharmacology from psychotherapy, family therapy may be the right modality at the right time. At the very least, putting aside the power of a family intervention by itself, the family systems approach is an efficacious way to increase medication compliance.

5. **Sequencing.** The next issue is to sequence the modalities effectively and efficiently. As a first step (usually), a working therapeutic alliance must be established. Medication should be prescribed only after the therapeutic alliance is in place. Simultaneously, if appropriate, the family should be referred to the appropriate consumer group (e.g., National Alliance on Mental Illness, Mental Health Association, Alcoholics Anonymous, Depression and Bipolar Support Alliance). Psychoeducation for the patient (if cognitively able) and the family is a crucial early step. This means the systematic administration over time of information about signs and symptoms, diagnosis, treatment, and prognosis. Individual supportive therapy or family supportive intervention may begin at this point. Only later are dynamic individual or systemic family models used. Later, depending on response, rehabilitation is added to the equation.

Effective Family Intervention

Lam[8] has described seven components of effective family approaches to schizophrenia, but each of these approaches can be adapted to most psychiatric disorders:

1. A positive approach and genuine working relationship between the therapist and family
2. Provision of family therapy in a stable, structured format with the availability of additional contacts with therapists if necessary
3. A focus on improving stress and coping in the here and now, rather than dwelling on the past
4. Encouragement of respect for interpersonal boundaries within the family
5. Provision of information about the biologic nature of the illness in order to reduce blaming of the patient and family guilt
6. Use of behavioral techniques such as breaking down goals into manageable steps
7. Improvement of communication among family members

The essence of the family intervention, when combined with medication, is to educate the family about the disorder (e.g., signs and symptoms, causes, and biologic and psychosocial treatments); provide communication skills training to improve the quality of family transactions and reduce family tension; provide problem-solving skills training for managing family or illness-related conflicts and reducing family burden; and resolve dynamic and systems issues created by the disorder.

The essence of the pharmacologic intervention, when combined with the family intervention, is to normalize the illness (as with lithium in bipolar disorder) and to suppress symptoms in the individual. To summarize, somewhat paradoxically family therapy ultimately and indirectly can promote medication adherence, whereas medication can improve interpersonal function and adherence with family therapy.

Comparison of Therapy Formats and Strategies

Now that we have presented the techniques of family therapy, let us again compare family therapy to individual therapy and to group therapy (see Chapter 1), only this time by type of strategies used. Table 14.1 is an expansion of Table 1.1. It reveals the relevant similarities and differences, but the main issue is to note the most obvious difference—the unit with which the therapist is working: in individual therapy, an individual; in family therapy, members of the same family (broadly defined); and in group therapy, persons who are not members of the same family.

CLINICAL PRACTICE IMPLICATIONS

In this chapter, we try to speak to the most frequent questions trainees have about the intricacies of actually doing therapy. Obviously, not every situation is addressed—the key clinical pearl

Table 14.1 Comparison of therapy formats and strategies

	Strategies		
Therapy format	**Insight-awareness**	**Systemic-strategic**	**Experiential-existential**
Family	Confrontation of family interaction Clarification of interaction Interpretation of conflict	Psychoeducation Assignment of task Marking of boundaries	Empathic contact Exploration of present family experience
Individual	Confrontation Clarification Interpretation	Assignment of individual task Cognitive restructuring Role-playing Desensitization	Empathic contact Exploration of present individual experience
Group	Confrontation of group interaction Interpretation of group and individual transference	Role-playing Behavioral rehearsal Assignment of tasks	Empathic contact Exploration of present group experience

is to remember that family treatment involves "the family" (i.e., it is a way of thinking about a problem). That principle should help in finding solutions to so-called impossible treatment dilemmas.[9]

REFERENCES

1. Josephson AM. Reinventing family therapy: teaching family intervention as a new treatment modality. *Acad Psychiatry*. 2008;32:405–413.
2. Detre T. Some comments on the future of child and adolescent psychiatry. *Acad Psychiatry*. 1989;13:189–191.
3. Lewis JM. For better or worse: interpersonal relationships and individual outcome. *Am J Psychiatry*. 1998;155:582–589.
4. Rice D, Fey W, Kepecs J. Therapist experience and "style" as factors in co-therapy. *Fam Process*. 1972;11:227–238.
5. Hoffman L. *Foundation of Family Therapy: A Conceptual Framework for Systems Change*. Basic Books; 1981.
6. Committee on Confidentiality. Guidelines on confidentiality. *Am J Psychiatry*. 1987;144:1522–1526.
7. Sugarman S, ed. *Interface of Individual and Family Therapy: Family Therapy Collection*. Aspen Publications; 1986.
8. Lam DH. Psychosocial family intervention in schizophrenia: a review of empirical studies. *Psychol Med*. 1991;21:423–441.
9. Zeanah CH, Berlin LJ, Boris NW. Practitioner review: clinical applications of attachment theory and research for infants and young children. *J Child Psychol Psychiatry*. 2011;52:819–833.

Although much overlap exists in the theory and practice of couples therapy and family therapy, for clarity's sake, we focus in this section on issues relevant to couples. In Chapter 15, we review the theory and therapy for couple dysfunction. In Chapter 17, we do the same for various forms of couple relationships. The reader must keep in mind the material from Chapters 2 to 5, which are focused on different forms of couples and marriage. For didactic reasons, we separate sexual issues from other couples issues and focus on couples and sex therapy in Chapter 16.

Section

V Couples Therapy

15 Dysfunctional Couples and Couples Therapy 193

16 Sex, Couples, and Sex Therapy 204

17 Couples and Families Breaking Apart: Separation and Divorce 215

15 Dysfunctional Couples and Couples Therapy

OBJECTIVES FOR THE READER

- To understand couples, marriage, and couples therapy in historical context
- To understand characteristics of distressed couples
- To be able to outline general guidelines for assessing couples
- To be able to outline strategies and techniques of couples therapy

For easier reading, we emphasize that the descriptors "couples" or "marital" are used nearly interchangeably in this chapter.

INTRODUCTION

Couples, both married and unmarried, form the essential subsystem of the nuclear family and a system in its own right. How this dyad functions and copes will determine in large measure how the family progresses over time. In Chapters 3 and 4, we considered how families function (and introduced the idea of dysfunction), with a special focus on how the couple coalition arises from the family of origin. In this chapter, we start with a historical perspective on marriage and then consider specific dimensions and patterns of dysfunction in the couple dyad in order to formulate couple therapy goals and strategies.

> *There is good data that couples therapy is effective for both heterosexual or same sex couples, in addition, "there is an ethical obligation to work with the partner should the relationship distress be present."*
>
> —*Reibstein and Burbach*[1]

MARRIAGE IN ITS HISTORICAL CONTEXT
COUPLES DIFFICULTIES, PROBLEMS, AND DYSFUNCTION
From a Dynamic Point of View
From a Behavioral Point of View
From a Systems Point of View
From a Psychiatric Illness Point of View
Couples' Development Dysfunction
COUPLES THERAPY
The Issue of Commitment—The Problem of Affairs
Evaluation of Partners

Goals
Strategies and Techniques of Intervention
A Model for Intervention Based on Patterns of Interaction
Individual Models
Strategies and Techniques
CLINICAL PRACTICE IMPLICATIONS

MARRIAGE IN ITS HISTORICAL CONTEXT

Before talking about couples in its variety of forms, we will take a look at marriage in its historical context. The marital relationship in all societies is a peculiar combination of the most idiosyncratic and intimate and the most culturally patterned of relationships. Each society varies in its emphasis on the external aspects of the marriage (e.g., the mechanism for the transfer of property and privilege and for management of paternity) and on the intimate aspects (e.g., the friendship, love, and sexual issues binding the couple). In general, the more Westernized the culture, the more free is marital choice and the more important are issues of love and intimacy. Even so, strong cultural sanctions within one's race or class remain.

Westernized marriages are today characterized by freedom to choose a spouse, equality in terms of marriage vows (although not necessarily of roles), emancipation from relatives, and an increased emphasis on intimacy. The issue of power inequality in relationships bound by love is complex.[2] Reasons for inequality in heterosexual couples include man's greater power in the culture, his greater physical strength, and the fact that marital choice often involves women marrying men who are older and more financially successful. Power differential is also found in LGBT couples and in fact, violence is common in lesbian relationships The CDC has stated that 43.8% of lesbian women reported experiencing physical violence, stalking, or rape by their partners. The study notes that, out of those 43.8%, two-thirds (67.4%) reported exclusively female perpetrators. Similarly, 61.1% of bisexual women reported physical violence, stalking, or rape by their partners in the same study with 89.5% reporting at least one perpetrator being male. In contrast, 35% of heterosexual women reported having been victim of intimate partner violence, with 98.7% of them reporting male perpetrators exclusively (Walters, Mikel L., Jieru Chen, and Matthew J. Breiding. The National Intimate Partner and Sexual Violence Survey (NISVS): 2010 findings on victimization by sexual orientation. National Center for Injury Prevention and Control, Centers for Disease Control and Prevention 648, no. 73(2013):6).[3]

Marriage is also distinguished among family relationships by its voluntary nature. That is, although you can never truly be an exparent or an exchild, it is possible to be an exspouse, to choose to sever the relationship. The voluntary nature of the relationship lends to it a particular complexity that is central to treatment.

The treatment implication for the clinician working with couples both married and unmarried, is that treatment is effective for heterosexual or same-sex couples. "In addition, there is an ethical obligation to work with the partner should relationship distress be present."[1]

COUPLES DIFFICULTIES, PROBLEMS, AND DYSFUNCTION

As we suggested in Chapters 3 and 4, some periods of couples dysfunction are inevitable in any long-term relationship. The burden of carrying intimate, social, and parenting roles means that people will inevitably clash over some aspects of life. It is common for long-term relationships to undergo periodic stages of crisis and reorganization. Problems occur when couples lose faith in the marriage or lose a sense of respect and warmth/intimacy for each other. Partners who have had poor role models, who have had a childhood of loss and violence, or who are poorly suited to each other by style or inclination may have increasing problems as time goes by.

A number of theories, not mutually exclusive, attempt to explain how couples become conflicted to the point of impairment. Although certain models may explain marital or couple conflict, they do not by themselves predict dissolution. The decision to dissolve a relationship is determined not only by the amount of conflict but also by a set of societal issues—the prevailing attitudes toward divorce and how easy it is to obtain, issues regarding money, the presence of children, and the individuals' assessment of whether life would be better single. Many couples in severe conflict remain together for complex reasons, living separate emotional lives without divorcing. Certainly, for children, the experiences of divorce and of living in a high-conflict home are both poor arrangements. Many high-conflict couples also have a great deal of positive intensity and passion for each other. Many low-conflict couples are indifferent to each other. John Gottman,[4] who has extensively researched divorce prediction, lists criticism, contempt, defensiveness, and stonewalling which lead to intense marital negativity, as highly predictive of divorce. Although certain models may explain marital conflict, they do not by themselves predict divorce.

Individuals come to marriage with the legacy of their several-generation family of origin plus the beliefs and role models of their parents. This means they carry with them firm ideas about what marriage should be like, how men and women should behave, and what behaviors signify love and respect.

From a developmental point of view, there remain unresolved needs and demands left from a childhood invested with deeply ambivalent feelings of love and hate. In the process of mate selection, a partner may be attractive partly because they promise rediscovery of an important lost aspect of the subject's own personality or because they offer the chance to redo an unfinished conflict with a parent. When the couple joins, they make a contract, in which each partner assumes they and the other partner will each do certain things. Some of these assumptions are conscious and shared (e.g., you will care for the children and I will work); some are not shared; and some are secret, even from the self. For example, a person may marry to get away from home or may believe that as long as they act like a good child their spouse will act like a good mother. Mate selection, of course, is also determined by less dynamic reasons such as physical attractiveness, family demands, financial considerations, timing, and luck. As Lewis[5] has pointed out, relationships fail "when either the person who is more powerful feels unrewarded for that responsibility, or the person with lesser power feels that they've had enough of that relatively powerless situation."

Treatment involves increasing the intensity of the affective bonds and repairing the inevitable disruption of those bonds. That is "each spouse must have someone who listens to our experience (i.e., the 'narratives') and helps to sort them out. The prerequisites include a genuine and reciprocal liking for each other, mutual respect, a two-way valuing and affirmation."[5] Lewis suggests that couples need to learn conflict management mechanisms, including techniques to prevent isolation. Couple communication style (i.e., how people talk to each other) is a critical variable in affecting couple satisfaction and function. To help prevent disconnections, the therapist must teach intimate communication (focusing on how to explore difficult issues and increase empathy).

Let's now examine couple dysfunction through the lens of various psychotherapy models.

From a Dynamic Point of View

Many individuals who need assistance with couple/marriage conflict seem to have a rigidity in their personalities that forces them to deny or be blind to the existence of certain aspects of themselves. If they are confronted with a similar aspect of the partner's personality, they will ignore it or not accept it. Such people may project onto the partner aspects of their own personality with which they are uncomfortable. They are therefore prevented from seeing the problem clearly or seeking alternative solutions. Often third parties are used to deflect conflict between the partners.

Gender differences in needs and communication often make marital problems more complex. In traditional marriages, men are more likely to wish for deference, to wish to deal with their problems by themselves first before talking about them, and to see sex as a way of solving problems. Women are more likely to wish for verbal intimacy and task equality, to prefer handling problems by discussion and feeling talk first rather than moving immediately to solutions, and to prefer sex after intimate connection has been re-established. Women tend to experience the emotional burden of the relationship as falling on themselves. Men tend to see themselves as more responsible for the family's finances even when the wife is working. Therefore, in a fairly high number of cases, the woman will find herself emotionally pursuing and sexually unhappy; the man will find himself criticized for his need to be less emotional even though he has been trained to control most of his feelings. Obviously, many individuals do not fit these traditional gender stereotypes.

As couples struggle over different ways of behaving or different and ambivalent needs, each person may see the other as unhelpful or bad and begins to become angry, thus creating a cycle of distress.

From a Behavioral Point of View

Distressed couples engage in fewer rewarding exchanges and more punishing exchanges than do nondistressed couples. Distressed couples are more likely to reciprocate each other's use of negative reinforcement and eventually go on the offensive by increasing the level of punishment regardless of the stimuli. Distressed couples are likely to attempt to control each other's behavior through negative communication and the withholding of positive communication. They strive for behavior change in the other by aversive control tactics, that is, by strategically presenting punishment and withholding rewards.

From a Systems Point of View

From a systems point of view, the solution becomes the problem—that is, more aversive control (e.g., silence or attack) produces more aversive behavior in the spouse rather than the longed-for connection. In addition, triangles may form to deflect conflict, so that children, friends, parents, or lovers are drawn into the marital conflict.

From a Psychiatric Illness Point of View

Having a spouse with a serious illness, such as anxiety disorder, mood disorder, or substance abuse, puts strain on the couple/marital relationship. The couple/marital interaction before, during, and after the onset of the symptoms in the spouse is influenced by numerous factors and varies greatly across dyads. It is false to assume that in all cases the interaction between the spouses brought on, caused, or even helped trigger the mental disorder and symptoms. Whatever the symptoms in one spouse, the relationship of symptoms to the couple/marital interaction is on a continuum and can take any one of the following forms:

- The couple/marital interaction neither causes the symptoms nor stresses the psychologically vulnerable spouse.
- The couple/marital interaction does not stress the vulnerable individual, but after the onset of symptoms, the marital interaction declines and becomes dysfunctional, thus causing more distress.
- The couple/marital interaction acts as a stressor that contributes to the onset of symptoms in a vulnerable spouse.
- The symptoms can be explained totally as under the control and function of the interactional patterns between the spouses.

The therapist meeting a new couple therefore can entertain a range of ideas that may help illuminate and explain the couple's distressing circumstances. In the next section, we offer guidelines for assessing and treating couples. Although these guidelines do not cover all couples' problems and situations, they represent a general set of ideas that therapists may apply to the specifics of many couple/marital issues.

Couples' Development Dysfunction

Dym[6] has described how couples' relationships evolve over time.

Members of couples are influenced by past and present relationships and tend to form ties that have a distinct character that emerges through regular cycles of conflict and resolution. Dym draws attention to broad, normative changes in couples, characterizing these developmental shifts as periods of expansion, contraction, and resolution. For example, in the early, expansive years of a committed, romantic relationship, the lives of two are, in a sense, woven into one, moving from "I" to "we."

Dym describes a predictable stage of contraction and a feeling of betrayal in the next years of the relationship, in which members of the couple reconnect with a need for an "I." This desire can be marked by experiences of doubts, fears, and insecurities, and many couples retreat from their established routines. Partners may find themselves feeling out of sync with their own personal ambitions, describe themselves as feeling trapped or lonely, and believe they are progressing at different tempos from each other. Stormy times may ensue with bitter conflict and blame. During the resolution stage, couples may resort to compromise, negotiation, or even a more radical restructuring of their relationship in an effort to make room for both the individual and the relationship. This cyclical movement from expansion to contraction to resolution repeats several times over the course of the relationship. Dym notes that many couples have what he calls a home base where they tend to reside, in terms of the sense of "we," "I," or "working on it." A home base is the point in the cycle of expansion and contraction at which the couples find themselves most often. For many couples, patterns of commitment, intimacy, and passion interact over time.

COUPLES THERAPY

Marital or couples therapy can be defined as a format of intervention involving both members of a dyad in which the focus of intervention is the problematic interactional patterns of the couple. Its similarities to family therapy are so numerous that the differences have often been overlooked. **The focus of couples therapy is on the dyad and its intimate emotional and sexual aspects, whereas family therapy is usually focused on issues involving behavior of a child or adolescent and the interactions between parents and children.** In family therapy, one can discern triangles involving various family members, whereas in couples therapy, triangles in the family must be inferred and triangulation in the here-and-now interaction must involve the therapist (because only two family members are present). In couples therapy, although the children may be invited during the initial assessment or later for specific issues, usually only the spouses attend the sessions. Couples therapy is distinguished by the peer relationship of the participants, the ever-present questions of commitment, and a need to carefully attend to gender issues. In general, even if behaviorally focused, couples therapy must attend particularly to the feeling level, with the goals being positive feeling between the partners and more reasonable behavior.

The Issue of Commitment—The Problem of Affairs

Infidelity is one of the most difficult problems to address in couple therapy, most likely because it involves a traumatic relationship event that alters the ways in which couples process information about each other and established behavioral patterns. However, the first step is to assess what the couple's understanding of fidelity means. Some couples accept affairs as a normal part of their relationship but they may have specific parameters about, for example, where the affair takes place and who knows. For most couples however, affairs are unacceptable and is a common reason for attending therapy. Affairs occur in relationships at the rate of 40% for men and 20% for women.

Coop Gordon and colleagues[7] present a three-stage treatment designed to address the cognitive, behavioral, and emotional sequelae of affairs that integrates cognitive-behavioral and insight-oriented strategies with the literature on traumatic response and forgiveness.

- Step one: Dealing with the impact
- Stage two: Exploring context and finding meaning
- Stage three: Moving on

For more details, see Coop Gordon K, Baucom DH, Snyder DK. An integrative intervention for promoting recovery from extramarital affairs. *J Marital Fam Ther.* 2004;30(2):213–231.

Evaluation of Partners

With the obvious modification of focusing mainly on the marital dyad, the outline for family evaluation we proposed in Chapter 6 can be used for the evaluation of a couple seeking assistance with their troubled relationship. This involves obtaining data on the current point in the couple and family life cycle, why the couple comes for assistance at this point in time, and each partner's views of the marital problem. In formulating the marital difficulty, the evaluator will want to consider the couple's communication, problem solving, roles, affective expression and involvement, and behavioral expression, especially in sexual and aggressive areas. The clinician will also want to evaluate gender roles, cultural and racial issues, and power inequities resulting from gender, class, age, or financial status. It is critical to ask about alcohol and substance misuse, general health, reproductive issues, and intimate partner violence. Even if the partners do not mention their children as a problem, it is wise to spend some time developing a sense of how the children are doing, whether there are favorites or problems with any of them, and whether the children are being pulled into couple conflicts. The clinician should ascertain whether a diagnosable psychiatric illness is present in either partner.

Several areas, included in the above-mentioned general categories, deserve special evaluation attention. Such areas include each spouse's commitment to the marital union and the couple's sexual life. Assessment is complicated when one spouse is keeping commitment doubts or extramarital sex secret. Conjoint and individual assessment interviews with each partner may be needed. Infidelity or serious commitment questions change the character of the couple therapy from one of how the couple manages to whether or not the couple stays together.

The complicated issue of how the therapist can get information about the degree of commitment and ongoing marital affairs, as well as other private information, can be handled in various ways. We recommend that as part of the marital evaluation the therapist hold one individual session with each partner after the first or second conjoint session. These sessions are usually considered confidential. However, the therapist may reserve the right not to continue treatment unless the spouse tells the partner relevant information, such as about an ongoing affair or HIV-positive status. The therapist may give the partner a few weeks or an extra session to plan for this disclosure but is not obligated to do therapy in situations in which such a secret makes therapeutic work impossible. Although some therapists prefer not to know certain secrets, it is our belief that to proceed with therapy in the face of an overwhelming secret as if it did not exist is futile. If the information (e.g., incest, violence, alcohol abuse) is known to the couple but is kept secret from the therapist at the wish of the erring partner, it is also best that the therapist hear it early, in private session, and find a way to bring it into the couples work.

It is often difficult to determine whether couples therapy is the treatment of choice and whether other therapy should be given concurrently or sequentially. For example, one partner may need concurrent medication or may be having enough other problems with work, their parents, or their own personality difficulties that no energy is left for couples work. In general, couples who come in for therapy together should be given evaluation, support, and perhaps education—plus a clear picture of how the couple's issues connect with the individual issues. If appropriate, partners may be sent for concurrent individual therapy or may be asked to have individual therapy first and return for couples work later.

The couples therapist may do individual work concurrently or work on individual issues in the couples setting. Some clinicians recommend that the same therapist not do individual work with only one partner and then do the couples work, because the therapist tends to become more bonded to the person with whom they do the individual work. Others believe that the advantage of one therapist knowing the systems' issues—that is, doing both the individual and the marital therapy—outweighs this disadvantage. As of now, we recommend it as an option.

Couples in which active violence has been present are not candidates for couples work unless the therapist believes that the couple can hold to a clear contract that no violence will occur during the therapy.

Goals

The mediating goals of couples therapy that uses an integrative model include the following: specification of the interactional problems, recognition of mutual contribution to the problems, clarification of marital boundaries, clarification and specification of each spouse's needs and desires in the relationship, increased communication skills, decreased coercion and blame, increased differentiation, and resolution of marital transference distortions. Final goals of the marital intervention may involve resolution of presenting problems, reduction of symptoms, increased intimacy, increased role flexibility and adaptability, toleration of differences, improved psychosexual functioning, balance of power, clear communication, resolution of conflictual interaction, and improved relationships with children and families of origin.[8] Couples therapy is often conceived of as a relatively brief therapy (though it need not be), usually meeting on a once-weekly basis, with a focus on the marital interaction. Sometimes bringing in the parents or children of one or both spouses may be beneficial for addressing issues affecting the marriage. The major indication for marital intervention is the presence of marital conflict to which both parties contribute, but other indications include symptomatic behavior such as depression or agoraphobia in one spouse.

We discuss specific guidelines in Section VII. If the couples therapy seems to consistently escalate conflict, then the goals should be reevaluated.

Strategies and Techniques of Intervention

Like family therapy in general, couples therapy uses strategies for imparting new information and opening up new and expanded individual and marital experiences, psychodynamic strategies for individual and interactional insight, communication and problem-solving strategies, and strategies for restructuring the repetitive interactions between the spouses. As the divisive spirit of earlier schools of psychotherapy recedes and a sense of pluralism and clinical pragmatism grows, clinicians will attempt to integrate the various strategies into a coherent treatment approach that can be adapted to individual couples. We advocate an integrative marital therapy model that uses psychodynamic, cognitive-behavioral, and structural-strategic strategies of intervention.

A Model for Intervention Based on Patterns of Interaction

Although couples may exhibit conflict over specific content issues, such as handling finances, spending time together, and reconciling individual and family needs, the therapist is usually confronted with repetitive patterns of interaction that will likely become the focus for treatment. For example, in one couple, the wife may try to explain something important to her husband about her need to feel emotionally connected to him; he reacts negatively to her tone of voice (saying he feels criticized) and retreats; she responds by suggesting that he is simply pushing her away and feels unloved; and so on. This pattern of pursuit withdrawal might well occupy the attention of the therapist, who notices that it occurs irrespective of the particular topic of conversation.

Other patterns involve either complementarity or symmetry in relationships.

In complementary relationships, the overfunctioning of one member may invite the underfunctioning of the other (e.g., responsible–irresponsible, nurse–patient). Because the pattern is reciprocal, the pattern description can be reversed; that is, the underfunctioning of one member may invite the overfunctioning of the other. In symmetrical relationships, the therapist encounters a power struggle in which each member is engaged in asserting their own position in order to gain the one-up position or to avoid feeling one-down.

As we said previously, Marital history and the presence of psychiatric illness will influence the planning of intervention. For example, if one spouse has major depression with no clear precipitating stressful life events, the marital interaction could be a chronic stressor and contributor to the condition. Marital therapy in this situation could well be a preferred mode of intervention. In contrast, if the spouse has a bipolar illness and experiences a manic episode, and the marital interaction was good prior to the episode, psychoeducational intervention with the couple may be in order with little or no attention to the ongoing marital interaction.

Sometimes couples have chronic histories of unresolved and unrelenting conflict. Other couples are in a state of transition, perhaps moving from the initial expansion stage of their marriage to the inevitable crisis related to the reevaluation of the contraction stage. In either case, clarifying the couples' process, that is, their reoccurring patterns of behavior, represents the starting place for couples therapy. We discuss how to interrupt these patterns in a later section.

Individual Models

Once the therapist understands the couple's specific problem and has defined it as a pattern that each partner helps to maintain, the goal is to find out what keeps the couple from making needed changes. It can generally be assumed that patterns are developed from the partners' individual models of marriage, learned in their families and in prior relationships and by their own traditions of relating to each other as a couple. In considering historical models, the therapist might suppose that each member of a couple brings their own images or model of how intimate relationships should proceed. The therapist can collect and organize historical data through the use of a genogram, the three-generational family tree that depicts the family's patterns regarding either specific problems or general family functioning (see Chapter 7). The genogram technique suggests possible connections between present family events and the prior experiences that family members have shared (e.g., regarding the management of serious illnesses, losses, and other critical transitions), thereby placing the presenting problem in a historical context.[9,10] The construction of a genogram early in treatment can provide a wealth of data that offers clues about the couple's pressures, expectations, and hopes regarding the marriage. This pictorial way of gathering a history allows each partner to learn about beliefs or themes that characterize their family background.

Based on the couple's own idiosyncratic experiences as individuals, the therapist can then try to help them understand how their own preferred patterns (which may relate to earlier family models) have limited their ability to adapt and change. The predictability with which they will respond to unmet needs and disappointments can be pointed out supportively so that the partners begin to understand the specific ways they each reenact the same process over and over again. If this is all the couple knows, they may become despondent at recognizing the limitations of their emotional–behavioral repertoire. However, with support and active interventions, the couple's therapist can begin to help the couple conduct experiments with each other aimed at expanding their ways of relating.

Strategies and Techniques

Like family therapy in general, couples therapy uses an array of techniques meant to create new experiences and new understanding for the couple. Although each school of couples and family therapy advocates its own emphasis on particular aspects of the change process (e.g., changing the couple's beliefs or cognitions, changing behavioral sequences, increasing differentiation, expanding emotional awareness), some relatively enduring characteristics can be identified among most marital therapies. The focus should be primarily on the interpersonal distortions between the couple and not on the couple–therapist transference. However, negative transference distortions toward the therapist must be addressed quickly and overtly. There are three strategies in this focused, active treatment of marital discord:

1. The therapist interrupts collusive processes between the spouses. The interaction may involve either spouse failing to perceive positive or negative aspects of the other (e.g., cruelty, generosity) that are clear to an outsider or it may involve either spouse behaving in a way aimed at protecting the other from experiences that are inconsistent with the spouse's self-perception (e.g., the husband working part time views himself as the breadwinner, but the wife works full time and manages the checkbook to shield her husband from the reality of their income and finances).
2. The therapist links individual experience, including past experience and inner thoughts, to the marital relationship.
3. The therapist creates and gives tasks that are constructed (a) to encourage the spouses to differentiate between the other's intent and the effect of their behavior, (b) to bring into awareness the concrete behavior of the partner that contradicts past perceptions of that partner, and (c) to encourage each spouse to acknowledge their own behavior changes that are incompatible with the maladaptive ways they have seen themselves and has been seen by the marital partner. These tasks also help to make the couple's narrative more positive. The last task is the most important. In the initial stage of marital treatment we ask that each partner focus on what they want to change in themselves, not how they want the other spouse to be different. Gurman's[8] integrative marital therapy model assumes that effective marital treatment does not artificially dichotomize individual and relationship change; rather it focuses on both. The model assumes that not all of one spouse's behaviors are under the interactional control of the other spouse, and even behavior with obvious relationship to the marital interaction is not completely under relational control. Furthermore, Gurman[8] asserts that the adoption of a systems perspective does not preclude attention to unconscious aspects of experience. Self-perceptions are the mechanisms that power the behavior-maintaining aspects of interpersonal reinforcement.

In Gurman's integrative model, the goals of assessment are to evaluate three related domains: "the functional relationships between the antecedents and consequences of discrete interactional sequences; the recurrent patterns of interaction including their implicit rules; and each spouse's individual schemata for intimate relationships. In the initial stage, alliances must be developed early between the therapist and each marital partner, with the therapist offering empathy, warmth, and understanding. The therapist must also ally with the couple as a whole and learn their shared language and their different problem-solving styles and attitudes"[8] (p. 434).

Behavioral techniques, including giving between-session homework, in-session tasks, and communication skills and problem-solving training, can help marital partners reintegrate denied aspects of themselves and of each other. However, the focus is not on behavioral change alone, because overt behavior is seen as reflecting the interlocking feelings and perceptions of each spouse. Ideally, the process of treatment should allow each partner to consider what they want to change in themselves as opposed to how they want the other spouse to be different; to safely explore new beliefs, feelings, and behaviors; and to experiment with new patterns of interaction that are unfamiliar and even anxiety provoking.

> *"Topics at issue between couples typically remain the same over many years. Psychoeducation is most helpful when it enables couples to label as entirely normal their continuing efforts to grapple with the same set of issues over a lifetime."*
>
> *—Lebow (1999, p. 172)*[11]

Beginning therapists sometimes feel more at ease when they have a set of questions that can help them to organize the session and the overall structure of the treatment. Table 15.1 offers one model that has been successful for advanced trainees (D. Rait, unpublished manuscript).

Table 15.1 Guidelines for interviewing couples—The process

Questions	Rationale
Can you tell me about yourself? As individuals? As a couple?	Joining, forming an alliance with each member and the couple, creating a safe place
What brings you here? How do you understand the problem? What feelings does it elicit for each of you?	Developing an interactional problem focus
How does the problematic pattern actually work? Can you show me how it works?	Observing by staging an enactment
How did this pattern originate? How did you create it?	Placing the problem in context of their relationship, families of origin, and individual development
How have you maintained this pattern? What have you done to keep it going?	Placing the pattern or problem under their joint control
Tell me about what you believe should be happening	Revealing myths, stories, ideas, and expectations about love, sexuality, marriage, and closeness
In what other ways is the pattern currently reinforced? What do your family and friends believe is the problem?	Reflecting how jobs, extended family members, and friends contribute to the pattern's resilience
Is this pattern always occurring or are there exceptions?	Demonstrating how pervasive the pattern is (i.e., whether it is chronic or related to a life transition)
What have you done to try to change the pattern?	Trying to avoid redundancy by inquiring about solution behavior
Have your efforts to change the pattern made things better or worse?	Looking at the problem as attempted solutions
What has been the influence of this problem in your lives?	Looking for the influence of the problem over their lives
How motivated are you to change the pattern now?	Assessing individual's and couple's motivation
What would happen if you succeeded in changing the pattern?	Anticipating possible consequences of change, both positive and negative
What patterns of relating have you created that you want to keep?	Identifying and honoring assets and resources
Are you ready to make a change? How about trying something different?	Preparing the couple for exploring new patterns of interaction

The table includes sample questions with the specific rationale for each set of questions. After the interview, the therapist is then free to track themes (always keeping an interactional focus), invent tasks and experiments designed to provide new experiences for the couple, and evaluate the changes that occur or do not occur as a result of the couple's efforts to change their patterns of interaction.

CLINICAL PRACTICE IMPLICATIONS

In a nationwide survey of family therapists, couple problems were identified as the most common presenting problem seen in their practices.[12]

Couples therapy also represents the most common pathway for many trainees to initially explore the field of couple and family therapy. At the same time, there is little question that developing the skills needed to work successfully with couples who present with a wide range of difficulties requires an understanding of how normal couples' relationships change over time, how problems emerge and are maintained, and how focused marital treatment can alleviate distress and dysfunction. The rewards are great when therapists can assist couples in recognizing and shifting the patterns that inhibit their abilities to live rich, intimate lives together.

REFERENCES

1. Reibstein J, Burbach F. An increasingly convincing case for couples therapy. *J Fam Ther.* 2013;35:225–228.
2. Goldner V, Penn P, Sheinberg M, Walker G. Love and violence: gender paradoxes in volatile attachments. *Fam Process*. 1990;29:343–364.
3. Walters ML, Chen J, Breiding MJ. The National Intimate Partner and Sexual Violence Survey (NISVS): 2010 Findings on Victimization by Sexual Orientation. Atlanta, GA: National Center for Injury Prevention and Control, Centers for Disease Control and Prevention. 2013.
4. Gottman J. *Why Marriages Succeed or Fail*. Simon & Schuster; 1994:68–102.
5. Lewis JM. For better or worse: interpersonal relationships and individual outcome. *Am J Psychiatry*. 1998; 155:582–589.
6. Dym B, Glenn ML. *Couples*. Guilford; 1993.
7. Coop Gordon K, Baucom DH, Snyder DK. An integrative intervention for promoting recovery from extramarital affairs. *J Marital Fam Ther.* 2004;30(2):213–231.
8. Gurman A. Integrative marital therapy: toward the development of an interpersonal approach. In: Budman S, ed. *Forms of Brief Therapy*. Guilford; 1981:415–457.
9. McGoldrick M, Gerson R. *Genograms in Family Assessment*. WW Norton; 1985.
10. Shorter E. *The Making of the Modern Family*. Basic Books; 1977.
11. Lebow JL. Building a science of couple relationships: comments on two articles by Gottman and Levenson. *Fam Process.* 1999;38:167–173.
12. Rait D. Family therapy practice survey. *The Family Therapy Networker*. 1988;1:52–56.

16 Sex, Couples, and Sex Therapy

OBJECTIVES FOR THE READER

- To be able to illustrate the connections between sexual problems and other family problems
- To understand the relationship between couples therapy and sex therapy
- To understand techniques of sex therapy and how they can be included in couples therapy

For easier reading, we emphasize that the descriptors "couples" or "marital" are used nearly interchangeably in this chapter.

INTRODUCTION

Sometimes specific problems in sexual functioning affect the couple's relationship. In this chapter, we look at issues of couples' sexuality and the evolving ways in which couples and sex therapy can be combined. Although DSM-5 (American Psychiatric Association, 2022[1]) and most of the early sex therapists make a dichotomous distinction between sexual function and dysfunction, sexuality is probably best thought of as a set of experiences on a continuum of satisfaction. It is possible, for example, to have a sexual life in which sexual arousal and orgasm occur, but the experience feels passionless and boring. The same functioning couple could have more passionate and exciting sex after therapy. It is possible to have an erotic sexual experience even if dysfunction is present (e.g., the male partner cannot achieve erection because of a physical illness) but the couple uses other methods of sexual expression. It is possible to have a good sexual experience even if there are serious arguments between the couple about the frequency or type of sexual practice.

It has been estimated that 50% of American marriages have some sexual problems. These problems can be divided into *difficulties* (such as inability to agree on frequency), which are clearly dyadic issues, and *dysfunctions*, which are specific problems with desire, arousal, and orgasm. Dysfunctions may be organic or psychological or a combination of both and may be lifelong or acquired, generalized or situational. They may be deeply embedded in relational power or intimacy struggles or may be the only problem in an otherwise well-functioning relationship. Although most family therapists believe that there is no uninvolved partner when one member of a couple presents with sexual dysfunction, that is different from saying that the relationship itself is the cause of the dysfunction. The family therapist's job is to ascertain as best as possible the etiology of the problem and to choose the most effective therapy, whether medical, individual, or relational. It is also within the therapist's purview to enquire about whether the couple would like to improve a technically functional but not very satisfying sexual relationship, in the same way that the therapist can offer to increase intimacy in a couple that wishes personal growth.

> The family therapist's job is to ascertain as best as possible the etiology of the problem and to choose the most effective therapy, whether medical, individual, or relational, or some combination.

DIAGNOSIS—SYSTEMS ISSUES
SOME PARAMETERS OF SEXUAL FUNCTION
ASSESSMENT OF SEXUAL DISORDER
TREATMENT
- Lack of Desire
- Erectile Disorder
- Premature (Early) Ejaculation
- Painful Intercourse/Female Orgasmic Disorder
- Sex Addiction and Pornography

OTHER ISSUES RELATED TO SEXUALITY AND COUPLES
- The Spectrum of Sexuality
  - *Overview*
  - *Marital Issues in Gay or Bisexual Individuals*
- Sexual Functioning After Rape or Sexual Abuse
- Sexual Problems After Medical Illness
- Sexual Problems in the Elderly

CLINICAL PRACTICE IMPLICATIONS

DIAGNOSIS—SYSTEMS ISSUES

Sexual dysfunction or dissatisfaction is primarily caused by a psychiatric disorder (although depression and anxiety may often decrease sexual desire). It is commonly caused by ignorance of sexual anatomy and physiology; negative attitudes and self-defeating behavior; anger, power, or intimacy issues with the partners; or medical conditions. Male erection problems have contributing physiologic causes and are amenable to medical treatment. It is important to remember that people vary enormously in the importance they place on the sexual, or erotic, in their lives. For example, according to Laumann and Michael,[2] about one-third of the people surveyed for their book had sex at least twice a week, about one-third a few times a month, and the rest had sex with a partner a few times a year or not at all. In general, when sex is not part of a marriage over a long period of time, the relationship has less vitality and life. However, even well-functioning relationships may have periods in which sexuality is much less a part of the couple's lives (such as after the birth of a child or during a family crisis). Different people have different tolerances for such periods.

SOME PARAMETERS OF SEXUAL FUNCTION

Healthy sexual functioning can be thought of as resulting from relatively nonconflicted and self-confident attitudes about sex and the belief that the partner is pleased by one's performance. In such a situation, a reinforcing positive cycle can be activated. When either partner has doubts about their sexual abilities or ability to please the other, the partner's sexual performance may suffer. This self-absorption and anxiety will characteristically produce a decrease in sexual performance and enjoyment and can lead to an inability to have sex or orgasmic difficulties. Couple or individual difficulties might then follow. A vicious circle may be activated, with worries being increased, leading to increasingly poor sexual performance.

Because each person is vulnerable to the other during sex, it is difficult to have sex when one is angry or not in a mood to be close (although some people can block out other feelings and keep the sexual area of their lives more separate). In addition, people who feel abused, mistreated, or ignored in a relationship are less likely to want to please their partner. For partners who feel that they have no voice in the relationship, lack of desire is sometimes the only way they feel able to manifest displeasure.

Couples that continue in marital or individual treatment for long periods of time can resolve some of their marital problems but can still experience specific sexual difficulties in their marriage. These difficulties may be reversed dramatically after relatively brief periods of sex therapy, even though such problems may have proven intractable following long periods of more customary psychotherapy. Sexual functioning that is suffering because the partners do not want to be close is not likely to respond to sex therapy unless other issues are also addressed.

Usually, when a married couple has a generally satisfactory relationship, any minor sexual problems may be only temporary. Resolution of sexual problems in a relationship, however, will not inevitably produce positive effects in other facets of a relationship.

Couple and sexual problems interact in various ways:

1. **The sexual dysfunction produces or contributes to secondary couple discord.** Specific strategies focused on the sexual dysfunctions would usually be considered the treatment of choice in these situations, especially if the same sexual dysfunction occurred in the person's other relationships.
2. **The sexual dysfunction is secondary to couple discord.** In such situations, general strategies of couples treatment might be considered the treatment of choice. If the marital relationship is not disrupted too severely, a trial of sex therapy might be attempted because relatively rapid relief of symptoms could produce beneficial effects on the couple's interest in pursuing other marital issues.
3. **Couple discord co-occurs with sexual problems.** This situation would probably not be amenable to sex therapy because of the partners' hostility to each other. Couple therapy would usually be attempted first, with later attention given to sexual dysfunction.
4. **Sexual dysfunction occurs without couple discord.** This situation might occur when one partner's medical illness has affected their sexual functioning, forcing the couple to learn new ways to manage the change. Another example might be when one partner has had a history of sexual abuse or a sexual assault that creates anxiety related to the sexual experience. Although individual therapy can be helpful in these situations, couples therapy can be especially useful in creating a safe place to address painful feelings and anxious expectations and to provide education and guidance for couples undergoing these transitions.

> When sexuality functions well in a marriage, it's a positive, integral component. However, when sexuality is dysfunctional or nonexistent, it plays an inordinately powerful role, robbing the marriage of intimacy and vitality.[3]

ASSESSMENT OF SEXUAL DISORDER

The therapist needs to evaluate carefully all of the couple's interactions and to conduct a physical assessment if dysfunction is present. If the basic couple appears to be a sound one but the couple experiences specific sexual difficulties (which may also lead to various secondary couple consequences), the primary focus might be sex therapy *per se*. In many cases, however, specific sex therapy cannot be carried out until the relationship between the two partners has improved in other respects. The sexual problems may clearly be an outgrowth of the couple difficulties. When marital problems are taken care of, the sexual problems may be resolved readily. It may be difficult to disentangle couple from sexual problems or to decide which came first. The priorities for therapy may not always be clear.

Aside from substance- or medication-induced sexual dysfunction, the other sexual dysfunctions are gender specific. The three female dysfunctions are female sexual interest/arousal disorder, female orgasmic disorder, and genitopelvic pain/penetration disorder. As for males, the four diagnoses are male hypoactive sexual desire disorder, delayed ejaculation, erectile disorder (ED), and premature (early) ejaculation.

In order to meet the criteria for a diagnosis of one of the sexual dysfunctions, an individual must be symptomatic for a period of 6 months (except for substance/medication-induced sexual dysfunction). The disorder must cause significant distress and classified as mild, moderate, or severe. Subtypes for sexual dysfunctions in the DSM-5 include "lifelong versus acquired" and "generalized versus situational."

According to DSM-5, the disorder should not be better explained by the effects of a "nonsexual mental disorder, a consequence of severe relationship distress (e.g., partner violence) or other significant stressors." Finally, to make the diagnosis of one of the sexual dysfunctions, the disorder should not be due to the effects of a substance or other medical condition. If the sexual problem is attributable to another medical condition (i.e., endocrine problem, trauma to spinal cord or genital area, peripheral neuropathy) then no psychiatric diagnosis is given.

Once a sexual dysfunction has been diagnosed, the clinician should indicate the presence and degree of medical and nonmedical "associated features." According to DSM-5, these may include "(1) partner factors (e.g., partner sexual problem; partner health status); (2) relationship factors (e.g., poor communication, discrepancies in desire for sexual activity); (3) individual vulnerability factors (e.g., poor body image; history of sexual or emotional abuse), psychiatric comorbidity (e.g., depression; anxiety) or stressors (e.g., job loss; bereavement); (4) cultural or religious factors (e.g., inhibitions related to prohibitions against sexual activity or pleasure; attitudes toward sexuality); and finally (5) medical factors relevant to prognosis, course, or treatment."

Let us briefly review the sexual dysfunctions:

- Substance/medication-induced sexual dysfunction: Some common causes are alcohol, amphetamines, cocaine, sedative–hypnotic medication, and antidepressants.
- Female sexual interest/arousal disorder: Absent or reduced interest/arousal related to sexual activities, thoughts, encounters, cues, etc.
- Male hypoactive sexual desire disorder: Persistent deficient or absent sexual thoughts, fantasies, or desires.
- ED: The failure to obtain or maintain erection during partnered sexual activities.
- Delayed ejaculation: A marked difficulty or inability to achieve desired ejaculation during partnered sexual activities.
- Premature (early) ejaculation: Persistent or recurrent pattern of ejaculation during partnered sexual activity within 1 minute following penetration or before the individual wishes it.
- Female orgasmic disorder: Delay, infrequency, or absence of orgasm or reduced intensity of orgasm sensations.
- Genitopelvic pain/penetration disorder: Difficulties with vaginal penetration during intercourse, pain during intercourse, fear or anxiety about pain or penetration, or contraction of pelvic floor muscles during sex.

Many people have more than one dysfunction (e.g., hypoactive sexual desire disorder plus orgasmic disorder), and often both members of a couple will have a dysfunction (e.g., premature

Table 16.1 Assessment of sexual problems

I. Definition of the problem
   A. How does the couple describe the problem? What are their theories about its etiology? How do they generally relate to their sexuality, as reflected in their language, attitudes toward sexuality, comfort level, and permission system?
   B. How is the problem a problem for them? What is the function of the problem in their relationship system? Is the relationship problem the central problem? Why now?

II. Relationship history
   A. Current partner.
   B. Previous relationship history.
   C. Psychosexual history, including information about early childhood experiences, nature of sexual encounters prior to the relationship, sexual orientation, feelings about masculinity and femininity.
   D. Description of current sexual functioning, focusing on conditions for satisfactory sex, positive behaviors, specific technique, and so on. Who initiates sex, who leads, or do both? How does the couple's sexual pattern of intimacy and control reflect or compensate for other aspects of their relationship?

III. Developmental life cycle issues (births, deaths, transitions).

IV. Medical history, focusing on current physical status, medications, and present medical care, especially endocrine, vascular, metabolic.

V. Goals (patients' and therapist's viewpoints): The task is to examine whether goals are realistic and what previous attempted solutions have yielded.

ejaculation in the man and hypoactive desire in the woman). It is important to understand the sequencing of the onset of the dysfunctions in order to understand how they influence each other. As we have said earlier, many sexual problems are not dysfunctions but are relational-based dissatisfactions.

Specific techniques have been devised for eliciting a sexual history and for evaluating sexual functioning. The marital therapist should become familiar with these techniques and obtain experience in their use. Just as many individual therapists shy away from enquiring about their patients' sexual histories, some marital therapists still are not well informed about their patients' sexual experiences. Anxieties arising from their own discomfort about such material, or from their lack of a conceptual frame of reference, handicap their ability to acquire and use sexual data. Table 16.1 lists the minimum requirements for a systemic assessment of sexual difficulties.

Leiblum and Rosen (2006)[4] provide a thorough discussion of assessment techniques for each specific sexual problem. For readers interested in family-of-origin work, a sexual genogram is useful.[5] The sexual genogram questions are as follows:

- What are the overt/covert messages in this family regarding sexuality/intimacy? Regarding masculinity/femininity?
- Who said/did what? Who was conspicuously silent/absent in the area of sexuality/intimacy?
- Who was the most open sexually? Intimately? In what ways?
- How was sexuality/intimacy encouraged? Discouraged? Controlled? Within a generation? Between generations?
- What questions have you had regarding sexuality/intimacy in your family tree that you have been reluctant to ask? Who might have the answers? How could you discover the answers?
- What were the secrets in your family regarding sexuality/intimacy (e.g., incest, unwanted pregnancies, extramarital affairs)?
- What do the other "players on the stage" (i.e., extended family members or [sometimes] close family friends) have to say regarding the aforementioned questions? How did these issues, events, and experiences affect them? Within a generation? Between generations? With whom have you talked about this? With whom would you like to talk about this? How could you do it?

- How does your partner perceive your family tree/genogram regarding the aforementioned questions? How do you perceive theirs?
- How would you change this genogram (including who and what) to reflect what you wish had occurred regarding messages and experiences of sexuality/intimacy?
- Were there inappropriate sexual behaviors by family members, such as sexual fondling of children by relatives or detailed sexual discussions in the presence of small children?
- Are any family members gay? How were they treated at home? Could one express nonsexual love for same-sex people?

In addition, a medical workup should be ordered for couples in whom the problems may have an organic component. This is particularly true for men, for whom small physiologic changes in potency may produce anxiety that exacerbates the problem.

Children should not be present when the therapist takes the partners' intimate sexual history. The process of taking a sexual history should be handled with care and regard for each person's level of comfort. What type of language should be used when discussing sexual topics? Obviously, the therapist should not use terms that would be offensive or uncomfortable for either the therapist or the couple. At the same time, care must be taken to avoid using bland generalities that fail to elicit specific sexual information. Frankness is encouraged, and when a patient's response is vague, the therapist needs to follow up with more specific questions. The therapist should use simple language or use the simplest technical sexual term with which the patient is comfortable. Some patients will misunderstand technical terms. For others, the therapist's use of the vernacular may be inappropriate. The problem faced in the choice of language is itself an indication of our general cultural discomfort with sexuality. The therapist's own use of a particular sexual vocabulary can be a model to help the marital partners feel comfortable in communicating with each other more openly.

TREATMENT

Clinical treatments have been developed for many common sexual dysfunctions and the focus is to restore sexual functioning and pleasure. All patients should initially receive a full general medical workup to rule out any underlying medical conditions that may be causing the sexual dysfunction. Remember, the same patient may be affected by both psychological and physical factors.

Lack of Desire

For men and women, sexual desire decreases as they age. Treatment for lack of desire is a multistep process. Clinicians can help patients identify negative attitudes and beliefs about sex, explore the origins of those ideas, and find new ways of thinking about sex. The focus then shifts to behavior change and the clinician also works to address any relationship problems that might exist. As we write this in 2024, there are effective medications, approved by the FDA for female desire disorder.

Erectile Disorder

One of the primary psychological causes of ED is performance anxiety. Therapy focuses on decreasing anxiety by taking the focus off intercourse. Sex therapists often use "sensate focus" exercises to treat ED in addition to other sexual dysfunctions. The exercises start with nonsexual touching and encourage both partners to express how they like to be touched. The goal is to help both partners understand how to recognize and communicate their preferences. For aging men with physical problems, physicians may prescribe medications (sildenafil, vardenafil, or tadalafil) or devices (penile prosthesis, vacuum pump).

Premature (Early) Ejaculation

Several techniques may be used in sexual treatment to facilitate this. Basically, the sexual activity with the partner is stopped just prior to the point where the man senses ejaculation is imminent. Then, the man either receives no stimulation or the head of the penis is squeezed by the partner. The goal of both approaches is to decrease arousal. Before the man loses his erection, the sexual activity is resumed until the man again signals the partner to stop. With this start–stop procedure, the man and his partner both gain a greater sense of control and the problem diminishes. Anxiety plays a role in premature ejaculation. Therefore, psychotherapy frequently helps. Other treatments include selective serotonin reuptake inhibitor (SSRI) medications and 1% dibucaine (anesthetic) ointment applied to the penis.

Painful Intercourse/Female Orgasmic Disorder

Many sex therapists prescribe the use of vaginal dilators and utilize biofeedback. Treatment can also focus on progressive muscle relaxation and cognitive behavioral therapy (CBT) by examining underlying beliefs that may be contributing to the pain. Female orgasmic disorder should be similarly treated. Since women differ in their responses to genital stimulation, each patient should be encouraged to explore her responses to a range of forms of stimulation (e.g., clitoral, vaginal, etc.).

Psychological causes should be explored and treated (e.g., anxiety, performance anxiety, guilt). Obviously, effective communication between sexual partners is pivotal to successful sex. Reassurance and encouragement from the therapist may be helpful. Some problems may be due to a lack of knowledge about sexual functioning. In these cases, books on normal sexual function may be recommended prior to psychotherapy.

Treatment of psychosexual disorders, in the form developed by Masters and Johnson,[6] consisted of a thorough assessment of the partners and the relationship, education about sexual functioning, and a series of behavioral (i.e., sensate focus) exercises. The model was based on three fundamental postulates: (1) a parallel sequence of physiologic and subjective arousal in both genders; (2) the primacy of psychogenic factors, particularly learning deficits and performance anxiety; and (3) the amenability of most sexual disorders to a brief, problem-focused treatment approach. The sensate focus exercises were designed predominantly for behavioral desensitization but also taught the individual partners about their own sexual desires and served to elicit relationship problems. In these exercises, the couple pleasures each other, alternating in the role of giver and receiver, first in nongenital areas, then genitally, then with intercourse. Intercourse is prohibited during the early stages to remove performance anxiety. There are also specific exercises for each of the sexual dysfunctions. Different authors have developed different exercises and ways of approaching them. For a complete description of these exercises, we recommend Kaplan,[7] LoPiccolo and Stock,[8] and Zilbergeld.[9] This method works best when ignorance, shame, or a specific dysfunction such as premature ejaculation is present. They are difficult to complete if the couple feels angry, resentful, or unloving toward each other. Many of the patients whom Masters and Johnson treated in the 1970s had issues related to sexual ignorance and inexperience. Four decades later, the increase in premarital sex and the proliferation of easily available articles and books on sexuality had decreased the number of these couples and allowed some couples with sexual dysfunction to work on their issues at home. Recent studies of couples seeking sex therapy have shown that a higher proportion have concomitant complicated marital problems than those treated by Masters and Johnson.

Some writers, particularly Schnarch,[10] have focused on cognitive and emotional issues in sexuality, especially on the meanings attached to a particular act and the level of intimacy involved. While the field has learned a great deal about the more behavioral and organic issues related to arousal and orgasm, it is important to rethink other aspects of sex—such as eroticism, passion, mystery, and dominance or submission—that make the act itself meaningful. This is particularly true in areas of sexual boredom or situational lack of desire. These therapists do not use rigidly staged exercises but focus on the couple's relatedness during sex; however, they may suggest specific homework to help a couple focus on a particular aspect of their sexuality. The presence of organic factors must be considered. Couples wishing personal growth in the area of sexuality need to be pushed past their comfort zone to areas of greater intensity and feeling, rather than simply being helped to expand the variety of techniques used.

Sex Addiction and Pornography

Sexual compulsions or sex addictions can wreak havoc on a couple. Individuals with this condition can spend an inordinate amount of time pursuing sexual encounters to the detriment of their personal life, occupational functioning, financial well-being, and even physical health. In such cases, one partner's unceasing compulsion to think about, talk about, and have sex may be very wearing on the other partner, especially because a key component of this problem is that such persons become extremely anxious if sex is denied. Sexually compulsive persons may present with multiple affairs or with constant demands on the other partner. Most people who have affairs do not have a sexual compulsion, however. Some therapists use a 12-step addiction model, with group therapy; some treat it as a compulsion with individual therapy and medications. Couples therapy is still a critical component part of treatment, to educate the couple, to deal with couple dynamics that are part of the problem, and if multiple affairs have taken place, to discuss the viability of the marriage.

Mrs. A had problems with anger during adolescence, generally because she felt neglected by her busy parents. She had a period of intense sexual activity during adolescence, which was related to her looking for affection through sexuality; she reported that she had no sexual problems during this time. Through twice-a-week individual psychotherapy in her 20s, she worked through these problems, married Mr. A, and had a child. Mr. A was a kind but rather distant man who soon after the marriage made a series of career moves that made him extremely busy. For the first 2 years, there were no sexual problems, but then marital problems developed, and Mrs. A's desire decreased. Mr. A then became more sexually demanding. Frequency and enjoyment of sex for both partners were decreased markedly. Mrs. A refused to have sex, saying that she was too upset. When they occasionally had sex, however, both were orgasmic.

Mr. and Mrs. A had been raised in traditional backgrounds and had been taught that sex should not be discussed. Although both partners had previous sexual experiences, they were unable to talk about their sexual problems. Mrs. A also began fantasizing about other men. Although fantasies of other partners are not unusual, Mrs. A's fantasies occurred only when she was particularly angry at her husband.

Whereas at one time individual psychotherapy for Mrs. A might have been the treatment of choice, the therapist decided to use both marital therapy and sex therapy. Marital therapy helped to open communication between the couple. It was discovered that Mrs. A was feeling very abandoned by her extremely hardworking husband and feeling that she was being ignored as she had been in her childhood. In addition, she was angry at her husband for not helping with child-rearing responsibilities. Her fantasies about other men, which seemed to be a way of wishing for the original affection she craved, were upsetting her and making her wonder if she loved her husband. She experienced further withdrawal at Mr. A's inability to insist on her connecting with him emotionally before he demanded sex.

The couple was encouraged to deal more directly with their differences and with the disappointments underlying their anger. Issues related to each partner's family of origin were brought up. Roles were restructured as Mr. A took over more of the child-rearing responsibilities. As the marital relationship improved, their sexual problems decreased. The couple was also given a series of sensate focus exercises in which they were asked to focus on giving and receiving pleasure. They were encouraged to talk with each other about their sexual wishes and to pay attention to the connection between themselves while being sexual. They also discussed deepening their nonsexual physical connection.

OTHER ISSUES RELATED TO SEXUALITY AND COUPLES

The Spectrum of Sexuality

Overview

Family therapists should be adequately educated in the area of human sexual orientation and sexual identity. The terms themselves are confusing. *Sexual orientation* is another way of indicating an individual's tendency to be attracted to one or both sexes. *Sexual identity* is one's sense of oneself as male or female. Sexual orientation, like most psychological phenomenon, is not an absolute. One may be sexually attracted to the opposite sex, the same sex, or both. Sexual orientation falls along a continuum, with completely homosexual and completely heterosexual preferences falling at the extreme ends, and many gradations in between.

Observations of human sexual behavior, emotional attachments, erotic fantasies, arousal, and erotic preference have suggested that sexual orientation and sexual identity are not static; both may fluctuate over a person's lifetime.

> Sexual orientation and sexual identity are not static; both may fluctuate over a person's lifetime.

Marital Issues in Gay or Bisexual Individuals

Many individuals who are gay or bisexual spend some years of their lives in heterosexual marriages. Many such people are able to function well heterosexually, changing their sexual focus when they realize that something appears to be missing or that their level of desire and love is greater for their own sex. Some have low levels of sexual desire in the marriage and pursue affairs. Because there may be a great deal of love and affection between the marital partners, the discovery that one member is gay is very painful, and the desire to remain in the marriage may be strong on one or both sides. The couple must decide how to handle the situation, that is, whether to divorce, whether to remain in the relationship and allow for alternative sexual behaviors, or whether the gay person can remain monogamous in the marriage and give up expressing the other parts of themselves. Therapy can help the couple clarify alternatives and make decisions. Unfortunately, even with the most loving spouses, the most common outcome is divorce, but this is not the only possible choice.

Sexual Functioning After Rape or Sexual Abuse

Rape and sexual abuse are acts of violence that may seriously affect the victim's ability to respond sexually in a relationship. Both are likely to produce symptoms of posttraumatic stress disorder, with anxiety and flashbacks occurring when sex is begun, even with a loved partner. Decreased sexual desire or sexual aversion is common, although some individuals with a history of early sexual abuse become indiscriminately sexual, considering themselves to be used merchandise and worth something only because of their sexuality. Some individuals maintain good sexual function but may be wary of intimacy. Some sexually abused individuals may go on to become abusers themselves in adulthood.

If a previously well-functioning adult has been raped, the sexual symptoms may be either relatively brief or long-standing, depending on the circumstances of the rape, the amount of physical damage, the vulnerability of the victim, and the partner's response. Because the partners of rape victims also have a complex set of feelings, including a wish to protect, a sense of shame, and murderous rage toward the rapist, they may or may not be able to respond empathically as the woman deals with the trauma and her own feelings. Couples therapy must be directed primarily toward helping the partners respond to each other emphatically and deal with the meaning of the trauma. Behavioral desensitization exercises may decrease sexual pressures enough to make sex more comfortable.

Sexual Problems After Medical Illness

Adults diagnosed with cancer, diabetes, heart disease, prostatitis, HIV, or substance use disorders may face special sexual challenges because of the underlying disorder, its treatment, or the effect of the illness on the couple's relationship. Two types of problems can occur. In one type, the illness can have a specific effect on sexual functioning. For example, surgery for prostate cancer may produce erectile dysfunction. This can now generally be treated medically with sildenafil; sometimes permanent dysfunction is unavoidable. Close communication with the patient's urologist is necessary. The therapist should also help partners expand their repertoire of sexual behaviors that do not involve intercourse. In the second type, sex is still possible, but the couple is anxious that having sex will injure the patient. The classic example is sex after a heart attack. There is no evidence that sex with a known partner in familiar surroundings is problematic for the heart. The couple should be advised to resume sex as soon as any reasonable exercise is permissible.

Likewise, erectile dysfunction may be the predictable side effect of certain antihypertensive medications. Narcotics, such as heroin, barbiturates, and alcohol, have a similar effect. Obviously, addictive drugs should be stopped or efforts made to change necessary medications. Many of the newer antidepressants, especially the SSRIs, can decrease sexual desire and slow orgasm.

In general, the treatment of choice is to lower the dose or change the antidepressant, although adjunctive pharmacologic therapy is sometimes helpful in reducing these side effects. Serious illness of any kind, and treatment for certain illness such as cancer, may leave the person with no sexual interest. In such cases, the couple may have to live with the situation, and the therapist's task is to help the couple decide the best way to handle the situation within the marital relationship. Similarly, surgery, chemotherapy, or radiation for cervical, ovarian, or prostate cancer can reduce sexual desire and performance. HIV and AIDS should alter a couple's approach to sex, and the therapist must recommend safe sexual practices.

Sexual Problems in the Elderly

With the rapid growth in the number of older people in the population, interest has increased in their psychiatric and sexual problems. The family therapist can help couples realize the following:

1. Advancing years are not a contraindication to sexuality and sensuality.
2. Older men may achieve erection and orgasm more slowly and may not necessarily ejaculate each time they have intercourse. Older women may have a shorter excitement phase, and their orgasms may be less intense, with slower vaginal contractions. Both partners, however, can still have a regular, ongoing sexual life.
3. Medications for desire and erectile problems can be effective and should be prescribed to treat the problem.
4. The couple should make efforts not to decrease their general level of affection and nonsexual physical connection.

Even after an elderly patient has experienced a severe disability, such as a stroke, their sexual life can still be maintained. The couple can be aided in adjusting to changes of sexual functioning by a thorough discussion of what positions and techniques are still possible.

CLINICAL PRACTICE IMPLICATIONS

Sexual issues are intimately and unpredictably intertwined with a couple's functioning. Couples with sexual dysfunction in one or both partners should be evaluated carefully, and the clinician should decide whether to add specific sensate focus exercises to the ongoing couples therapy and medication if appropriate. If the clinician chooses to do so, they must be sure to obtain adequate training or supervision.

SUGGESTED READINGS

We strongly recommend for the reader who is interested in a full discussion of new issues and treatment of systemic sex therapy, please see the special issue of the Journal of Family Psychotherapy.

Hertlein KM. Special issue: systemic sex therapy. *J Fam Psychother.* 2009;20:95–302.

REFERENCES

1. American Psychiatric Association. *Diagnostic and Statistical Manual of Mental Disorders*. 5th ed. American Psychiatric Publishing; 2022.
2. Laumann EO, Michael RT. *Social Organization of Sexuality*. University of Chicago Press; 1994.
3. McCarthy BW. Marital style and its effects on sexual desire and functioning. *J Fam Psychother.* 1999;10:1–12.
4. Leiblum S, Rosen R. *Principles and Practice of Sex Therapy.* 4th ed. Guilford; 2006.
5. Berman E, Hof H. The sexual genogram—assessing family of origin factors in the treatment of sexual dysfunction. In: Weeks G, Hof L, eds. *Integrating Sex and Marital Therapy: A Clinical Guide*. Brunner/Mazel; 1987:37–57.
6. Masters W, Johnson V. *Human Sexual Response*. Little, Brown; 1966.
7. Kaplan HS. *The Sexual Desire Disorders: Dysfunctional Regulation of Sexual Motivation*. Brunner/Mazel; 1995.
8. LoPiccolo J, Stock W. Treatment of sexual dysfunction. *J Consult Clin Psychol.* 1986;54:158–167.
9. Zilbergeld B. *The New Male Sexuality*. Bantam; 1992
10. Schnarch D. *Passionate Marriage*. WW Norton; 1997.

17 Couples and Families Breaking Apart: Separation and Divorce

OBJECTIVES FOR THE READER

- To learn the principles of diagnosis and treatment of separated, divorced, single-parent, binuclear, blended, and other family forms
- To learn treatment goals and techniques with these family forms

For easier reading, we emphasize that the descriptors "couples" or "marital" are used nearly interchangeably in this chapter.

INTRODUCTION

In Chapters 4 and 5, we discussed the functioning as well as some of the difficulties that separated, divorced, single-parent, binuclear, and blended families commonly experience and cope with. Some families, because of the multiplicity of stressors, poor coping, or psychopathology, are not able to deal with the situation and therefore seek help. In this chapter, we discuss the assessment and treatment of these families.

SEPARATION
- Separation Leading to Divorce
- Communicating the Issue of Divorce to Children
- Immediate Issues
- Therapy for Families Facing Divorce

DIVORCE AND POSTDIVORCE TREATMENT
SINGLE-PARENT AND BINUCLEAR FAMILIES
BLENDED FAMILIES (STEPFAMILIES)
- Goals
- Evaluation and Treatment

COHABITING COUPLES
SERIAL RELATIONSHIPS
CLINICAL PRACTICE IMPLICATIONS

SEPARATION

The process of separation can be an experiment on the part of a couple that is experiencing stress, or the first step in a process leading directly to divorce. We describe in the next section in this chapter separations in which the couple is definitely ending the relationship. Trial separations in which the couple (neither spouse is having an affair) still expresses interest in rebuilding the marriage can be a chance for the therapist and the couple to do serious work. In general, separations are to be avoided when possible, as the best therapy can usually be done when the partners are in constant contact. Separations may be unavoidable or preferable when high conflict, violence, or severe substance use disorders are present or when a person who married young feels as if they have no separate identity and needs to be alone for a period of time. During a trial separation, the couple should be encouraged to have ongoing couple therapy and to have planned and scheduled times to be together during which they have some pleasant experiences and some serious talks. They should be encouraged not to date others during the separation. Some therapists suggest that each partner should also be in individual therapy during this time because part of the problem involves individual issues that are hard to address in conjoint work. Others believe that individual therapy is necessary only in certain situations. For example, when emotions are extremely intense, separate individual therapy for one or both partners, or group therapy, may be indicated to cool down a contentious relationship while marital therapy is proceeding. It is also worth mentioning that separation and divorce increase the risk of depression, more significantly in men than in women.[1] This may also require individual therapy or medication. Separation may involve couples without children or couples with children of any age. Arrangements for children must be made. This may or may not necessitate a legal separation agreement. The therapist also needs to evaluate the relationships among the parent(s), other caregivers, and the children.

When a couple separates, the family therapist can help uncover the problems that prevented the partners from living together successfully on a sustained basis. **The primary task for the marital therapist is to remain *neutral* on the decision as to whether to separate or to stay together.** Having said that, the experience of the family clinician suggests that rebuilding a once-functioning relationship may be less difficult than finding and building a new one (although initially and/or in anger, it may seem easier to walk away). In some situations, both couples and their therapists give up too quickly, whereas in others all parties hold on too long. We recommend avoiding the extremes and, when appropriate, making reasonable attempts to hold together a relationship that the therapist evaluates as having once been, and having the potential to be, satisfying and functional for *both* partners. Not everything can be changed, but some things can be improved, and the therapist needs to be realistic in helping the husband and wife to accept parts of themselves that cannot be changed. It is critical, however, that the therapist not be the only one in the system trying to hold together the relationship. The decision to separate or to stay together must be made by the couple, not the therapist.

The primary task for the marital therapist is to remain neutral on the decision as to whether to separate or to stay together.

Couples that separate because one partner is having an active affair present a more difficult situation. The couple and the therapist must decide whether therapy is possible and whether ongoing contact between spouses is preferable. With highly ambivalent spouses, the one having the affair may move repeatedly between the relationships in a way that is distressing for everyone. (We know of one couple in which the husband returned to his home and then moved out more than 11 times over the course of 1 year. Another couple's separation continued for 8 years with multiple affairs and reconciliations before the wife finally gave up and refused to take back her husband.)

Such separations leave everyone, including the children, in limbo and should be time limited if possible. Guidelines for the departing spouse regarding time spent with the children and financial arrangements should be spelled out carefully. Legal separation should be considered to prevent financial problems and to protect against later charges of abandonment, although not all couples find this necessary.

Separation Leading to Divorce

If the couple has decided that divorce is inevitable, a different approach applies.

The imminent dissolution of the family as it was produces violent feelings of abandonment, grief, and loss in family members, regardless of their age (it has been said that every divorce is the death of a small civilization). Although it has always been assumed that divorce is easier after children have left home for college or work, even adults in their thirties or forties are often deeply upset by their parents' divorce. The parents and siblings of each spouse may also experience a variety of feelings, including anger and loss. Obviously, the partners who are initiating the divorce may have other feelings as well, such as relief, but loss is always present.

We discussed a number of issues related to divorce in Chapter 4. The most immediate of these issues have to do with finding separate living arrangements, dealing with children, and redistributing money. In general, men will have the least experience dealing with issues related to the children, and women the least experience with and the most fear related to issues of money. If the husband has left parenting primarily to his wife, he must learn quickly how to relate to his children when he is alone, and he must be actively encouraged to see them frequently and regularly and to be in contact with his wife about sharing parenting. If the wife has assumed that her husband will protect her financially, she may, even in current times, be woefully ignorant about finances and without much earning power. In her panic, she may initiate an unnecessary legal battle over money. Alternatively, she may be so sure that her husband will protect her (or may feel so guilty if she thinks the divorce is her fault) that she will not protect herself and the children financially by fighting hard enough. Another critical issue at this time is how long should the couple live in the same house. If there are children at home, they should be given a few weeks to adjust to the situation; that is, one of the parents should not move out immediately after the divorce is announced.

Remaining together for months after divorce has been chosen is often destructive to both parties, although couples in poor financial situations, or in those where neither is willing to leave the family home, have done this. The therapist needs to be very active during the early phases of separation to make sure the children are cared for and not used by the parents as pawns. The therapist should help the couple in making coherent, not emotionally driven, decisions in areas such as the redistribution of money. It is usually best to postpone any major decisions, such as selling the house or giving up one's job, until the dust settles. Even if legal divorce has not been initiated, both partners need to seek legal advice about local divorce laws. We strongly advise mediation rather than adversarial legal procedures whenever possible.

After a couple has decided to divorce, they often drop out of therapy. They should be encouraged to remain in treatment at least long enough to plan their initial moves; that is, telling the children and their families of origin, making preliminary financial arrangements, and discussing how to handle the physical separation. Some couples may want to review the course of the marriage to further understand what went wrong, but for most couples, their emotions are too intense at this time. One or both partners may request individual therapy; sometimes a support group for separating and divorcing partners is also helpful. If the couple has been seen conjointly, it may be helpful to refer the spouses to different therapists rather than have the former couples therapist do the individual work. In other cases, the couples therapist may continue with one member (or rarely both). If only one person is seen by the original couples therapist, the other may feel that it is unfair, but some spouses are relieved when their former mate continues in therapy. It is almost impossible for the couples therapist to see, individually, both members of a divorcing couple, because the therapist then becomes privy to information about legal and custody battles from both sides. In addition, the spouses may see the former couples therapist as a link to the other or as favoring the other and may not be able to engage fully in their own work.

Communicating the Issue of Divorce to Children

Telling the children about impending separation is usually a traumatic event for the parents. It is useful to remember that, as with many other issues, this is a process and not a single event. Initially, most children hear very little other than divorce is impending. Children do not really know what separation will mean for them until they have gone through the experience, and they usually do not know what questions to ask at first. The parents must discuss the divorce with the children repeatedly in the ensuing weeks, as plans are made. The parents must convey the following information to the children, either all at once or over time:

"We are getting a divorce. That means we won't be living together. We will always be your parents, and we both love you. That does not change. You will not have to choose between us." (This may or may not come true, and the therapist must help the couple keep the children out of the middle.)

"You did not cause this divorce and could not have prevented it. As time goes on, we will need to keep talking about what is happening with all of us, both the feelings and the changes in our lives. We will talk about what is happening with us, and you need to talk about what you need. You can also talk to your friends and whoever else it would help to talk to."

The children need to be told, as simply as possible in broad strokes, the reasons for the divorce. Teenage children in particular want a reasonable amount of information. If one of the parents is having an active affair, it is not unusual for one or more of the children to already be aware of it. Children tend to overhear conversations and know what is going on with their parents to a larger extent than parents are aware. It is very difficult to keep secret the major reasons for the divorce. Because children today usually have friends whose parents are divorced, there is less stigma and more knowledge than a generation or two ago. However, no child wants the details of their parents' sexual or intimate lives. No child wants to sit in judgment as to which parent is at fault. Children need to be reminded that at the time of their birth, their parents loved each other and that they wanted children. This can help alleviate the children's fear that they were in some way responsible for the divorce.

Children are appropriately also concerned about the details of their daily lives—for example, who will care for me, who will pick me up at school, where do I keep my pets, will I have to leave my house. For most children, their house and their neighborhood are crucial parts of their sense of self. They need to be reassured that regardless of the living arrangements, they will be considered and cared for. It is generally best for both parents to be present when the initial announcement is made, so that everyone hears the same information. Private talks later are also necessary and appropriate, because each parent must now learn how to parent alone. Parents need to check with each other before conveying potentially explosive information about financial changes or about an affair partner. Talks should be informational and not about the badness of the other parent.

Immediate Issues

The level of conflict during the initial year of living apart varies greatly depending on whether the divorce is sudden or long in the planning, whether one spouse opposes it, and what the level of conflict was like before the separation. Regardless of how long separation was anticipated, the many ensuing changes in feelings and life structure make the situation difficult. If the couple has a fair amount of goodwill left, or if one partner is so guilty that they agree to almost anything, many decisions can be made quickly. Most often, each decision is complex and will be struggled over.

The early months of the separation are likely to cause irrational feelings and behavior toward the ex-spouse, regardless of how rationally the person is behaving with children or work.

For many people, the first months in particular are a "crazy time," when everything feels upside down. The therapist's job is to keep both partners grounded, allowing them to retell the story over and over, to find some answer to the questions "How did this happen?" and "Am I still a good person?"

For the couple, mediation is often helpful in solving problems. The more the couple can make decisions themselves with a mediator's help, rather than using the judicial system, the better. However, if this does not work, it may be helpful to the couple if the therapist supports the process of finding and working with lawyers. For many people, divorce represents their first experience with the legal system. They may be overwhelmed and unable to be an advocate for their own interests with the lawyer.

Family conflict may escalate during the year after divorce, although it may decrease in high-conflict families. If the parents are having a difficult time they may temporarily find their parental skills decrease, and they may become inconsistent, less affectionate, and less focused on discipline and continuity. Parental quarreling and mutual denigration can result in the children becoming anxious, feeling that they must take sides or, in the case of school-age and early adolescent children, completely cutting off the absent parent. The risk of delinquency is believed to be greater if the parents separate or divorce than if a parent dies. The parameters of marital discord that seem most toxic for children are prolonged marital disputes, parental pathology that impinges on the children's functioning, and the child's lack of a good relationship with either parent. Rapid changes in lifestyle and finances are stressful for everyone and add to the frustration. However, things improve in many families, particularly when the parent who is leaving has been violent, alcoholic, or emotionally abusive. When fathers have left the active parenting to mothers, they may improve their parenting when they have the children by themselves. And many families do very well after an initial period of disruption.

Therapy for Families Facing Divorce

Common treatment alternatives for families facing divorce could include (1) no formal treatment, (2) marital therapy with discussion about the children, (3) family treatment with both ex-spouses and the children, or (4) therapy with the children and only one parent on issues that parent has with the children. Family therapy must have a careful agenda focused primarily on practical matters—for example, what are the living arrangements, or how do the parents handle emergencies, discipline, and child transfers between parents.

Central issues include what the children need; whether they are caught between the parents; and whether they have been asked to report on parental activities, ask one parent for money for the other, and so on. Therapy must be focused clearly on problems with the children and not on rehashing the marriage. Although the same therapist can see each parent alone with the children, they must also have knowledge and respect for the other partner. A therapist who begins working with the custodial parent and children after the divorce, and does not speak to or meet the noncustodial parent or consider that person's concerns, is likely to worsen the struggles between the spouses. Psychoeducation, including recommending books like *The Difficult Divorce*,[2] is a good reference book for therapists working with couples that have no ability to compromise or deal with each other. For the children alone, intervention is also possible but not mandatory. It may include a children's support group or individual therapy. It is also important to inform others who have contact with the children (especially at their schools) that the parents have divorced.

A difficult issue is that of introducing children to their parents' new love relationships. Children may not want to meet a parent's new lover, particularly if the lover was an affair partner for whom the parent left the marriage. Even if the children are ready, the ex-spouse may be furious about having the children meet the affair partner, whom they may see as immoral or evil. However, if the children are to have a relationship with both parents, they must eventually find some way to deal with the new lover, at least with regard if not affection. The therapist must help the family deal with the realities of the situation, although if a great deal of animosity is present, it is generally wise to wait at least a few months after the separation before introducing the new person. New relationships are gradually introduced to the children especially when the relationships are potentially serious ones. If possible, live-in status should be reserved for partners with whom marriage is planned; otherwise, their ambiguous status in the house may lead to real problems with the children. Sleepover status is a highly emotional topic, and no clear guidelines are obvious in most situations. A good rule of thumb is that new partners should not sleep over unless the relationship has reached a relatively committed status.

DIVORCE AND POSTDIVORCE TREATMENT

The presence of divorce should not lead one to think of only pathologic sequelae, because an intact, conflict-ridden family can be more detrimental to children than is a stable home in which the parents are divorced. As such, divorce can be a positive solution to a destructive family situation. This seems to be especially true in the presence of a rejecting, demeaning, or psychiatrically ill parent. Most adults report positive feelings about their parents' divorce when surveyed years later and eventually conclude that their parents made the right decision. Adult children have different attitudes toward their mothers and fathers, however, and a majority of the children had at least some "very negative" feelings about their mothers. A lesser number harbored such feelings about their fathers. A crucial issue for divorce therapy is the fact that a majority of adult children report that their mothers maligned their fathers, whereas, only 12% said their fathers spoke critically about their ex-spouses. This must be seen in the context that most mothers were custodial parents who were doing most of the parenting without spousal support.

As to the long-term effects of the divorce process, research is complex and somewhat contradictory. The problem is that no study has been done comparing those parents who divorce with those who are discordant and contemplating divorce but stay together or with those who are discordant but never contemplated divorce. In one of the earliest and best-known studies, Wallerstein[3] suggested that some children of divorced families have strong feelings about it even 10 years later. She conducted a systematic follow-up study of a small sample of children of divorce (with no control subjects) and found that (1) three in five felt rejected by at least one of the parents; (2) in at least half the families both parents remained angry; and (3) as expected, children conceptualize and feel differently about the divorce, depending on their age. She suggests that divorcing parents apologize for the pain they are causing their children, express their own sadness so as to allow children to express their feelings about the ending of the relationship, and give children concrete details about future plans as soon as possible. Her age-specific comments include:

1. For the adolescent: Try not to lean on the child for support—do not get lost in one's own needs to the detriment of helping the adolescent deal with their own needs.
2. For children aged 9 to 12 years: The angriest child tends to take sides and act as if they understand the issue even though they may understand very little. This child needs to be told that the parent's fight is a battle in which they should not get involved.
3. For younger children: The important thing to remember is to reassure the child that they will still have both a mother and a father. Abandonment can be a central issue for younger children. For preschoolers, continued, ongoing contact from both parents on a regular and frequent basis is best.

It must be kept in mind that these comments are generalizations. For example, although fear of abandonment is preeminent in younger children, older children and adolescents often experience similar feelings. Additionally, family stressors often cause children to regress emotionally and behaviorally to earlier stages of development. Thus, a prediction of the predominant issues caused by divorce is best made on a case-by-case basis.

Many authors have issued strong challenges to the idea that divorce is inevitably harmful, pointing to the fact that at least 50% of divorced partners have amicable relationships and to the positive functioning of nontraditional families for both parents and children. Ahrons[4] reviews this literature and describes the process of creating a functional divorce. An organization begun in 1997, the Council on Contemporary Families, has begun working to collect this research and disseminate it and to consider ways of exploring the needs of contemporary nontraditional families.

SINGLE-PARENT AND BINUCLEAR FAMILIES

"Single-parent" families may include a variety of people in the parenting system.

A parent with legal custody of the children may be living with their parents, a lover, or a friend. Even if the noncustodial parent visits infrequently, he (usually it is a he) may still be very important in the children's lives. Alternatively, the single parent and children may form a tightly self-contained unit. In binuclear families, both biologic parents are responsible for childcare. Although the general rules of family therapy apply to all families, single-parent and binuclear families experience additional issues.

Hierarchy is a complex issue in single-parent families. A grandparent may take over a majority of the child-rearing duties, especially if the single parent and children are living in the grandparent's house. A lover may feel that they should take over disciplinary duties without any clear mandate to do so. Because the custodial parent may be overwhelmed by a combination of work and household duties, one or more of the children may act as companion to the parent or surrogate parent to younger children. In other cases, the family may operate with a high level of democracy, with all children sharing more of the power and responsibility than in a two-adult household. It is important that the therapist consider the possibilities for health inherent in nontraditional models rather than assume that the only possible functioning family is a mother who is totally head of the household. However, if conflicts occur, it should be clear that the custodial parent has final say in the matter.

Children must not be overburdened with parenting responsibilities, but they are capable of taking on a reasonable share of the chores when it is obvious that help is needed. For many children, a single-parent family is one in which their contribution is needed and welcomed.

> If conflicts occur, it should be clear that the custodial parent has final say in the matter.

In therapy, it is important to speak to all family members rather than only to a parent or one child. If the family is living with grandparents, it is important to include the grandparents in at least some of the meetings. The therapist must be willing to work with the family to determine the best system available, rather than assuming the parent must carry the entire burden himself or herself.

If the custodial parent has no supports, they are prone to depression and demoralization. The therapist's job is to help the parent form a functioning support system rather than to try to be the support system. In binuclear families, the central issue involves the multiple systems in which the children must operate. Not only must the parents collaborate on clear rules for the children, but if one or both parents remarry, the new spouses also will be involved.

In single-parent families, the launching of the children, particularly the oldest, is often problematic because they have been such crucial supports for the parent and the younger children. Sometimes the oldest child becomes briefly symptomatic immediately before they are ready to leave for college, as a way of testing whether it is safe to go.

BLENDED FAMILIES (STEPFAMILIES)

For the majority of divorcing spouses, at least one will remarry, forming a blended family or stepfamily. A study of responses to stepfamily therapy provides valuable insights into what 280 remarried couples found to be most helpful in their stepfamily therapy.[5] Besides responses that commented on the importance of therapist warmth and good basic skills, couples reported four specific types of interventions that were particularly helpful: (1) validating their feelings and normalizing stepfamily dynamics and issues, (2) supplying psychoeducation, (3) reducing their feelings of helplessness, and (4) helping them strengthen their couple relationship. Respondents were also asked to list any therapeutic elements that were not helpful to them. Nearly 50% of the negative comments concerned the therapist's "lack of knowledge about stepfamily issues and dynamics."

Goals

We suggest the following goals for therapists working with remarried couples with children:

1. To consolidate the remarried couple as a unit and their authority in the system, helping the two adults to understand and develop a *modus operandi* to further their romantic love requirements and their necessity to parent.
2. To consolidate the parental authority in the system among biologic and stepparents, with the formation of a collaborative co-parenting team.
3. As a corollary to the preceding goal, to help children deal with and minimize the continuation and exacerbation of loyalty conflicts between their two biologic parents and between each biologic parent and the corresponding stepparent.
4. To facilitate mourning of the nuclear family, former partner, old neighborhoods, friends, and way of life. A period of mourning prepares the way to accept and to grow with the new reality of the stepfamily.
5. To be sure, there is a secure place for the children's development and to maximize the potential within both family systems. It is hoped that the two systems can be synergistic at the same time that the children learn there is more than one way to deal with many life situations.
6. To accept and integrate the children's need for individuation from both families and for more peer involvement. At the other extreme, some children may prematurely develop great peer involvement if they cannot find appropriate love and nurturance in the household systems of either biologic parent. One approach may be to strengthen the bond and acceptance of the children in one if not both family systems.
7. To help family members accept and tolerate their differences from some idealized nuclear family model. These differences include the following:
   a. Lack of complete control of money and income.
   b. Shared responsibility for children; some lack of control (e.g., when the child is in the other parent's home).
   c. The reality that children may neither like nor love a stepparent and vice versa.
   d. Different feeling to the families. The stepfamily will not feel the same to a participant as did their former nuclear family. There are different levels of bonding and different characters playing different if seemingly similar roles; these latter roles need clarification for all involved.
   e. Different rules and expectations likely to exist in the two homes. Flexibility is necessary for the children to navigate situations that do not meet their own wishes.
   f. Difficulty in living in a stepfamily structure. Sometimes the stepfamily is more complex, more persons are involved, models and guidelines are less clear, and every stepfamily is in a sense a pioneer family; however, the stepfamily system can be regarded and promoted as an enriching one, enabling the children to avail themselves of more diverse parental and interactive models.

Evaluation and Treatment

Stepfamilies need to be evaluated and treated in a context of awareness of appropriate stepfamily norms (see Chapter 4). Using a nuclear family model can lead stepfamily members to pursue unrealistic goals with unfortunate consequences.

In this section, we discuss some issues related to stepfamilies and the implications of these issues for therapy (Table 17.1).

The complexities and intricacies of stepfamily relationships appear to require a systemic perspective even when the therapist is working with a single individual from a stepfamily (i.e.,

Table 17.1 Differences between stepfamilies and nuclear families; therapeutic implications

How stepfamilies differ from nuclear families	Therapeutic implications
Stepfamilies and nuclear families have different structural characteristics.	The therapist must evaluate the family using stepfamily norms; a nuclear family model is not valid.
There is little or no family loyalty in stepfamilies.	Initially, seeing the family members together may be unproductive.
Before integration, stepfamilies react to transitional stresses.	The first focus needs to be on the transitional adjustment process, not on intrapsychic processes.
Society compares stepfamilies negatively with nuclear families.	There is a basic need for acceptance and validation as a worthwhile family unit.
Stepfamilies experience a long integration period with predictable stages.	The stage of family development is very important in the assessment of whom to see in therapy.
There is no breakdown of family homeostasis in stepfamilies; equilibrium has never been established.	With normalization and education, stability can emerge from chaos and ignorance of the norms.
Stepfamilies have complicated suprafamily systems.	The complications of the family need to be kept in mind during therapy. Drawing a genogram helps.
Stepfamilies have experienced many losses for most individuals.	Grief work may be necessary.
Stepfamilies involve preexisting parent–child coalitions.	Developing a secure couple relationship is essential. Many times, permission is needed to do this.
A solid couple relationship does not signify good stepparent–stepchild relationships.	Steprelationships require special attention, separate from the couple relationship.
The balance of power differs in stepfamilies and nuclear families.	Stepparents have very little authority in the family initially; therefore, discipline issues need to be handled by the biologic parent. Children have more power, which needs to be channeled positively.
There is less family control in stepfamilies, because there is an influential parent elsewhere or in memory.	Appropriate control can be fostered to lessen the anxiety engendered by helplessness.
Children have more than two parenting figures in stepfamilies.	There is a need to think in terms of a parenting coalition, not a parenting couple.
Ambiguous family boundaries exist in stepfamilies, with little agreement as to family history.	These losses and stresses may require attention.
Initially, stepfamilies have no family history.	Members need to share their histories and develop family rituals and ways of doing things.
The emotional climate is intense and unexpected in stepfamilies.	Empathy with other family members can be encouraged by understanding the human needs that are not being met: to be loved and appreciated, to belong, and to have control over one's life.

Used with permission of Taylor & Francis Group LLC - Books from Visher EB, Visher JS. *Therapy with Stepfamilies. Brunner/Mazel;* 1996:41–42; permission conveyed through Copyright Clearance Center, Inc.

outside the system).[7] The therapist must think in terms of the family, no matter who or how many family members they are treating. This approach is also important when the stepfamily has multiple problems. In addition to other types of interventions (e.g., for drug abuse, chronic illness), dealing with stepfamily dynamics and issues can reduce tensions, thus giving family members more energy to deal with other difficulties.

The question of whom to see in therapy is important. It can be detrimental to see the new couple and the children together in the same session before the couple has arrived at the stage of family integration in which the spouses have some ability to be supportive of each other and to work together on family issues. Seeing the couple alone is an important way to demonstrate the importance of the couple and to help the two individuals to strengthen their relationship. Some therapists have meetings with all those involved with the children (i.e., ex-spouses, lovers, stepparents). Unfortunately, with preexisting parent–child alliances, the parent who has remarried often feels it is betraying to these relationships to form a strong new couple bond. However, children need the family stability and modeling that can come from association with a unified, well-functioning couple.

Even when the couple is working well together, step relationships do not necessarily develop spontaneously. The family may need inclusive family therapy to work out these relationships. Communication and having special one-to-one times between parents and children, and between stepparents and stepchildren, can be important in building and maintaining relationships. For children in stepfamilies, this approach can reduce the loss of more exclusive parental attention and can foster communication and bonding between stepparents and stepchildren.

The balance of power does not reside initially with the couple in stepfamilies. The stepparent joins the biologic parent and their children but has no authority as far as the children are concerned. Many remarried biologic parents make the error of expecting the stepparent to take on a disciplinary role with the children. Research indicates that the stepparent needs to take on the co-manager role slowly; meanwhile, the biologic parent needs to become, or remain, the active parenting adult with their children and also needs to require civil behavior in the household. These steps can create a climate in which step relationships can develop and stepparents can begin to take on a co-management role with the biologic parent. With young children, this may take 1 to 2 years[8]; with older children it usually takes longer.[9]

Many stepfamily adults need psychoeducation about discipline and roles for stepparents. Adults are relying on their previous experiences in their families of origin and former marriage(s). Therapists can help these adults share these expectations, join them by understanding their positions, and help them to pursue more realistic stepfamily goals. If the couple is reluctant to change unproductive patterns, they may be willing to try a different approach for 3 or 4 weeks as an experiment. Frequently, positive experiences change the family dynamics so that continuing change is supported. Finally, when the stepparent is alone with the children, the biologic parent's authority needs to be delegated to the stepparent, as one delegates authority to a babysitter or other caregiver, by bringing the family together and letting the children know the stepparent is in charge when only that adult is present.

A great deal of the complexity in stepfamilies comes from the fact that there are more than two parenting adults in the children's lives. With a biologic parent in another household, there may be three or four parenting adults if both parents are remarried, and children may be living part of the time in each of these two households. When parents feel insecure, they tend to fear loss of their children's love to the other parent and perhaps to that parent's new partner. Another concern is the loss of control and sense of helplessness that arises because of the mere existence of the other household, and the therapeutic task can become one of helping the couple build an adequate boundary around its household and learn to respect the boundary around the other household. Gates in the boundaries are needed for the children so that they can come and go comfortably. Adults often need help controlling the things they can control in their own household and letting go of concern about situations in the other household. Gaining control and accepting the limits of their influence is helpful in reducing the feelings of helplessness that remarried adults may feel.

Forming a parenting coalition of parents and stepparents can be difficult, but with help it is possible.[10,11] Ordinarily this requires the new couple to develop a solid, secure bond before they are emotionally able to form a working relationship with the children's other household. The lesser the hostility between the households, the fewer the loyalty conflicts for the children and the greater the satisfaction for the adults. In some situations, it can be helpful to bring the adults together to work on issues involving the children. Bringing them together in therapy becomes a possibility when each parent has formed a strong bond with their new partner. The therapist needs to make direct, personal contact with each household, state clearly the purpose of the joint meeting, and then make certain the agenda of the session does not include potentially explosive areas unconnected with the present welfare of the children. Older children may need to be included when their situation is being discussed.

The emotional climate in stepfamilies is often intense, particularly during the early stages of stepfamily integration. A helpful way to conceptualize the reasons for this intensity is to understand and recognize the inability of new stepfamilies to meet three very basic human emotional needs: (1) to belong to a group, (2) to be cared about and loved by a few special people, and (3) to have some control over one's life.

Because of all the changes and unfamiliarity in the household, stepfamily members can feel out of control, not accepted by the new people in their lives, and as though they do not belong in this unfamiliar group. Parents who have remarried frequently fear the loss of their children, whom they love and by whom they are loved. Stepparents in particular feel unloved, alienated from the group, and with little control. Children are upset by their lack of control over all the losses and events occurring in their lives.

For therapists, then, the basic task is to help family members gain an understanding of these basic emotional needs so that they can have empathy for everyone in the family and be understood in return. The family members need to find ways in which to communicate, to fill in history with one another, and to further accelerate the sense of control and belonging by developing rituals and predictable day-to-day ways of doing things. Being cared about requires the building of relationships. This takes time and positive shared memories, both on a one-to-one basis and as a family unit.

Many stepfamilies that come for therapy need the therapist to validate their feelings and the worth and viability of their families, to normalize the situations that arise in such families, to find ways to deal effectively with the challenges, and to find support for the new couple relationship. With this assistance, stepfamilies can work toward satisfactory integration, deal more effectively with disruptive situations, and bring satisfaction and happiness to the adults and to the children.

COHABITING COUPLES

Cohabitation, once seen as pathology, sin, or nonconformity, is now a common developmental phase for young people who are developing intimacy or for older people after divorce. About 50% of marrying couples have lived together for some time before marriage. Cohabiting couples that come for therapy are most likely to present with the need to determine the future of the relationship.

Therapy consists of clarifying each partner's position and helping the couple think through what would have to occur in order to make the relationship go forward (or end). Each partner can be asked to take the other's position—that is, the less committed partner could explain why marriage would be a good idea, and the more committed one why it would be better to breakup. Often, when pressed, the uncommitted partner can finally admit that they have no intention of changing, or the more committed one can admit that if they do not get married, and soon, they will leave. Faced with the real possibility of ending the relationship, one or both partners may change their positions. If both partners are unhappy, the therapist should initiate a careful exploration of the relationship, in the same way the therapist would with a married couple.

Other couples enter therapy seeking help with communication, sexuality, or children and are clear that the question of commitment is not an issue. The therapist should proceed as if this were true, although commitment issues may surface later, and a high index of suspicion is wise.

SERIAL RELATIONSHIPS

Even if a person has previously been in multiple relationships, they may enter treatment for a specific relationship at a specific time either alone or with the partner. **The critical questions are whether the person has been making the same set of mistakes each time or has been making new ones, and whether they have grown developmentally.** A common pattern is as follows:

A man marries first a woman whom his parents approve of and who seems "safe," then someone totally different, of a different religion or race. Finally, around age 40, he figures out who he is and what he wants and marries someone who is like him culturally and is interesting to him emotionally. Similarly, a woman might marry cold, abusive men until she decides that she is worth something and then marries someone who respects her. A less hopeful pattern is a person who marries two or three people in succession, each with the same serious problem, such as alcoholism, violence, or mental illness. The therapist's job is to help the person work on their own development, enough to make healthy choices in the future.

CLINICAL PRACTICE IMPLICATIONS

These are difficult situations, and it is hard for us to make guidelines. Our advice is to be flexible in the context of what evidence-based data on such families is available with the objective of improving family functioning for all family members. This is easy for us to say, the devil for the therapist is in the details of how to work out these situations.

In any case, the task of the family clinician is to set goals and treat with classical family techniques depending on the particular needs of the family.

SUGGESTED READINGS

The following two books are highly recommended for the lay public.

Ahrons CR. *We're Still Family*. HarperCollins; 2009.

REFERENCES

1. Weissman MM, Bland RC, Canino GJ, et al. Cross-national epidemiology of major depression and bipolar disorder. *JAMA*. 1996;276:293–299.
2. Isaacs M, Montalvo B, Abelsohn D. *The Difficult Divorce: Therapy for Children and Families*. Basic Books; 1986.
3. Wallerstein J. *Second Chances*. Ticknor and Fields; 1988.
4. Ahrons CR. *The Good Divorce*. HarperCollins; 1994.
5. Pasley K, Rhoden L, Visher EB, et al. Stepfamilies in therapy: insights from adult stepfamily members. *J Marital Fam Ther*. 1996;22:343–357.
6. Visher EB, Visher JS. *Therapy With Stepfamilies*. Brunner/Mazel; 1996:41–42.
7. Sager CJ, Brown HS, Crohn H, et al. *Treating the Remarried Family*. Brunner/Mazel; 1983.
8. Stern PA: Stepfather families: integration around child discipline. *Issues Ment Health Nurs*. 1978;1:49–56.
9. Papernow P: *Becoming a Stepfamily: Patterns of Development in Remarried Families*. Jossey-Bass; 1993.
10. Visher EB, Visher JS. *Old Loyalties, New Ties: Therapeutic Strategies with Stepfamilies*. Brunner/Mazel; 1988.
11. Visher EB, Visher JS. Parenting coalitions after remarriage: dynamics and therapeutic guidelines. *Fam Relat*. 1990;38:65–70.

We discuss in this section the differences in evaluation and treatment made necessary by the presence of a psychiatric disorder or other special problem in a family member. In Chapter 18, we discuss how the family is affected and how to use family intervention when one member has a psychiatric disorder. In Chapter 19, we examine how treatment techniques must be modified for special but common situations such as the problematic family in which aggressive, abusive, or suicidal behaviors are frequent. In Chapter 20, we go on to discuss how family behavior can be organized around acute or chronic mental illness and why the therapist must be aware of the typical patterns and responses of families in these situations. We also discuss treatment in settings such as the psychiatric hospital or the community mental health center, in which these problems are (or should be) managed from a family perspective. Chapter 21 asks the family therapist to consider how medical and psychiatric illness affects the family and how specific family characteristics influence the course of medical illness. In order to achieve this understanding, the family therapist must expand the traditional family assessment interview to include clarifying questions. Medical illness may cause the family to feel overwhelmed with practical and emotional challenges. In such situations, the family therapist can provide a therapeutic space for family reflection. Regarding specific family interventions, family research demonstrates the effectiveness of family interventions such as family inclusion approaches, family psychoeducation, and systemic family therapy.

Section

VI Family Treatment When One Member Has a Psychiatric Disorder or Other Special Problem

18 Family Treatment in the Context of Individual Psychiatric Disorders 231

19 Family Treatment in the Context of Other Special Problems—Violence to Self and Others 264

20 The Family and Treatment of Acute and Chronic Psychiatric Illness 284

21 Working with Families in the Medical Setting 302

18 Family Treatment in the Context of Individual Psychiatric Disorders

OBJECTIVES FOR THE READER

- To be aware of family interaction patterns associated with individual psychiatric disorders
- To know the indications for, and techniques of, family intervention in combination with other treatment methods in specific psychiatric disorders

For easier reading, we emphasize that the descriptors "couples" or "marital" are used nearly interchangeably in this chapter.

INTRODUCTION

In this chapter, we demonstrate how family, individual, dynamic, and physiologic issues intersect in various mental disorders, and how family therapy is conducted when a family member has a specific disorder. We concentrate on those diagnoses in which we believe family issues are most often part of the total picture. We also propose treatment guidelines and strategies for each disorder.

If the identified patient has a specific major psychiatric diagnosis, treatment will usually include individual therapy and, most often, medication. In most instances, treatment is also indicated for the family problems and interactions accompanying these conditions. Some of the family problems may be related to the etiology of the individual illness, some may be secondary to it, others may adversely affect the course of the illness, and still others may not be connected at all. For example, if schizophrenia has developed in a spouse early in the marriage, the therapist's attention must be directed not only to treatment of the mental illness but also to the nature of the marital interaction, including its possible role in exacerbating or ameliorating the illness. If a major psychiatric disorder occurs in one family member, attention must be paid to the family's ability to cope with the illness. For example, a child may respond to their mother's severe depressive illness by becoming a caretaker to younger siblings, at risk of their own development, or the child may begin "acting out." The cardinal symptoms of depression like lowered mood, anhedonia, and irritability will cause marital stress. Conversely, the depression may have been symptomatic of severe marital or family stress.

Family interventions for many psychiatric disorders are one component of a multimodal prescription, but those interventions may be crucial to success.

THE FAMILY MODEL AND INDIVIDUAL DIAGNOSIS
SCHIZOPHRENIA
Rationale
Treatment Considerations
Patients with Schizophrenia Living with or Supported by Families of Origin
Patients with Schizophrenia Who Are Married, with or without Children
MOOD DISORDERS: BIPOLAR DISORDER
Rationale
Treatment Considerations
Psychoeducational Marital Interventions
Other Specific Psychosocial Interventions
MOOD DISORDERS: PERSISTENT DEPRESSIVE DISORDER AND MAJOR DEPRESSIVE DISORDER
Rationale
Depression in Adolescents and Young Adults
Depression in Partnered or Married People
Depression in Parents
Depression in Middle-aged and Older Adults
Treatment Considerations
BORDERLINE PERSONALITY DISORDER
Rationale
Borderline Adolescents and Young Adults at Home
Borderline-Partnered and Married People
Treatment Considerations
ANXIETY DISORDERS
Rationale
Panic Disorder and Agoraphobia
Treatment
OBSESSIVE-COMPULSIVE DISORDER
Rationale
Treatment
POSTTRAUMATIC STRESS DISORDER
Rationale
Treatment
DEMENTIA, AMNESIA, AND OTHER COGNITIVE DISORDERS
Rationale
Treatment Considerations
EATING DISORDERS
Rationale
Treatment Considerations
SUBSTANCE-RELATED DISORDERS
Rationale
Assessment and Treatment Guidelines
Children of Alcoholic Parents
PSYCHIATRIC DISORDERS OF CHILDHOOD
Intellectual Disability
Treatment
Autism Spectrum Disorder
Rationale
Treatment
Attention-Deficit/Hyperactivity Disorder

Rationale
Treatment
Oppositional Defiant Disorder and Conduct Disorder
Rationale
Treatment
Anxiety Disorders
Mood Disorders
Rationale
Treatment
Childhood Obesity
CLINICAL PRACTICE IMPLICATIONS

THE FAMILY MODEL AND INDIVIDUAL DIAGNOSIS

In medicine, psychiatry, and related fields, the traditional focus of healing and treatment has been on disease and disorder. Diagnosis as a rubric implies a model that includes signs and symptoms, etiologic theories, treatment, and prognosis. For some family therapists, any kind of labeling of the individual is inappropriate, because it locates the problems in the individual while ignoring the role of family members and other environmental conditions and stimuli. **We subscribe to a broad psychosocial model in which the individual and family model interacts.**

This chapter will discuss how the existing research informs clinical practice. We will be highlighting many individual disorders but use schizophrenia as a prime example.

SCHIZOPHRENIA

Rationale

From the early days of the family therapy movement, clinicians have had a fascination with schizophrenia and the families of patients with the disorder. Over the last five decades, the family approach has changed dramatically in this area, relating to these most seriously ill patients and their family interactions.

Early family theorists were interested in the family's role in the etiology of schizophrenia. These writers emphasized concepts such as the schizophrenogenic mother,[1] faulty boundary setting, and family interactions such as double bind,[2,3] pseudomutuality,[4] and schism and skew.[5] Current conceptualizations have been influenced by subsequent research concerning the multiple factors in the etiology of schizophrenia. **Schizophrenia is now understood to be a brain disorder with strong familial links. Specific brain area functions show abnormalities.** The familial aggregation of persons with schizophrenia appears to be largely from genetic causes.[6,7] Changes in brain function may precede adolescence. A vulnerability–stress model of schizophrenic episodes was proposed in the 1980s,[8] emphasizing individual deficits (e.g., information-processing deficits, autonomic reactivity anomalies, social competence, and coping limitations) in combination with stressors (e.g., life events, family environmental stress, substance abuse as it affects the brain). This model still seems relevant to the development of psychotic episodes (see Fig. 18.1).

A number of historical and scientific trends have contributed to the development of the psychosocial interventions recommended today for families of persons with schizophrenia. One trend is the development of the construct of expressed emotion. In 1962, a team of British investigators reported that patients who returned to live with their families after psychiatric hospitalization were more prone to rehospitalization than those patients who went to boarding homes and hostels after discharge.[9] To explore these interesting leads, this group developed a semistructured interview to quantify the family environment to which the patient would return.

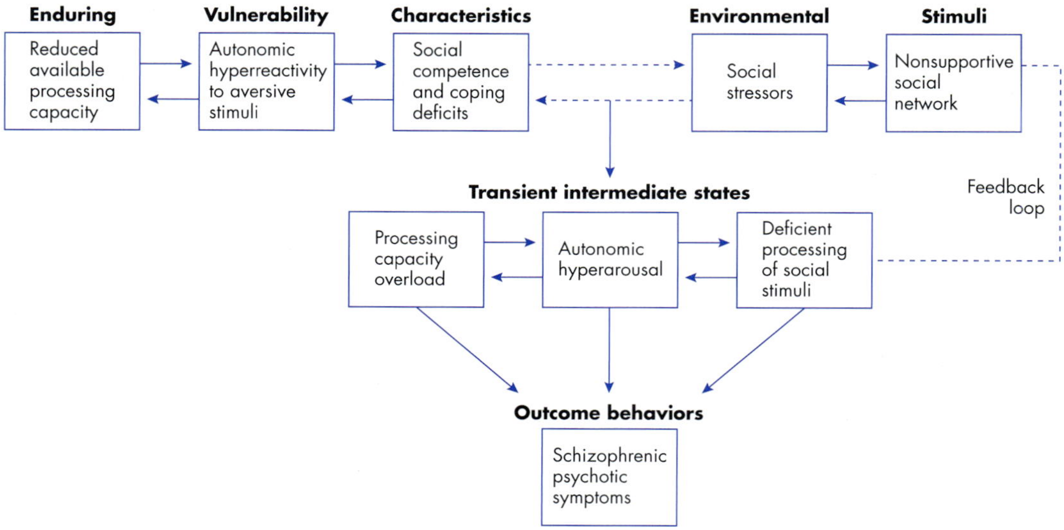

Figure 18.1 A tentative, interactive vulnerability–stress model for the development of schizophrenic psychotic episodes. (*Source:* Nuechterlein KH, Dawson ME. Information processing and attentional functioning in the developmental course of schizophrenic disorders. *Schizophr Bull.* 1984;10(2):160–203.)

This instrument, the Camberwell Family Interview, provides measures of what these researchers have termed **expressed emotion, which is primarily an index of the family's criticism of, and overinvolvement with, the identified patient.** Although researchers commonly refer to high expressed emotion families, it is important to understand that the rating of expressed emotion is based on observations made of a single cross-sectional interview of one family member and the patient.[10] In subsequent years, it has been found both with British and American samples that the percentage of patients in families with high expressed emotion who relapse, or are rehospitalized, is significantly higher than the percentage in the low expressed emotion families. For example, patients with schizophrenia that were in high-EE families experienced a relapse rate of 58% as compared to only 16% in low-EE families.[11]

The concept of expressed emotion has been dissected further. In the long term (i.e., after the acute episode), emotional overinvolvement is associated with a better social outcome in patients because it is part of the increased care that these disabled patients need (and desire).[12] The concept of expressed emotion may be detecting excess stress in the environment of the person with schizophrenia; however, much more needs to be learned about how the patient may contribute to this family response, how expressed emotion changes over time, and how it varies across cultures. Somewhat parenthetically, "expressed emotion" has been found important in understanding and preventing relapse not only in schizophrenia but also in both mood disorders and eating disorders (see later in this chapter).[13]

This work has led to very specific family therapeutic approaches concerning schizophrenia. Influenced by such work, researchers have put together treatment packages with the specific goals of reducing familial hostility and over-involvement in the acute phase. These studies will not only provide data on a potential intervention strategy but also might provide experimental evidence that expressed emotion indeed has some causal relationship to the course of the illness. This work has been carried on in the United States and in England.[14] This therapeutic approach has been used with chronic schizophrenia on an outpatient basis,[15] with more acutely ill schizophrenia in inpatient settings,[16] and in brief therapy immediately after hospitalization.[17] We describe the outcome studies for schizophrenia and family interventions in Chapter 24.

Treatment of major psychoses	=	Medication	+	Family intervention	+	Individual intervention	+	Consumer group support

Figure 18.2 A quality treatment equation.

Treatment Considerations

In an important follow-up of formerly hospitalized patients with schizophrenia, who had partially recovered—they were asked what had made the difference. They all said, "The key was a relationship with a personal family or friend who believed in them, who talked to them, and who was committed to staying with them".

Modern family interventions have been based partly on the concept of expressed emotion and partly on the increasing evidence that schizophrenia is a disease of the brain. Children with a genetic predisposition to schizophrenia appear to be more sensitive to environmental influences (i.e., parents, peers, poverty) than children who do not have a genetic predisposition.[6] The shift in caretaking burden to families after the deinstitutionalization movement of the 1950s and 1960s led to the rise in the family advocacy movement. Families demanded services for their family members and themselves that did not blame them for the illness. **Because families may perceive the concept of expressed emotion as a form of blaming, an alternative term that appreciates the complexity of this phenomenon is "expressed exasperation."**

Family therapists acknowledged that traditional family therapy techniques were not working and had caused many family members to complain and revolt (i.e., they did not want to be treated by family therapists, preferring biologically oriented professionals).

A number of guidelines exist for the treatment of schizophrenia using a family approach. **The family approach has shifted dramatically from the early conceptualization of the family as part of the problem to the family as part of the treatment team. First and foremost, the family intervention must be combined with medication**. Figure 18.2 provides a quality treatment equation (i.e., the elements of what must be done for most Axis I disorders). Second, different formats of family intervention must be used at different phases of the illness (Table 18.1). Third, the approach must be mostly psychoeducational rather than systemic but can shift in later phases of the illness.

As we discuss in Chapter 20, during acute episodes when the patient is psychotic and may need hospitalization, contact is not only helpful to the family but is also beneficial for later collaboration with treatment personnel.[20] The family is involved from the first contact. The main focus is psychoeducational—to teach the family about the symptoms, diagnosis, treatment, and prognosis with and without treatment and about the family's role in management.[21] The family therapist should take a positive, interested, supportive, undemanding, and noninterpretive stance toward the family during this phase. The acute psychosis may last for several weeks or months, during which time hospitalization or crisis intervention may proceed with the use of antipsychotic medication. Conjoint family meetings with the patient during this period may be contraindicated

Table 18.1 Alternative formats for psychoeducational family treatment

Individual family unit[15,17]
Individual family plus relatives' groups[14]
Relatives-only groups[14]
Multiple family groups[18]
Parallel patient and relatives' groups

Source: Reprinted with permission from Goldstein MJ. Psycho-education and family treatment related to the phase of a psychotic disorder. *Int Clin Psychopharmacol.* 1996;11(Suppl 2):77–83.

as being too stimulating for an acutely psychotic patient but sometimes yield helpful information about family patterns during the psychotic phase. Family meetings with the patient for psychoeducational purposes should be started early and the family referred to the National Alliance on Mental Illness (NAMI) that sponsor family- and peer-based education programs. One such program that is widely disseminated is the Family-to-Family Education Program (FFEP) which is designed specifically to help families cope with having a family member who has severe mental illness. These programs are generally free of charge and are available in many communities.

During the subsequent stabilization phase, when symptoms are subsiding, the family's feelings (e.g., guilt, anger, worry) are more likely to emerge. In this phase (lasting 3 to 9 months), the patient's florid symptoms give way and expose negative symptoms such as lack of initiative and apathy. At this point, the family needs further information and support in dealing with the chronic condition. The psychoeducational approach should be started early and continued during this phase. The approach consists of individual meetings with the family, educational workshops with other families, family support groups, and so on.[22]

Individual sessions focus heavily on concerns of a particular family, whereas family groups and workshops focus on more generic issues linked to the diagnosis. As the illness becomes stabilized and the clinical team moves into the maintenance phase, multifamily psychoeducational groups become more important. This is probably because other families that are coping with the same kinds of problems are extremely helpful to the individual family that has a member with schizophrenia. Lucksted et al.[23] conducted a controlled study of individual versus multifamily groups and found that the multifamily group format is more efficacious than the individual format for some types of families (e.g., Caucasian). B. McFarlane (personal communication, 1998) has developed an excellent list of "family guidelines" for families of patients with chronic schizophrenia:

Here is a list of things everyone can do to help make things run more smoothly:

1. GO SLOW. Recovery takes time. Rest is important. Things will get better in their own time.
2. KEEP IT COOL. Enthusiasm is normal. Tone it down. Disagreement is normal. Tone it down too.
3. GIVE EACH OTHER SPACE. Time out is important for everyone. It is okay to reach out. It is okay to say "no."
4. SET LIMITS. Everyone needs to know what the rules are. A few good rules keep things clear.
5. IGNORE WHAT YOU CANNOT CHANGE. Let some things slide. Do not ignore violence.
6. KEEP IT SIMPLE. Say what you have to say clearly, calmly, and positively.
7. FOLLOW DOCTOR'S ORDERS. Take medications as they are prescribed.

Take only medications that are prescribed.

8. CARRY ON BUSINESS AS USUAL. Reestablish family routines as quickly as possible. Stay in touch with family and friends.
9. NO STREET DRUGS OR ALCOHOL. They make symptoms worse.
10. PICK UP ON EARLY SIGNS. Note changes. Consult with your family clinician.
11. SOLVE PROBLEMS STEP BY STEP. Make changes gradually. Work on one thing at a time.
12. LOWER EXPECTATIONS, TEMPORARILY. Use a personal yardstick.

Compare this month to last month rather than last year or next year.

Not everything can be accomplished with psychoeducation. Tables 18.2 and 18.3 cover issues relevant to patients experiencing their first psychotic break and what can and cannot be taught in psychoeducation. Some sessions must be directed to family dynamics. Adding family intervention cannot replace adequate medication. Schooler et al.[24] found convincing evidence that the

Table 18.2 Special issues in carrying out psychoeducational family programs with patients experiencing their first psychotic break

Diagnostic ambiguity
Presence of striking affective features
Need to acknowledge diagnostic uncertainty
Education cannot be as specific as with chronic patients
Impact on family different compared with chronic cases
No previous experience with psychosis
Acuteness of episode more mystifying
Limited readiness of patients and relatives to seek support outside family

Source: Reprinted with permission from Goldstein MJ. Psycho-education and family treatment related to the phase of a psychotic disorder. *Int Clin Psychopharmacol.* 1996;11(Suppl 2):77–83.

standard dose of medication is the best dose strategy, in comparison with a low dose or a targeted medication strategy, and that adding family intervention is insufficient to lower a particular dose.

Should family intervention always be described during the acute phase? Glick et al.[16] randomly assigned 84 schizophrenic patients either to an inpatient family intervention plus medication in the context of standard hospital treatment or to medication and standard hospital treatment without family intervention. They found positive effects for female patients with schizophrenia and their families at discharge and at 18-month follow-up for those who received the family intervention. Male patients were unaffected or did worse, probably either because the brain disease was worse than in females or because females have been socialized to be more compliant with treatment (both with family therapy and with medication) and therefore do better than males. Perhaps women are more responsive to family environment improvement. This is also true in couple's therapy for depression (i.e., women did better, men did worse). In summary, where possible, family intervention should start as early as possible.

Patients with Schizophrenia Living with or Supported by Families of Origin

Because the majority of schizophrenia symptoms, including first psychotic break, occur in the late teens and early 20s, the majority of young patients with schizophrenia will be unmarried and living and/or supported by their families of origin. For these families, the onset of symptoms is cause for enormous fear, helplessness, and guilt over whether they have damaged their

Table 18.3 Factors affected and not affected by a brief family education program

Factors affected	Factors not affected
Feeling of support from the treatment team	Information retention
Family's sense of responsibility for the illness	Perception of symptoms Interactions with patient
Understanding of the illness	Burden from illness
Awareness that the patient's behavior is not intentional	Hope for the future Hours per week spent with patient
Rejection of the patient	

Source: Reprinted with permission from Goldstein MJ. Psycho-education and family treatment related to the phase of a psychotic disorder. *Int Clin Psychopharmacol.* 1996;11(Suppl 2):77–83.

child. Early individual therapists and early family therapists blamed the family for the child's schizophrenia. Individual therapists often kept families ignorant of the treatment process, and family therapists burdened the family with the full responsibility for the child's recovery. Many of these families were doubly traumatized. Current assumptions are that although families are not responsible for the illness, they can aid in (or derail) the recovery process and need to be given as much information as possible, while being supported in the huge burden of caring for their child and mourning the loss of the child's healthy self and possible future. The current state of health care has increased the burden on families, who can no longer rely on the health care system to respond adequately to psychotic symptoms and who can seldom get a child hospitalized unless violence to self or others has occurred. Because schizophrenia has a large genetic component, it is important to consider the mental health of other family members and their ability to support or contain the manifestations of illness. Chronic illness in a child can exacerbate marital conflict, and because marital conflict may amplify stress at home, the parental unit also must be evaluated.

Multifamily psychoeducation groups are designed to inform, teach, and empower family members with information about the disease and kinds of psychosocial interventions that can worsen symptoms in the identified patient.[25]

> Families need to be given as much information as possible, while being supported in the huge burden of caring for their child and mourning the loss of the child's healthy self and possible future.

One of the most complicated issues with these families is a decision about when the child is well enough to leave home to work or live on their own. Parents who are understandably concerned about their offspring managing alone in an apartment may be labeled incorrectly as enmeshed; in contrast, parents can infantilize children who could manage in the world with help. For these families, the process of leaving home can be complicated and protracted, with many attempts before some form of independent living is managed.

Landeen et al.[26] found that siblings of patients with schizophrenia have a special need for information and benefit from workshops with other well siblings. This is because of the emotions they commonly experience—guilt, fear, shame, and anger. Without some help, their most common defense is flight from the family and emotional constriction.

Patients with Schizophrenia Who Are Married, with or without Children

Although the rate of marriage among patients with schizophrenia is lower than that of the general population, many do marry and have children. Many of these are patients with periods of relatively good functioning between psychotic breaks. Some patients develop symptoms after marriage. The spouse of such a patient lives with the constant anxiety that another episode will occur, plus the oddness or difficulties with intimacy characteristic of the majority of these patients. Isolation and stigma also take a toll. Because some patients attempt self-medication with alcohol or other drugs, intoxication or addiction is a concern. Violence during psychotic episodes may occur. The rate of separation or divorce is quite high among individuals with schizophrenia.

Children faced with psychotic parents who cannot care for them, or parents whose thinking is far from consensual reality, face a series of problems growing up. A parent who changes suddenly from a loving caretaker to a helpless or dangerous being is an enormous source of fear for a child. If the healthy spouse cannot tolerate the situation and becomes emotionally absent or leaves the family, very young children may become caretakers for their ill parent. If the family cannot explain to the child what is happening, or insists that everything is normal, the child's own grasp of reality is compromised. Needs of offspring of patients with schizophrenia and other serious mental illnesses have also received increasing attention at family organizations such as NAMI. We recommend referral to such organizations in almost all cases.

The therapist must evaluate the family and the family's support system, make sure children are provided for and adequately informed, and ensure that the family is supported in its functioning. The therapist must approach the family with a supportive, nonblaming attitude. Families will blame themselves and need help to become constructive participants in the management of patients with schizophrenia.

In summary, the psychiatrist should serve as advocates for the family while providing psychoeducation. The clinician should listen to families and treat them as equal partners in treatment planning while exploring family members' expectations of treatment for the patient. Families should be encouraged to expand their social network and be referred to organizations like NAMI for support. Each family has strengths and limitations in being able to support the family and the clinician should be prepared to address feelings of loss, help resolve family conflict, and improve communication and problem solving. Planning for moments of crisis is of utmost importance.

MOOD DISORDERS: BIPOLAR DISORDER

Rationale

Bipolar disorder (BD) is a severe, recurrent, and usually chronic mental disorder that affects approximately 1% of the U.S. population. Patients with this disorder are characterized by depressive, manic, hypomanic, or mixed mood states. While pharmacologic treatments are first line, psychosocial interventions can improve symptoms and interpersonal functioning in bipolar patients. A range of family factors are implicated in the onset and course of bipolar disorders. These include dysfunctional early relationships with parents, high expressed emotion in families, family conflict, and lack of social support.

> Medication treatment alone is almost always not sufficient in the treatment of bipolar illness. Social support, including family interventions is key.

Rates of medication nonadherence among bipolar patients are as high as 53%. Patients who are at higher risk of medication nonadherence include those living alone, having unstable and unsupportive families, a more complex treatment regimen, and higher numbers and cost of medications.

Even when taken in adequate doses, medication may have a limited effect on impaired social function, and even with medication, psychosocial stress may provoke relapse and recurrence. Research demonstrates the need to specify more precisely the critical psychosocial variables that mediate medication compliance and, therefore, medication effectiveness.

Because psychosocial stress is an important determinant of relapse and recurrence in major affective disorders, it needs to be addressed both theoretically and pragmatically in the development and evaluation of treatment models. Although the characterization of high levels of expressed emotion as a response or adaptation to the stress of caretaking is not fully clear, the usefulness of expressed emotion as a predictor of relapse and rehospitalization in schizophrenia and unipolar depression is now well established.

Work with bipolar or manic patients shows that expressed emotion, along with affective style, predicts clinical outcome at 9 months postdischarge.

The first manic and depressive episodes are likely to occur in young adulthood, when patients are beginning to establish their own lives. Patients with BD are more likely than patients with schizophrenia to maintain good personality function between episodes; bipolar patients also marry more often and divorce less often than those with schizophrenia. If episodes are mild, the disorder may not be diagnosed. If episodes are severe, they are likely to wreak havoc on the family, especially in the manic phase when the patient's judgment is impaired and they may spend the family's money, lose jobs and friends, or become irritable, angry, and paranoid. Severe depression brings the possibility of suicide. The family must be involved, particularly in monitoring early symptoms and promoting medication adherence.

Because of genetic inheritance and because children of bipolar parents may experience chaos and parental loss periodically in the family, they are highly vulnerable to psychiatric disorders in adulthood. They may show early signs of bipolar illness that may not be understood and treated unless the family is evaluated. Bipolar patients who are not in the acute phase, or cyclothymic patients without frank psychosis, often have personality issues and subsyndromal symptoms. Individual and couples therapy is often helpful when the patient is in remission or maintained on medication. Consider the following case example:

Mrs. A, a 50-year-old married mother of eight children, experienced her first psychiatric disturbance 8 years earlier. At that time, a depressive episode characterized by profound lethargy, weeping and sadness, inability to complete minimal household tasks, and eventual withdrawal to bed led her to outpatient treatment with tricyclic antidepressants for a period of 2 years, with little change. The depression had occurred soon after the marriage of Mrs. A's oldest child and only daughter. A full-blown episode of mania led to an extended hospitalization, which lasted 1 year. During that time, Mrs. A was treated unsuccessfully with various antidepressants, including monoamine oxidase inhibitors, carbamazepine, and lithium carbonate. Since being discharged from the hospital, Mrs. A has continued to cycle unrelentingly, with periods of hypomania lasting 2 weeks and alternating with similar-length periods of severe depression. She is currently taking low doses of lithium and carbamazepine, which have altered the severity of the episodes slightly but not changed their frequency.

The history obtained from Mr. A presented a premorbid picture of an energetic and intellectual woman who was resourceful and well liked in the community where the family lived. Mrs. A's father, who committed suicide when she was age 16 years, and her paternal grandfather had histories of pronounced mood swings and are assumed to have had bipolar illness. The paternal grandfather lived in the family home until his death, and Mrs. A vividly recalled the profound effect this model of depression and hypomania had on her childhood.

By the time family therapy began, Mr. and Mrs. A's older children had assumed responsibility for cooking the meals, managing the shopping and the laundry, and generally attending to the needs of the younger children so that they were properly dressed and sent to school. During the first four family sessions, all of the children were present. They discussed the resentment they felt when their mother's mood switched from depression to hypomania, especially the resentment of her attempts in the first few days of mood elevation to reestablish her standards and control. They felt that she was oblivious to what was happening in the family and explained that her unavailability during a depression, when they had to be responsible, was experienced as abandonment.

Mr. A was noted to be quite passive. It became clear that despite resenting their mother's seeking to reclaim control during the first hypomanic days, the children nonetheless preferred her to be hypomanic, when fantasies could be acted out, no limits were set, and the children were swept along by Mrs. A's infectious high spirits.

During hypomanic periods, Mr. A perceived his wife as untrustworthy, a spendthrift, and neglectful of him and the children. He also seemed to prefer the hypomanic phase, which is unusual because many bipolar spouses prefer the period when the patient is depressed and less active. Mr. A resented his wife's threats of divorce, which occurred invariably during her hypomania and were linked to her lack of access to money and credit cards, which Mr. A controlled.

He experienced comfort and gratification from the high energy level and the excitement of Mrs. A's hypomanic phase. He was pleased by the increase in sexual activity and was excited by Mrs. A's plans and ideas, which though sometimes bizarre were perceived as sound and reasonable enough to be tolerable.

While Mrs. A was in the hospital, the family was seen weekly. After that, Mr. A and the children came in only when there was a marital- or family-focused problem or when they felt a need for support during a particularly trying episode. Mrs. A continued as an outpatient in individual therapy for many years. Over time, the sessions focused on the despair she felt about her relentless illness, her losses, and her sense of being a useless person. In individual sessions, she articulated conflictual and ambivalent feelings, areas that became available because of the family work. During good periods, she would talk about the possibilities that she could reintegrate and become a functioning person again. With two exceptions, she remained out of the hospital. One hospitalization entailed a brief stay when she was admitted for reevaluation of her medication. The other occasion, also brief, occurred when the therapist who had treated Mrs. A and her family throughout this period announced her departure from the area. Shortly afterward, Mrs. A had an episode in which she smashed and destroyed objects in her house, and the therapist was summoned in the middle of the night. Mrs. A insisted that the destructiveness had nothing to do with the coming loss of the therapist—that it merely represented anger felt toward Mr. A, who happened to be away on a business trip. Needless to say, this painful incident was also invaluable in the psychotherapy in working through the termination.

Mrs. A continues to have cycles and remains severely impaired by her illness; however, the marriage is intact and the children are coping relatively successfully in high school and college and have dealt well with the possible heritable aspects of the illness. Mrs. A continues to take her medication, which at best alleviates her symptoms only slightly, and has begun therapeutic work with a new and interested therapist.

Treatment Considerations

The combination of psychosocial interventions with medication treatments can be useful in BD. The growing research on the medication treatment of this crippling disorder is in sharp contrast to the relative absence of research on crucial behaviors associated with seeking treatment and the outcome of treatment, such as medication adherence, symptom monitoring, and stress management.

Intensive family interventions are most effective when family-associated stress is elevated or when persistent manic or hypomanic symptoms are the primary targets of treatment.[27]

A combination of inpatient psychosocial and pharmacologic treatments can result in improved work and social functioning in bipolar patients.[28,29] Clarkin et al.[29] randomly assigned bipolar patients and their families to either standard acute inpatient treatment or standard treatment, plus inpatient family intervention. The family treatment was brief (approximately six sessions) and included a psychoeducational component. Goals included accepting the reality of the illness, identifying precipitating stresses and likely future stresses inside and outside the family, elucidating family interactions that produce stress on the patient, planning strategies for managing or minimizing future stresses, and bringing about the family's acceptance of the need for continued treatment after hospital discharge.

Patients receiving inpatient family intervention showed less symptomatology at discharge. There was no rehospitalization of patients in either treatment group at 6 months after discharge. However, at 18 months, significantly fewer patients from the inpatient family intervention group had been rehospitalized (2/12) compared with the standard treatment group (4/8) ($P < .05$). Work or primary role functioning was significantly better for inpatient family intervention patients at both 6 and 18 months. Social role functioning was significantly better for the inpatient family intervention patients at 6 months.

Reviews of these psychoeducational treatment programs[19] have identified two common features: (1) They all aim to ameliorate the course of the illness and reduce relapse rate rather than to cure the condition, and (2) they try to attain these goals via clearly defined types of family intervention that are largely educational in nature.[30] Psychoeducational interventions are those aimed at obtaining the family's help in working with the patient, educating the family as to the nature of the illness and what can be expected, and helping the family to modify stressful interaction patterns.

Although the exact mechanism of relapse is unknown, expressed emotion is regarded as a form of psychosocial stress with biologic implications for at-risk patients.[31] It is postulated that when patients experience increased levels of stress, in which family behavior is experienced as emotionally threatening, a surge of cortisol from the adrenal gland stimulates dopaminergic and glutamatergic neurotransmitter systems, ultimately contributing to psychiatric relapse.[31] In one study of bipolar patients,[32] the determining factor in relapse was not the patients' rating of the severity of the criticism, but rather their rating of how distressed they were because of the criticism. Interestingly, patients who reported that their relatives became more upset by their criticisms had less severe depressive symptoms at follow-up. This suggests that the stress was the patient's cognitive sense of criticism as a threat.[32]

Psychoeducational Marital Interventions

For the family therapist we suggest an approach called psychoeducational marital intervention. It is based on the belief that the following four variables mediate outcome: (1) medication compliance, (2) engagement in the psychoeducational marital intervention treatment, (3) change in spousal negative attitudes, (4) and increase in problem-solving skills. Clarkin et al.[33] conducted a controlled study of psychoeducational marital intervention and found that this treatment may be most useful with patients who have more severe illness and have a personality disorder. Less severely ill bipolar patients without personality disorder may respond adequately to medication without the need for family intervention.

Other Specific Psychosocial Interventions

Behavioral family management is a treatment for patients who have recently been hospitalized for an episode of mania. It is based on a home-centered psychosocial treatment for schizophrenia.[34] The treatment includes psychoeducation, communication skills training, and problem-solving skills training. Although definitive trials of behavioral family management have not been completed, preliminary evidence suggests that the treatment approach, in concert with adequate pharmacotherapy, leads to a substantial decrease in relapse rate. Miklowitz. (2016)[35] reported a pilot study of the effect of family therapy and psychoeducation (in addition to pharmacologic and milieu treatment) on patients with BD. Patients who were assigned randomly to the family therapy group (compared with a control group) had lower rates of family separations, greater improvements in the level of family functioning, higher rates of full recovery, and lower rates of rehospitalization for 2 years following family treatment. In recent years, Miklowitz et al.[32] demonstrated that family-focused therapy (FFT) was helpful to patients during the depressive phase of bipolar illness. FFT is an evidence-based treatment for BD that focuses on psychoeducation around the disease, as well as building upon communication skills as well as problem solving strategies. This treatment has been found most effective for high-expressed emotional relatives of patients with BD. For outcome data regarding FFT in adolescents with BD, please see Chapter 24.

In summary, medication and family psychoeducational intervention is crucial. Whether systemic family therapy in the prevention phase is useful remains to be tested. Family intervention in BD should focus on helping families to decrease expressed emotion and improve problem-solving skills while developing strategies to deal with relapse.

MOOD DISORDERS: PERSISTENT DEPRESSIVE DISORDER AND MAJOR DEPRESSIVE DISORDER

Rationale

Where an association exists between family conflict and depressive disorders, it can be understood in a number of possible ways[36,37]:

- Family stressors may elicit or precipitate depressive symptoms in a biologically vulnerable individual.
- Family stress or the lack of a sufficiently supportive intimate relationship may potentiate the effects of other environmental stressors.
- Depressive symptoms may trigger maladaptive behaviors and negative responses from family members, thus eliciting conflict.
- Subclinical depression or characterologic traits, behavior patterns, and so on may potentiate family discord, which tends to trigger a depressive episode.

A major depressive disorder may develop, slowly or quickly, in a person with previously good mood and social functioning. These patients may progress to complete inability to function at home or work. Although these depressions sometimes remit spontaneously after several months, most last 6 to 12 months untreated. Appropriate treatment, usually including medication, will restore function quickly in most patients. Research has indicated that depression is in many cases a relapsing problem. If multiple episodes occur, the patient may develop personality changes and social maladjustment.

In patients with persistent depressive disorder, a slow course of depressed mood, lack of concentration, sleep disturbance, and so on occurs over a period of months. These patients may have an intact or mildly impaired ability to function. They receive diagnoses and treatment less often than those with more severely impaired function. Shyness, low self-esteem, and anxiety or a depressive personality style may precede either a major depressive disorder or dysthymia.

Depression in Adolescents and Young Adults

Undiagnosed depression is a major cause of adolescent suicide and alcohol and substance use problems. Because adolescents are trying to separate from their parents they may be reluctant to share their distress, see a therapist, or accept treatment. Depression in adolescents may occur without obvious cause, especially in children with a family history of depression, or it may occur secondary to family factors such as parental divorce, alcoholism, or conflict; parental mental illness; or child abuse or neglect. Because the peer system is so important and the teen's identity shaky, difficulties in love relationships are particularly likely to precipitate depressive episodes, especially if the adolescent has a history of parental loss or neglect.

Serious depression in young adults can also seriously compromise the launching process. If a child believes they are needed at home to protect a parent, depression provides an excuse to be home instead of out in the world. Even if the parents are ready for the child to leave, the child may be overwhelmed by the choices inherent in setting up a home and life of one's own and may require more parental support. In those who complete the launching successfully, difficulties in love relationships (especially for women) and work relationships (especially for men) may precipitate depression in vulnerable people.

Depression in Partnered or Married People

Depression in marriage is a common outgrowth of the complex nature of the relationship. The fact that two out of three depressed people are women has led to considerable questioning about the role of hormones; the role of female role conditioning for passivity, caretaking, and low self-worth; and the role of chronic stress and discrimination as precipitants for depression.

Because women are particularly attuned to relational contexts and draw much of their self-worth from intimate relationships, marital and family dysfunction or overload are particularly likely to generate depressive symptoms in a vulnerable woman. Verbal and physical abuse especially are likely to lead to depression. Severe environmental stress—such as job loss leading to alcohol intake in one or both partners, a very ill child or parent who requires care, or multiple interpersonal losses—can lead to depression. Men who become depressed within marriage sometimes present with masked depression, in which they become irritable and withdrawn but deny sadness or feelings of poor self-worth. At other times, they may present a classic depressive triad (i.e., I am bad, the world is bad, and it won't get better).

How depression in one partner affects the marital interaction has been clarified.[38] The depressed person gives and receives aversive stimulation (i.e., irritable or negative responses) at higher rates than do other family members. Depressed partners and mates engage in negative exchanges more frequently than do nondistressed normal couples. In social situations, depressed people tend to avoid others, which is associated with the tendency for others to avoid them. This further narrows their interaction field and leads to problems at work and with friends, putting additional stress on the marriage. Systemic patterns commonly seen in depressed couples include the following:

- *Both partners are depressed.* Often one partner is more angry and the other more sad. Neither has time nor energy to care for the other. This pattern often occurs when there has been severe family trauma such as the death of a child.
- *One partner is depressed, and the other is the caretaker.* The depressed person is labeled incompetent, helpless, and in need of cheering up and support. They are allowed to avoid unwanted activities because of the depression. The caretaker may be angry or take on the role of saint or superperson. Because both of these roles involve many positive attributes, they may be hard to give up.
- *One partner is demanding, coercive, and abusive, and the other is depressed.* This pattern is common in abusive relationships. The depression is often a response to the abuse and control; it may also mask the anger that, if expressed, would lead to more abuse.

Depression in Parents

Considerable evidence indicates that a mother depressed enough not to respond empathically to her infant puts the infant at some risk. Because the infant is dependent on the parent's ability to return nonverbal cues, a parent who cannot do so may cause the infant to give up on the possibility of response. Depressed persons have less energy for their children and are more apt to be less encouraging and more irritable and unavailable. In addition, they model a depressive world view and low self-esteem. Female children of depressed mothers are particularly likely to become caretakers in the home. The marital discord found in families with a depressed mother may have a larger negative effect on the child than does the parent's mood disorder itself.

Depression in Middle-aged and Older Adults

Because depressive episodes become more frequent as people age, many middle-aged and older people with previously adequate functioning develop depression secondary to life stresses or losses. Middle-aged depression may be a factor in midlife divorce, as one partner blames their sadness on the spouse and determines to leave. Major depression or dysthymia may also be the result of divorces, especially for middle-aged women whose primary job was homemaking and who did not want the divorce. Retirement is another cause of depression, particularly in men. When older adults become depressed, they are often a burden on their adult children, who may respond with a mixture of guilt and anger or who may refuse to help at all. This can often affect all generations of the family system, including the grandchildren.

Treatment Considerations

The temporal and functional relationships between depression and aspects of family interaction have important implications for the design and implementation of family treatment of depressive disorders. Family conflict is often reported as the primary precipitant in episodes of clinical depression. In such cases, family therapy would be indicated for treatment of the interpersonal problems, often directed at reducing the frequency of aversive communications between partners, inducing more frequent mutual reinforcement, and modifying distorted cognitive and perceptual responses to the partner's behavior.[39] Antidepressant medication can be combined with these therapies for symptom relief without risk of compromising their effectiveness. If family conflict appears not to be a contributing factor in the depressive episode, the identified patient should be treated with appropriate medication and then reevaluated for psychotherapy. The addition of short-term supportive family therapy may be useful in helping to engage the patient in the recommended medication regimen.

With more severe depression in which the identified patient's function is severely impaired, a two-phase program of family intervention is needed. During the initial phase, psychopharmacological treatments are begun and short-term supportive family therapy is introduced to ameliorate the family's negative reactions to the symptoms (thus reducing secondary stress reactions) and to educate the patient and family as to the nature of the disorder, the recommended treatment, and strategies for coping with residual symptoms and possible relapse. The family can be helpful either directly to the patient or indirectly in maintaining its own homeostasis by early recognition of symptoms (especially hypomania); by monitoring the patient's mood; by being aware of early signs of medication toxicity such as nausea, vomiting, diarrhea, ataxia, and dysarthria; and by encouraging medication adherence. An objective family therapy helps the family develop new patterns necessary as a result of changes in the patient's role and function that stem from the illness and the medication.

Only after the florid symptoms have diminished and the patient and family have reached a plateau or relatively stable stage of adjustment can a second phase of therapy be initiated. Efforts to modify maladaptive communication patterns and problem-solving strategies, to deal with resistances, and to effect structural changes are best reserved for this phase of intervention. Consider the following case example:

Mr. B was a 46-year-old lawyer and his wife, Dr. B, was a 45-year-old physician. They had three children, aged 6, 9, and 12 years. The couple were referred for marital treatment (as a last resort) because of dissatisfaction with the marriage. The spouses saw divorce as the only solution. Over the previous year the couple's fighting (and mutual blaming), which dated to the beginning of their marriage some 20 years earlier, had intensified. Areas of conflict included money and childrearing. Mr. B's need for control of the relationship was evident in financial and parenting issues. To accomplish this, he would criticize his wife's attempts in both areas. For example, Dr. B would discipline the children, and Mr. B would say she should not have been so tough on them. When she did not discipline them, he would proclaim that she was negligent. The couple's history revealed that both had been brought up in Europe in what they described as chaotic households, with parents who fought more than their peers' parents. Each partner had a parent who experienced depressive episodes. The history of treatment attempts revealed that both husband and wife had had separate, classical psychoanalyses, which they described as "helpful but not enough to end the marital fighting." Both partners met criteria for a diagnosis of major depressive disorder, recurrent type.

When couples treatment started, Mr. B and Dr. B were extremely depressed, manifesting symptoms of loss of interest and pleasure, low self-esteem, and lack of energy. Treatment sessions centered on mutual blaming for each partner's symptoms. Three sessions led to no improvement. At that point, antidepressant medication was instituted. After 6 weeks, both partners experienced considerable improvement in mood and activity level. This change afforded the therapist two tactical advantages. First, with their mood and cognition improvements, the couple could conceivably begin to examine and alter behavioral interactions that might build a viable relationship.

Second, the therapist was now viewed as an expert who could prescribe tasks (e.g., taking the right medication) that were effective and thus was in a position to prescribe interpersonal tasks to change the previously described negative feedback systems such as Dr. B's control, Mr. B's criticism, and their resulting morass of further depression and lowered self-esteem. At this point, the therapist took advantage of this position by guiding the couple to interpersonal changes that led to further marital improvement.

The preceding case example illustrates how psychopharmacotherapy may enhance the efficacy of marital therapy. We also believe that marital therapy is likely to enhance psychopharmacotherapy in many depressive patients. Controlled studies have shown that psychosocial treatment with families can have significant effects on patient outcome. Well-controlled clinical research on unipolar depression has demonstrated that outpatient psychotherapy used in conjunction with pharmacologic treatments can improve patient functioning in the areas of social, family, and work adjustment. Jacobson and colleagues[40] treated depressed females and their spouses with cognitive-behavioral therapy, behavioral marital therapy, and a combination of the two. The results depended on the presence or absence of marital conflict. Without marital conflict, behavioral marital therapy was less effective than cognitive therapy in reducing depression. In contrast, when marital conflict was present, the two treatments were equally effective in reducing depression, but behavioral marital treatment was also effective in improving marital satisfaction. The combined treatment was the only treatment condition to reduce aversive behavior in the husband and wife and to increase facilitative behavior in the wife. On follow-up study,[41] relapse rates did not distinguish between the treatments. The nature of the husband–wife interaction related to relapse. Reductions in dysphoria in the husband and wife and increases in facilitative behavior in the wife during therapy predicted recovery. High rates of facilitative behavior in the husband at follow-up were associated with recovery. In one pilot study,[42] it was found that emotionally focused couples therapy was as effective as antidepressants in alleviating depression. For outcome data regarding behavioral marital therapy for depression, please see Chapter 24.

Keitner et al.[43] showed a clear association between better family functioning and recovery from major depression over the long term. Different aspects of family life respond differently to the depressive illness; no one family dimension was uniquely related to outcome.

In their study of adolescent depression, Brent et al.[44] compared cognitive therapy, individual supportive therapy, and systemic behavioral family therapy. All three treatments reduced suicidality and functional impairment, but cognitive therapy was more efficacious on a number of other parameters including credibility to the parents and more rapid relief of depression.

In summary, the overarching goals of family intervention in depressive disorders are to improve communication, improve family support, clarify family roles, reduce expressed emotion, provide psychoeducational support. In general, evidence suggests that family therapy combined with medication is better than either alone.

BORDERLINE PERSONALITY DISORDER

Rationale

A large body of research over the past decade provides strong evidence that borderline personality disorder (BPD) is a neurobiologic or brain disease.[45] Borderline patients experience significant problems pervasively in multiple aspects of life. Specifically, they suffer from unstable interpersonal relationships, unstable affects, an unstable sense of self, and poor impulse control (substance abuse, fighting, reckless driving, risky sexual behavior). These patients tend to use *splitting* as a defense mechanism and can quickly go from idealizing a clinician to devaluing the same clinician following a disappointment or misunderstanding. Borderline patients fear being alone and being abandoned and can suffer from major mood shifts throughout the day.

These patients are at high risk for self-harm (cutting and self-mutilation) which can be an outlet for expressing anger, self-punishment, and "to feel normal" in response to a dissociated state. They can feel very empty and can also present with quasipsychosis or "micropsychotic" experiences or dissociative states when very stressed. Patients can experience depersonalization (I am not real) and derealization (the world is not real). They can have unusual perceptions and experience nondelusional paranoia. Borderline patients are unable to tolerate the idea of being alone and can be very demanding and entitled. They can respond out of proportion to real or imagined abandonment and have difficulty controlling anger. There are very high levels of comorbid Axis I disorders including major depressive disorder, PTSD, and substance use disorders (SUDs). Many of these patients have a history of being invalidated, neglected, or abused as children. Early environmental experiences play a role in the etiology of BPD. A child, constantly threatened with abandonment, may grow to fear separations. Some patients may be more genetically predisposed to this disorder and biologic factors play a role, too (e.g., abnormal neurotransmitters, frontal lobe problems, and structural brain differences).

Borderline Adolescents and Young Adults at Home

Individuals undergoing a difficult adolescence may exhibit characteristics of BPD, including unstable and intense interpersonal relationships, identity disturbance, impulsivity and affective instability, feelings of emptiness, and inappropriate anger. In most teenagers, these characteristics alternate with periods of better function and a sense of developing self. BPD is generally not diagnosed until young adulthood, when it is clear that the symptoms do not represent a stage or a crisis but are a stable state. Young people with BPD are usually deeply involved in highly aversive and intense relationships with their families, involving early, ineffective, and protracted launching with inability to truly individuate. Relationships with peers and lovers are often intense and unstable, leading to rage or suicide attempts.

Borderline-Partnered and Married People

Borderline patients are likely to withdraw from others or engage in highly intense and dramatic relationships. Marriages are likely to be highly conflicted and unstable. In some couples, both spouses have BPD; in most others, one spouse has significant psychopathology. Borderline patients as parents run the gamut from reasonably functional to intrusive, hostile, and neglectful. Of note, the association between expressed emotion and patient outcome may be different for patients with BPD: one study did not find that relative's criticism and hostility predicted outcome. In fact, emotional overinvolvement predicted *better* clinical outcomes.[46]

Treatment Considerations

Psychotherapists have struggled for years to treat borderline patients, whose shifting symptom picture and difficulties with relating make a treatment alliance difficult. For some patients, medication management is essential to deal with psychotic symptoms and mood regulation. Individual therapy and medication are usually part of the treatment package. Magnavita and McFarlane[47] reviewed in detail the subject of the family and BPD.

One of the most effective treatments for borderline personality pathology is dialectical behavioral therapy (DBT). This intensive, evidence-based treatment consists of DBT skills group and individualized therapy. The treatment is also available for family members who can also benefit from learning the same DBT skills as the identified patient.

Family therapy is complex and depends on the family's situation. For example, if a young adult with BPD is living in a chaotic household, the entire family needs to be treated as the patient. In a family that is apparently running smoothly except for the identified patient, a decision must be made about whether to focus on basic psychoeducation (i.e., what can be expected, what types of support are sensible) or whether the patient is the truth teller or symptom bearer (e.g., in the case of a family that looks functional but in which the father has abused his daughters). In some families, whatever the issues or neglect of the early years, the rest of the family members have experienced good development and are now being overwhelmed by the demands of the borderline patient and by their own guilt. These families must be supported in setting limits on the amount of help they will give. Because borderline patients are at risk for suicide, the issues of risk must be discussed with the family at length.

Couples may have stormy relationships or may include one borderline spouse (usually the woman) and an apparently stoic or saintly caretaker. Therapy with these couples is slow and involves creating an atmosphere of support and consistency. These individuals try the therapist's tolerance and patience. The therapist must interview the children and consider their support system. Because many borderline women are single parents, particular attention must be paid to adequate support for the children.

In sum, clinicians should provide support to families of patients with BPD. Referring families to Family Connections (FC) sponsored by the National Education Alliance for Borderline Personality Disorder is a 12-week community-based BPD education program for family members. Research has shown that families who complete the program feel more empowered and experience less burden and grief.[48]

ANXIETY DISORDERS

Rationale

DSM-5 groups together the following anxiety disorders: panic disorder, agoraphobia, specific phobias, social anxiety disorder, generalized anxiety disorder, anxiety due to another medical condition, and substance/medication induced anxiety disorder.[49] Anxiety disorders can be treated with medication, cognitive-behavioral therapy including desensitization, or both. Many of these disorders have a far higher incidence in women, and family stress or the loss or disruption of close personal relationships often precipitates attacks. Most of these patients marry, and the considerable morbidity associated with anxiety disorders strains both marital relations and parenting practices. The symptoms are often deeply embedded in the family's way of operating, and the anxious person is sometimes a symptom bearer for the family. This is particularly true with panic disorder, generalized anxiety disorder, and agoraphobia. Consider the following case example:

Mrs. C, the mother of two young children, had low self-esteem and a family history of anxiety. Mr. C was a rather controlling husband who held a demanding academic job. After a number of years as a homemaker, Mrs. C decided to return to school to finish her degree. Mr. C was very unsupportive and declared that Mrs. C could go back to school only if she made all the child-care arrangements and continued to care for the house. After her first exam at school, on which she did adequately but not spectacularly, she became acutely anxious and subsequently depressed. For a number of weeks she was so consistently anxious that she could not function at home at all, forcing her husband to take over the household and childcare. Her anxiety could be construed in several ways: it expressed her rage at his unsupportiveness, it was a way of going "on strike" that he could not combat with logic, and it represented her hopelessness over her inability to either find the intimacy and support she wanted from her husband or do brilliantly at school to support her self-esteem. She was treated with a combination of antidepressants, antianxiety medication, brief couples therapy (her husband would not tolerate more), and supportive individual therapy over a period of 3 months. At the end of treatment, she was back at school, and her husband was functioning more supportively, grateful that he no longer had the full burden of the house.

Although the therapist in the preceding case example initially thought that the patient should be stabilized on medication before couples therapy was started, it was not until couples therapy had been initiated and the patient's husband had begun to take his wife's concerns seriously that the symptoms subsided. This has been true of the majority of patients seen in our practice. We recommend early evaluation of the entire family system with the rapid initiation of couples' work if it appears indicated.

Panic Disorder and Agoraphobia

Patients who suffer from panic disorder experience panic attacks that usually occur out of the clear blue and result in transient, acute, severe anxiety. Patients with this condition eventually get anxious about becoming anxious and begin to do things to try to avoid panic attacks (e.g., staying in the house all the time). The panic attacks cannot be due to another medical condition or substance use. The specifier *with panic attacks* is added to any DSM-5 diagnosis and can arise from a calm or an anxious state. This specifier is crucial to note in a patient's chart because it can be used as a marker for the prognosis or severity of a particular diagnosis. Agoraphobia is when someone fears or avoids certain situations like riding a bus, being in a crowded area (or open areas), or being outside of the home alone because of cognitions or thoughts that say "I won't be able to escape this situation if I suffer a panic attack or some other embarrassing or incapacitating symptom/s."

Of all the anxiety disorders, panic disorder and agoraphobia may be the most conducive to combined treatment. Agoraphobic individuals fear the recurrence of another panic attack, usually fearing to be alone or to go certain places. A variety of theories have been proposed to explain this disorder, including that family influences play an important role in its etiology. A mutually reinforcing system may exist in which the agoraphobic person is kept in a dependent state by a significant other, usually a spouse, to cover up the latter's anger and dependence. The symptom bearer finds a symbolic, dysfunctional way of communicating with and controlling the spouse (e.g., a wife who refuses to leave the house thus forces her husband to stay home and take care of her).

Does the removal of the agoraphobia in one spouse affect the adjustment of the other spouse? The answer is not simple. In a study of behavioral treatment in women with agoraphobia, there was no evidence of symptoms arising in the nonagoraphobic spouse.[50] In contrast, in a study of the marital interaction of 36 married agoraphobic women treated over a period of 3 years, 7 of the husbands displayed abnormal jealousy that adversely influenced the wife's response to treatment.[51] Improvement in the wives was associated with increased jealousy in the husbands. In a study of the husbands of 26 agoraphobic women, before and after intensive in vivo exposure treatment of the wives for agoraphobia, Hafner[52] found that most husbands had experienced transitory negative reactions including anxiety and depression. These negative reactions often coincided with large, rapid improvements in the most severely disturbed patients. Hafner suggested that negative effects were most likely in those men who were hostile, critical, and unsupportive of their wives and who had adapted to their wives' disability as part of a sex role–stereotyped view of marriage.

Treatment

Antianxiety and antidepressant agents are effective for panic disorder, agoraphobia, and social phobia. Couple therapy (or behavioral therapy) in combination with medication can be extremely effective. Individual behavior modification is not as effective as family behavior modification because it is easy to overlook the reinforcing nature of the interpersonal interaction.[52] This complicated treatment picture suggests that in some situations the patient with panic disorder can be successfully treated individually with behavioral interventions with no need for marital intervention. In other situations, however, especially when the spouse without panic disorder is hostile and has some investment in their partner's symptom picture, involving the spouse in the treatment may be necessary.

The addition of the spouse as a co-therapist in the behavioral treatment of the agoraphobic spouse may enhance the treatment effect for non-systems reasons. For example, Munby and Johnston[53] followed 66 agoraphobic patients 5 to 9 years after their involvement in a behavioral treatment. Patients who had a home-based program using the husband as a co-therapist fared somewhat better than those involved in programs that did not involve the husband. The authors suggest that this is because the patient and spouse learned to deal with the agoraphobic problem themselves with less need for further professional intervention.

Family interventions including panic disorder and agoraphobia involve enlisting family members to help identify and correct erroneous beliefs and realistically evaluate the probability of fears coming true. Furthermore, treatment should help reduce the emotional intensity of family interactions, reduce emotional overinvolvement, and negotiate adjustment in role expectations.

OBSESSIVE-COMPULSIVE DISORDER

Rationale

Obsessive-compulsive disorder has strong genetic roots. Obsessive-compulsive disorder describes anxious people who try to squelch their anxiety by thinking or performing rituals. The disorder places major burdens on the families of patients who have it, including physical, financial, and emotional burdens and marital and family problems. In addition, couples can share obsessive disorder. This results from individuals preoccupied with contamination and cleanliness who may be more likely to seek partners who share these characteristics with them or alternatively becoming more similar the longer they are married. Therefore, both should be treated.[54]

Treatment

Treatment consists of medication plus individual therapy. Family interventions to deal with disruption of family life are also much needed. If the family believes, and genuinely feels, that the patient is not motivated to change, excessive arguing and being drawn into the ritualizing behavior will result. The family's attempts to accommodate the patient's symptoms cause global family dysfunction and stress but are best viewed as the family trying to reduce the patient's anxiety. Psychoeducation is crucial so that the family's behavior can be reframed as its attempt to get along and to change the accommodating behavior, allowing the whole family to function better.[55] In addition to family therapy, workshops and support groups are helpful.

Family intervention in OCD can help to decrease accommodation to rituals, improve communication, as well as problem solving. Additionally, families can greatly help with exposure and response prevention.

POSTTRAUMATIC STRESS DISORDER

Rationale

When a person has been exposed to a severely stressful event that involves actual or threatened death, serious injury, or sexual violence, they may develop posttraumatic stress disorder (PTSD). The trauma can be: (1) directly experienced by the individual; (2) witnessed as happening to another; (3) learning the event happened to a loved one; or (4) work-related, with the extreme exposure to aversive details of horrific event (e.g., first aid responders repeatedly having to cleanup human remains, law enforcement repeatedly exposed to details of sexual abuse against children).

The four major symptom clusters for PTSD are:

- Intrusion symptoms (re-experiencing of the event), for example, sudden memories, dreams, or flashbacks related to the event.
- Heightened arousal, for example, reckless or self-destructive behavior, as well as sleep disturbances, hypervigilance, startle responses, or aggressiveness.
- Avoidance, for example, staying away from places, events, or objects that are reminders of the experience.
- Negative thoughts and moods or feelings, for example, individuals may be unable to experience positive emotions. They may feel a sense of blame toward themselves or others about the event. They may have markedly diminished interest in activities or an inability to remember major aspects of the event.

The *PTSD Dissociative Subtype* is when PTSD is observed with prominent dissociative symptoms. These dissociative symptoms can be either experiences of feeling detached from one's own mind, body, or experiences in which the world seems unreal, dreamlike, or distorted. These symptoms are exhibited by 15% to 30% of individuals with PTSD.

Treatment

The treatment for PTSD is psychotherapy, including cognitive therapy, exposure-based therapy, and eye movement desensitization and reprocessing therapy (EMDR). Cognitive therapies aim to alter the meaning and implications of the trauma. Exposure-based therapies involve systematic exposure and desensitization to trauma, while incorporating relaxation techniques. EMDR has been shown to be helpful in desensitizing patients to traumatic memories. Antianxiety and antidepressant medications are also occasionally helpful. Prazosin (an antihypertensive medication) has been found to be helpful to target nightmares. In more severe cases, antipsychotic medications may be used.

The symptoms are very distressing to the family and to the patient, and other members of the family can have violent reactions to a trauma befalling a loved one, including anxiety, depression, and PTSD (as a result of witnessing the trauma or the result). Couples and family therapy have been found to be helpful.[56] The therapist must evaluate the family and provide support and education about the disorder.

DEMENTIA, AMNESIA, AND OTHER COGNITIVE DISORDERS

Rationale

The most common of the cognitive disorders are those associated with presenile or senile brain disease or with chronic atherosclerotic brain disease. A variety of other syndromes (e.g., Alzheimer disease or cerebral vascular accidents) incapacitate patients and create problems for the family. Because these disorders are of slow onset, they are sometimes confused with depression or marital problems in the early stages. Chronic dementias are among the most painful issues that any family has to face. Because of the patient's cognitive deficits, family is crucial in providing the history necessary for the differential diagnosis.

Watching a loved one decline mentally, becoming incapacitated and confused while in good physical health, is an almost unbearable grief. The constant caretaking required drains a family of its resources—money, time, energy. Because many years may elapse between early symptoms and death, the family must manage a situation that worsens constantly over many years. For the person losing function gradually, the pain and anxiety are often severe. It is not surprising that some of these situations end in suicide or euthanasia.

Assuming that the illness occurs in a person with grown children and a spouse, the first questions are apportioning caretaking duties. These usually fall to the spouse first and then to the women in the family—daughters, daughters-in-law, sisters. Members of the extended family vary in their responses. **Often the ones farthest away, and least helpful, are the most critical of family care.** Decisions that must be made are many, from when to take away the car keys, to when the person needs constant care, to who is in charge of the nurses or caretakers, to whether the parent should be placed in a hospital or nursing home. Questions about whether a senile parent will be taken into the home of an adult child, particularly one with children still at home, are complex and there are no comfortable answers. Guilt and anger are often paramount. Often the child who had the worst relationship with the parent and the most unfinished business is left as caretaker, stirring up further anger over having to care for a parent who did not care for them.

Treatment Considerations

The family therapist's job is to assist the family members in working and making decisions together, to support them in getting adequate medical care, to encourage them to use the many uncoordinated helping agencies that are available, and to help them use well the time left with the loved one. Often many years of partial function are left, during which time the family can find ways to help the person compensate for their memory loss and remain part of the family. The therapist must also allow time for grief. Consider the following case example:

Mrs. D, a 60-year-old executive secretary, presented for a diagnostic evaluation because of memory loss. She gave a 3-year history of progressive inability to do her work because she was forgetting things and was irritable on the job (a marked change from her previous premorbid personality as a quiet, careful person). Her 65-year-old husband, Mr. D, quit his job in order to take care of her, and for several months, things went reasonably smoothly. However, her functioning continued to decline and she developed hallucinations, confusion, and paranoia. Medications did not help the situation. Multiple consultations suggested that Mrs. D had senile dementia due to vascular causes and recommended nursing home placement. Mr. D vehemently opposed this, saying that the illness was temporary and that he could not be away from his wife. His two daughters, one living in the same city and one several states away, were violently at odds. The younger daughter, who lived close by and saw her parents often, was very frightened by the situation and pushed for placement. The older daughter, who lived far away, and who had been the father's favorite, insisted that Mrs. D be kept at home to make Mr. D happy. Mr. D was also beginning to show signs of forgetfulness, and it was unclear whether this was due to depression over the wife's illness, sleep deprivation (his wife no longer slept much at night), or beginning organic brain disorder of his own.

The family therapist held a meeting that included the father, both daughters, and their husbands. The more distant daughter was asked to stay in her parents' house for several days to evaluate the situation, at the end of which she was far more aware of the problems her father faced. At the end of the several-session consultation, it was agreed that the two daughters and Mr. D would pay for 24-hour care in the parental home to keep Mrs. D at home as long as possible, with nursing home placement to be discussed again in 3 months or earlier if certain specified crises occurred. Mr. D was evaluated for depression and placed on a low dose of an antidepressant. With the antidepressant and the presence of another adult in the house, Mr. D was able to sleep. He was encouraged to return to work part time in order to have some respite from the situation.

In sum, the role of the family therapist is to support the loved ones and caretakers of the patient with dementia. It is often necessary to refer loved ones to their own therapists to properly grief the loss. Families should be encouraged not to criticize their loved ones for behavior that they are unable to control. Families should be encouraged to maintain their own individual self-care.

EATING DISORDERS

Rationale

Eating disorders affect individuals of all races, ethnicities, and socioeconomic backgrounds and there is an approximately 10:1 female to male ratio. Psychological anguish experienced by individuals and their loved ones is severe. Diagnosing an eating disorder can be difficult because many suffer in silence, do not seek treatment, and keep the behaviors very secret. The main types of eating disorders are anorexia nervosa (AN), bulimia nervosa (BN), binge eating disorder (BED), and avoidant restrictive food intake disorder (ARFD). Patients who do not fall neatly into the diagnostic categories of AN, BN, BED, or ARFD, often receive the diagnosis of eating disorder NOS (EDNOS). EDNOS is the most diagnosed eating disorder in clinical settings.

The key diagnostic findings for AN include loss of weight (usually with a BMI <18.5 or for moderate-to-severe cases, <17) and distortion of body image. Miscellaneous symptoms (most of which are secondary to weight loss) include anemia, amenorrhea, lanugo hair growth, bradycardia, QT abnormalities, osteoporosis, seizures, and delirium. There are two subgroups of AN: the *restricting type* with no purging or binge eating behaviors; and the *binge eating–purging type* who maintain low weight and engage in behaviors such as self-induced vomiting and/or misuse of laxatives, diuretics, or enemas. The incidence of AN is on the rise, probably due to social and cultural factors. Thin is beautiful in the United States and 1 in 200 girls at puberty are now thought to have AN. The disorder tends to occur more commonly in Jewish and Italian families. Middle and upper income families are at greater risk for having a child develop this disorder than are lower socioeconomic status families. The most common age of onset is during the adolescent years, and the illness may be preceded by a period of mild obesity and mild dieting. Many people with AN are noted to have above-average intelligence.

BN involves recurrent episodes of binge eating followed by some form of purging (including vomiting or increased exercise to atone for overeating) in patients who otherwise maintain a normal weight. To meet the criteria for BN, both binge eating and purging must occur at least once a week for 3 months. An important aspect of BN is that gross overeating is followed by shame and guilt. Preoccupation with body image is a key aspect of these patients as well. Patients who suffer from BN often have other co-occurring psychiatric disorders including mood and anxiety disorders, SUDs, or BPD. These patients tend to have problems with impulsivity in multiple spheres of life. Repeatedly inducing vomiting can lead to stomach and esophageal tears and these patients may have menstrual irregularities, nutritional deficiencies, and many other medical problems.

Treatment Considerations

The treatment of these patients should consist of behavioral modification to reinforce weight gain, and some combination of individual and family therapy. **Family therapy, specifically the Maudsley model, is particularly effective for teens and family members living in the same household.** When a patient's weight drops to a critical point, encouraging the individual to eat becomes of utmost importance. If the patient refuses, a nasogastric tube or intravenous hyperalimentation becomes mandatory. It is usually possible to prevent a patient with AN from dying from complications of the disease. A variety of interventions can be made to prevent starvation. There are no FDA-approved medications for AN, but medications may be used to treat any co-occurring psychiatric disorders.

Treatment for BN may involve treating electrolyte and acid/base abnormalities. Psychotherapy is crucial and cognitive behavior therapy (CBT) has been shown to be very effective especially in conjunction with medications such as the serotonin reuptake inhibitors (SSRIs). Interpersonal therapy, DBT, and psychodynamic therapy can also be effective. Encouraging patients to join self-help groups and peer support networks can also be helpful in recovery.

Therapy is tailored to the family's specific issues. Education about the illness is necessary. Even if the predominant type of therapy is family or individual, the therapist must weigh and medically monitor the patient and periodically check electrolyte balance, which can change rapidly in very ill patients and is a serious medical issue. Starvation produces difficulties in thinking that make therapy or living even harder. The question of when to hospitalize the patient is always an issue in very low–weight anorexic patients.

Hospitalization usually is a continuation of previous treatment. Sometimes a hospitalization provides the crisis needed for the patient and family to break through established patterns. Many models of therapy, including insight awareness, cognitive behavioral, and supportive, have been applied in the treatment of these disorders. Eating disorders are best approached with a treatment team, whether inpatient or outpatient, consisting of a nutritionist, internist, therapist, and an experienced supervisor or team leader.

Lock et al.[57] compared two active treatments (family and individual therapy) for adolescents suffering from AN. Participants who received family therapy showed greater improvement in percentile BMI and eating-disordered thinking at the end of treatment and higher remission rates at follow-up.

In one study, patients with AN with onset at or before age 18 years and with a duration of less than 3 years showed greater improvement 1 year after discharge from the hospital with family therapy than with individual psychotherapy; in contrast, older AN patients did better with individual therapy than with family therapy.[58] Patients in this study were not assigned to both family and individual treatment, a combination frequently used in practice. For bulimia, family therapy was reported as being helpful in a large case series.[59] Although no systematic studies of the approach exist, some patients have found Overeaters Anonymous and similar groups to be helpful in recovery, in part because of the networking, sense of connectedness to a group, and 24-hour-per day support against food cravings that they offer.[60,61] Controversy exists regarding the role of 12-step programs that do not address nutritional considerations and psychological or behavioral deficits when used as the sole intervention in the treatment of eating disorders.[62] For more outcome data on family interventions, please refer to Chapter 24.

The American Psychiatric Association practice guidelines strongly recommend family treatment for children and teens with eating disorders, and suggest that family assessment and involvement may be useful for older patients as well (https://www.psychiatry.org/File%20Library/Psychiatrists/Practice/Clinical%20Practice%20Guidelines/APA-Draft-Practice-Guidelines-Eating-Disorders.pdf).

In sum, clinicians should provide support to family of patients suffering from eating disorders and encourage them to receive specialized family-based interventions.

SUBSTANCE-RELATED DISORDERS

Rationale

The definition of addiction has been described by Koob and Le Moal as a "chronic relapsing disorder characterized by compulsive drug seeking, a loss of control in limiting intake, and the emergence of a negative emotional state when access to the drug is prevented."[63] Both genes and environment can significantly impact brain functioning and behavior and the neurotransmitter most extensively implicated in the development of addiction is dopamine. Most drugs of abuse affect the brain reward system and first induce the release of dopamine in the nucleus accumbens, followed by other limbic regions and the prefrontal cortex, which affects multiple neurotransmitters systems and leads to characteristic plastic adaptations.

To fully understand the effect of SUDs, the therapist must understand alcoholism and drug addiction as diseases that affect the entire family. The ways in which SUDs affect family members are varied and pervasive. SUDs can produce severe health problems in the individuals with these disorders and in other family members.

Most clinicians recognize the power of the family system in the etiology and maintenance of addiction. Most family therapy approaches recognize the life-threatening and progressive nature of the disease of alcoholism. In addition, most approaches are informed by the idea that addiction can generate family dysfunction.

Assessment and Treatment Guidelines

Because of the life-threatening quality of alcohol and drug dependence, it is necessary to assess the nature and severity of alcohol and drug use before constructing a treatment plan. Brief screening instruments such as the CAGE,[64] S-MAST,[65] and the Alcohol Use Disorders Identification Test (AUDIT)[66] can be useful tools to augment the initial assessment.

Another efficient, comprehensive assessment tool is the Addiction Severity Index.[67] It is useful for both clinical and research settings and provides a thorough review of alcohol and other drug use and a limited but useful review of related problems. Compared with other assessment tools, the Addiction Severity Index is relatively long and might be best used after a brief assessment has indicated a problem. The therapist must assess the patient's risk for suicide, violence, and other life-threatening factors such as co-occurring medical illnesses and impulsivity. Assessment of the ways in which family members have been affected by substance use should also occur in this initial evaluation.

Most individuals with SUDs resist engaging in treatment despite the negative consequences of their addictions.[68] People who misuse substances typically have calamitous effects on their families, who then need to reach out to mental health professionals for advice, support, empathy, and direction—yet family members often do not seek help. In the families of addicts, marital distress, social problems, financial woes, legal problems, criminality, aggression, and interpersonal violence commonly arise,[69] often leading to feelings of intense anger, sadness, anxiety, shame, guilt, and social isolation.[70] Providing support to families of addicts is crucial, along with getting the substance abuser into treatment.

Family-focused interventions can lead to positive outcomes for both the substance misuser and their family members. Alcoholics Anonymous (families group)/Narcotics Anonymous (families group) are good family-support groups. Family therapy, such as the Behavioral Couples Therapy (BCT) of Fals-Stewart, is very effective. BCT of Fals-Stewart is the family intervention with the strongest research support for treating SUDs. For more information on outcome studies regarding BCT for alcoholism, please see Chapter 24.

Community Reinforcement and Family Treatment (CRAFT) helps families to promote the engagement of addicted loved ones into treatment. Family members learn how to improve their communication skills in order to more effectively express their needs and also to reestablish good self-care. In one study, CRAFT encouraged two-thirds of treatment-resistant patients to attend treatment.[71]

Peter Steinglass and colleagues at the Ackerman Institute for Substance Abuse and the Family have developed an approach called systemic-motivational therapy (SMT), to address the current divide that exists between traditional substance-abuse treatment and family therapy. The model emphasizes therapist neutrality, the use of nonpathologizing language with patients and families, and family therapist collaboration. Both individual and family level beliefs about the role of substance use in the family life is explored. Additionally, for therapy to move forward an action plan must be agreed upon by all members of the family.[72]

In sum, SUDs can have a devastating influence on both the individual and the family. The importance of a nonjudgmental and caring approach when working with these families is paramount. Oftentimes, the clinician must refer the addicted individual to detox or rehab prior to meaningfully engaging in family therapy.

Children of Alcoholic Parents

Children who are living with an alcoholic parent face an environment that is unpredictable and often verbally or physically abusive. They are often told that what they are observing is something else (e.g., "Nothing's wrong with dad, he's just tired."). If there are several children, they will often be given or accept narrow and specific roles. One, usually the oldest, will be the overly responsible caretaker in the family (e.g., protecting siblings and the mother if the father is violent, or doing childcare and cooking if the mother is drunk and unavailable). One will often become "sad or bad," one the angry truth-teller, and one or more will hide out or become the family clown and cheerer-upper. Many children of alcoholic parents enter adult life with their thinking organized around unpredictability, distrust, survival, vigilance, hyperresponsibility, and isolation of affect. Most of the time at least one of the siblings also develops alcohol or substance abuse, and at least one becomes terrified of alcohol. Many children, especially the overly responsible caretaker, are at risk for later mood disorder. Often at least one of the children will marry an alcoholic individual. Children should be evaluated for depression and questioned about abuse. Many children benefit from Al-Anon. Adult children should at some time point in the therapy be referred to Adult Children of Alcoholics groups or literature.

PSYCHIATRIC DISORDERS OF CHILDHOOD

Intellectual Disability

One percent of the population has an intellectual disability (formerly known as mental retardation). In 35% of cases, a genetic cause can be found, and 10% are in the context of a congenital malformation syndrome (Downs syndrome, Edwards syndrome, Fragile X, Lesch–Nyhan, Prader–Willi, Angelman syndrome, cri du chat, fetal alcohol syndrome). In order to be diagnosed with an intellectual disability, the individual must have a very low IQ (usually below 70), in addition to impaired adaptive functioning (problems in communicating, self-care, interpersonal skills, etc.). In addition to the real problem of social development and functioning of the identified patient because of their possibly damaged biologic equipment, associated family reactions require attention. The family may feel antipathy, guilt, social isolation, or anxiety about caring for the child's usual health needs.[73] Family members may make the child with an intellectual disability a scapegoat to cover up unresolved conflicts between mother and father or between parents and children.

Treatment

Help must be focused on the identified patient's specific needs and on the family's attitudes and behavior. In addition to medication (if indicated), psychosocial treatments that provide support for the family's sense of loss and helplessness, education about the appropriate use of community resources, psychoeducation about mental retardation, and behavioral strategies for managing destructive behaviors are most likely to bring relief and success to these families.

Autism Spectrum Disorder

Rationale

Autism spectrum disorder (ASD) usually commences early in infancy and consists of abnormal development of social communication and social interaction, as well as an array of restrictive and repetitive behaviors (RRBs). If the impairment is limited to difficulty with verbal and nonverbal communication and no RRBs are present, then the individual is diagnosed with social communication disorder.

In both ASD and social communication disorder, language abnormalities can include echolalia (the child repeats verbatim what he has heard), mutism, pronoun reversals (e.g., the child uses "we" or "you" instead of "I"), and language delays. Typical responses to the environment include a pathologic need for sameness. Such children, for example, might become anxious if the furniture in their classroom is rearranged. Their social development is delayed or absent. They show very little interest in other people and are usually found to have delayed or aberrant social milestones in their developmental histories. For example, such children might demonstrate poor eye contact, no social outreach, very little smiling, and no interest in the communications of their parents.

Obviously, ASD is a devastating illness. It occurs evenly across all social strata and may be slightly more common in boys than in girls. Some associated conditions include congenital infections (rubella, cytomegalovirus, etc.), hepatic encephalopathy, and even massive head trauma, which could result in a clinical picture indistinguishable from ASD. Children who are congenitally blind have a greater chance of having autistic mannerisms than other children. Complex genetic patterns of inheritance may exist in this condition. Rett syndrome is seen in girls and consists of autistic behaviors, acquired microcephaly, and stereotyped hand movements.

ASD should no longer be considered simply a psychological disorder. Children with ASD have abnormal auditory-evoked responses, decreased nystagmus in response to vestibular stimulation, and an increased frequency of grand mal seizures prior to adolescence. This suggests that there are organic difficulties that are present in this condition. The prognosis varies depending on the amount of language development present in the child and the child's IQ. The higher the IQ, the better the language, and the better the prognosis.

Treatment

Treatment should consist of a structured educational program that includes behavioral modification encouraging social and language behaviors. Medications can be used in the case of severe impulsivity or dangerous behavior. The issues of loss for parents of a child with autistic disorder are monumental, and family therapy can provide a place for couples to talk openly about their sadness, helplessness, and anxiety. At the same time, family meetings are important in consolidating a plan for advocating for the child's needs (e.g., obtaining adequate educational and therapeutic resources), learning specific strategies for teaching the child and promoting language development, and building in time for parents to focus on their needs and practical needs of others in the family. Because ASDs can take a large toll on families, family support is viewed widely as crucial in terms of acute and long-term adaptation.

Attention-Deficit/Hyperactivity Disorder

Rationale

The prevalence of ADHD in children is between 5% and 11% depending on the age group. While ADHD has a strong neurobiologic basis, the precise cause is unknown. There are three specifiers of ADHD: predominantly inattentive presentation (easily distracted, forgetful, difficulty organizing, and problems with giving close attention to detail), predominantly hyperactive/impulsive presentation (fidgety, talks out of turn, has difficulty staying in seat), or combined type. ADHD children have difficulty with executive dysfunction and usually have difficulty in school and at home. They tend to suffer from lower self-esteem and may have impaired social adaptive functioning.

The majority of children with ADHD will continue to have ADHD symptoms into adulthood. Adults with ADHD usually report trouble with organization, planning, task initiation, and task completion. Overall, symptoms of inattention are much more prominent than frank hyperactivity although adults with ADHD often report a greater sense of internal restlessness.

Treatment

ADHD is often associated with discrete learning disabilities. The standard treatment is a combination of medication (usually a psychostimulant) and therapy for both the child and family. Although medication and tutoring can modify many of the symptoms, behavioral interventions in the classroom and in the home (e.g., structuring) should also be used to reduce stimulus overload and to help the child to develop greater self-monitoring and self-control. Family intervention is necessary to provide psychoeducation about ADHD (parents commonly blame each other or the child for what is primarily a pathophysiologic disorder), and instruction in behavioral techniques may be quite useful.[74] Consultation with the family is often crucial in alleviating a family crisis or long-term turmoil.

The less common situation results when the disorder continues through adulthood and involves a married couple. ADHD in adults has found new acceptance as a diagnosis, and more adults are taking stimulants for this disorder than ever before. As with children, multimodal treatments combining medication and therapy are the recommended approaches. With successful combined treatment, most patients notice that they are more productive at work and can spend more quality time with the family. Psychoeducation for spouses and other family members can be helpful in identifying realistic expectations for behavior, organization, and attention. Consider the following case example:

> *Mr. E, a 27-year-old man, met the DSM-5 criteria for ADHD, combined type. When treated with methylphenidate ER 20 mg/day, he experienced a marked decrease in target symptoms, and within 10 days of his starting the methylphenidate regimen, Mr. E and his wife noted a dramatic decrease in hostility, anxiety, and irritability. His attention span lengthened, and he was able to complete household projects that had been left unfinished for years. In his words, "I can never remember feeling so calm." He had previously taken low-dose neuroleptics and benzodiazepines without benefit. Mr. E, his wife, and the treatment team considered the treatment with stimulants to be successful. Although Mr. and Mrs. E were thrilled initially with Mr. E's improvement, they soon began to experience increased marital tension. Before Mr. E began to take stimulants, the couple's primary focus had been on his symptoms. With the initiation of medication and the subsequent amelioration of those symptoms, this focus was no longer relevant. The couple had previously communicated through arguments, affective storms, and at times outright physical aggression. While taking the methylphenidate, however, Mr. E found that his mood was less labile and hostile, and Mrs. E began to complain bitterly that she "couldn't get a fight out of him anymore." She sought marital separation. Outside the home, Mr. E expressed confusion over his newly acquired ability to "stop myself from hitting people—I have a few seconds now to think before I act."*
>
> *Although the target symptoms had diminished, Mr. E and his wife did not adjust readily to the change. In the absence of symptoms as a major focus in the marriage the couple were disarmed; their accustomed pattern of interaction was also disrupted.*[75]

The preceding case highlights the potential for a different set of difficulties to arise after the acute symptoms are resolved by medication. The partners have to relate to each other in different ways. Family therapy is an excellent adjunct to the treatment that not only helps the patient but also helps the couple to change. The same principle holds true for other mental disorders, when rapid changes in treatment occur.

Oppositional Defiant Disorder and Conduct Disorder

Rationale

Children with oppositional defiant disorder (ODD) demonstrate negative, defiant, disobedient, and often hostile behavior toward adults and authority figures. These children can be extremely stubborn and continually test limits by ignoring orders, arguing, and failing to accept blame for personal wrongdoings. ODD kids have very low frustration tolerance and are hostile toward others by deliberately annoying others or by verbal aggression. When behaviors start escalating to physical aggression, these children are usually diagnosed with conduct disorder (CD). Conduct disordered children are bullies to others, and can be physically aggressive to people and animals. They violate serious rules and can engage in deceit, theft, and destruction of property. Children with CD often develop adult antisocial personality disorder.

Treatment

Behavioral and structural interventions have been most successful in altering patterns of antisocial and oppositional behavior in children and adolescents. These treatments focus on the establishment of clear rules and consequences, a family structure in which the parents are in an executive position, the appropriate use of community resources, parent training in behavioral techniques, and attention to marital adjustment. Although resistance to treatment is especially prominent in these disorders,[76] results are generally supportive of family therapy.

Anxiety Disorders

Anxiety disorders in childhood are often treated with family and individual therapy, often in combination. Behavioral techniques in both family and individual treatment are especially useful. School phobias are ideal situations for family therapy. Commonly, when mother and child find it difficult to separate, there may be an underlying marital problem. With all types of phobias, treatment of the individual by behavior modification or medication should be considered, possibly using the parent as a cotherapist who assists with the behavioral techniques.

Mood Disorders

Rationale

Although we discussed mood disorders earlier in this chapter, we must add a caveat here. Depressive and bipolar disorders may start in childhood or more commonly in adolescence. Mood disorders that first appear in adolescence usually continue into adulthood—a fact that should be shared with the family. Otherwise, the patient and family will deny existence of the illness and focus mostly on the secondary family problems. In fact, Rueter et al.[77] reported that parent–adolescent–child disagreements predict the onset of both depressive and anxiety disorders (i.e., a direct relation among stress, symptoms, and onset of disorder). Consider the following analogy: in certain infections it is not the direct destruction of the cell by the virus but the response of the host that is responsible for producing the disease. Similarly, in psychiatry, certain behaviors are not pathogenic by themselves, but the response of the family system creates what we now call pathology.

Treatment

Recognition and prescription of medication combined with psychoeducation and family intervention (when indicated) provides the best basis for healthier individual and family coping. In fact, pharmacotherapy plus FFT has been found to be more effective than pharmacotherapy with brief psychoeducation.[27]

Childhood Obesity

Kitzman and Beech,[78] have reviewed the literature and found considerable evidence for effectiveness of family intervention. Treatment focuses on parental management of nutrition and exercise of obese children, but also parent–child relationship issues.

All childhood disorders benefit from a family-oriented approach. The clinician must establish both a positive therapeutic alliance with both the child and the parents. For outcome data and references, please see Chapter 24.

CLINICAL PRACTICE IMPLICATIONS

In the introduction to this chapter we broadly described the interactions between the family (and its issues) and the patient (and their psychiatric disorders). Throughout this chapter, we described the specific "rationale" for family intervention as well as "treatment implications" for the most common psychiatric disorders of adults and children.

The central, sometimes crucial outcome, teaching pearl is to "think family" when treating psychiatric illness. It has been consistently demonstrated that combining medication plus psychotherapy including "family intervention" is almost always more effective than either alone. The family should always be a member of the treatment team and we strongly recommend regular sessions of patients plus families for most mental disorders. In some situations, this is even true when the identified patient specifically asks the provider to exclude family members because the patient feels the family is toxic. In our experience, given the severity and functional impairment over a lifetime of most Axis I disorders, patients need the help of a significant other or family member.

For example, in the NIMH CATIE study of antipsychotic effectiveness, Glick et al.[22] found that regardless of which antipsychotic medication patients were randomized to, having a family which was "supportive and helpful" resulted in better therapeutic outcomes compared to those who did not have a family member with those characteristics. In short, quality treatment is usually accomplished by including the family over the lifetime course of the illness, rather than excluding them.

The combination of both judicious use of medication and family-oriented care can improve outcome for patients and help families to develop more resilience to be able to cope effectively with a loved one suffering from a mental illness.

SUGGESTED READING

Readers may want to consult this reference that focuses on the need to be aware of the latest literature in order to do competent family therapy.

Heru AM, Keitner GI, Glick ID. The neglected core competence. *Acad Psychiatry*. 2012;36:433–435.

REFERENCES

1. Fromm-Reichman F. Notes on the development of schizophrenia by psychoanalytic psychotherapy. *Psychiatry*. 1948;11:267–277.
2. Bateson G, Jackson DD, Haley J, Weakland J. Towards a theory of schizophrenia. *Behav Sci.* 1956;1:251–264.
3. Bateson G, Jackson DD, Haley J, Weakland JH. A note on the double bind—1962. *Fam Process*. 1963;2:154–161.
4. Wynne LC, Ryckoff I, Day J, et al. Pseudo-mutuality in the family relations of schizophrenics. In: Bell NW, Vogel FF, eds. *A Modern Introduction to the Family*. Free Press; 1960:573–594.
5. Fleck S. Family dynamics and origin of schizophrenia. *Psychosom Med*. 1960;22:333–344.
6. Wahlberg KE, Wynne LC, Oja H, et al. Gene-environment interaction in vulnerability to schizophrenia: findings from the Finnish adoptive family study of schizophrenia. *Am J Psychiatry*. 1997;154:355–362.
7. Swerdlow NR, Light GA, Sprock J, et al. Deficient prepulse inhibition in schizophrenia detected by the multi-site COGS. *Schizophr Res*. 2014;152(2–3):503–512.

8. Nuechterlein KH, Dawson ME. Information processing and attentional functioning in the development course of schizophrenic disorders. *Schizophr Bull.* 1984;10:160–203.
9. Brown GW, Monck EM, Carstairs GM, Wing JK. The influence of family life on the course of schizophrenic illness. *Br J Prev Soc Med.* 1962;16:55.
10. Heru A. Cultural research deconstructs the psychosocial construct 'expressed emotion'. *Br J Psychiatry.* 2021; 219(4):565–568.
11. Brown GW, Birley JLT, Wing JK. Influence of family life on the course of schizophrenic disorders: a replication. *Br J Psychiatry.* 1972;121:241–258.
12. King S, Dixon MJ. The influence of expressed emotion, family dynamics, and symptom type on the social adjustment of schizophrenic young adults. *Arch Gen Psychiatry.* 1996;53:1098–1104.
13. Butzloff RL, Hooley JM. Expressed emotion and psychiatric relapse: a meta-analysis. *Arch Gen Psychiatry.* 1998;55:547–551.
14. Leff JP, Berkowitz R, Shavit N, Strachan A, Glass I, Vaughn C. A trial of family therapy v. a relatives group for schizophrenia. *Br J Psychiatry.* 1989;154:58–66.
15. Falloon IR, Boyd JL, McGill CW, Razani J, Moss HB, Gilderman AM. Family management in the prevention of exacerbations of schizophrenia: a controlled study. *N Engl J Med.* 1982;306:1437–1440.
16. Glick ID, Clarkin JF, Haas GL, Spencer JH Jr. Clinical significance of inpatient family intervention; VII. conclusions from the clinical trial. *Hosp Community Psychiatry.* 1993;44:869–873.
17. Goldstein MJ, Rodnick EH, Evans JR, May PR, Steinberg MR. Drug and family therapy in the aftercare treatment of acute schizophrenia. *Arch Gen Psychiatry.* 1978;35:1169–1177.
18. McFarlane WR, Link B, Dushay R, Marchal J, Crilly J. Psychoeducational multiple family groups: four-year relapse outcome in schizophrenia. *Fam Process.* 1995;34:127–144.
19. Goldstein MJ. Psychoeducation and family treatment related to the phase of a psychotic disorder. *Int Clin Psychopharmacol.* 1996;11:77–83.
20. Glick ID, Clarkin JF. Family support and intervention. In: Sederer LI, Rothschild AJ, eds. *Acute Care Psychiatry: Diagnosis and Treatment.* Williams & Wilkins; 1997:337–354.
21. Alvarez-Himenez, et al. Risk factors for relapse following treatment for first episode psychosis: a systematic review and meta-analysis of longitudinal studies. *Schizophr Res.* 2012;139(1–3):116–128.
22. Glick ID, Stekoll AH, Hays S. The role of the family and improvement in treatment maintenance, adherence, and outcome for schizophrenia. *J Clin Psychopharmacol.* 2011;31:82–85.
23. Lucksted A, McFarlane W, Downing D, Dixon L. Recent developments in family psychoeducation as an evidence-based practice. *J Marital Fam Ther.* 2012;38(1):101–121.
24. Schooler NR, Keith SJ, Severe JB, et al. Relapse and rehospitalization during maintenance treatment of schizophrenia. The effects of dose reduction and family treatment. *Arch Gen Psychiatry.* 1997;54:453–463.
25. Moran M. Psychosocial interventions beneficial in schizophrenia. Psychiatry News. 2007.
26. Landeen J, Whelton C, Dermer S, Cardamone J, Munroe-Blum H, Thornton J. Needs of well siblings of persons with schizophrenia. *Hosp Community Psychiatry.* 1992;43:266–269.
27. Miklowitz DJ. The role of the family in the course and treatment of bipolar disorder. *Curr Dir Psychol Sci.* 2007; 16(4):192–196.
28. Clarkin JF, Haas GL, Glick ID, eds. *Affective Disorders and the Family: Assessment and Treatment.* Guilford; 1988.
29. Clarkin JF, Glick ID, Haas GL, et al. A randomized clinical trial of inpatient family intervention; V. Results for affective disorders. *J Affect Disord.* 1990;18:17–28.
30. Anderson C, Reiss D, Hogarty G. *Schizophrenia and the Family.* Guilford; 1986.
31. Hooley JM, Gotlib IH. A diathesis-stress conceptualization of expressed emotion and clinical outcome. *J Appl Soc Psychol.* 2000;9:135–151.
32. Miklowitz DJ, Wisniewski SR, Miyahara S, Otto MW, Sachs GS. Perceived criticism from family members as a predictor of the 1-year course of bipolar disorder. *Psychiatric Res.* 2005;136:101–111.
33. Clarkin JF, Carpenter D, Hull J, Wilner P, Glick I. Effects of psychoeducational marital intervention for bipolar patients and spouses. *Psychiatr Serv.* 1998;49:531–533.
34. Falloon IRH, Hole V, Mulroy L, et al. Behavioral family therapy. In: Clarkin JF, Haas GL, Glick ID, eds. *Affective Disorders and the Family: Assessment and Treatment.* Guilford; 1988:117–133.
35. Miklowitz DJ, Chung B. Family-focused therapy for bipolar disorder: reflections on 30 years of research. *Fam Process.* 2016;55(3):483–499.
36. Akiskal HS, Bitar AH, Puzantian VR, Rosenthal TL, Walker PW. The nosological status of neurotic depressions: a prospective three- to four-year follow-up examination in light of the primary-secondary and the unipolar-bipolar dichotomies. *Arch Gen Psychiatry.* 1978;35:756–766.
37. Akiskal HS, Hirschfeld MA, Yerevanian BI. The relationship of personality to affective disorders: a critical review. *Arch Gen Psychiatry.* 1983;40:801–810.
38. Haas G, Clarkin JF, Glick ID. Marital and family treatment of depression. In: Beckham E, Leber W, eds. *Handbook of Depression: Treatment, Assessment and Research.* Dorsey; 1985:151–183.

39. Prince SE, Jacobson NS. A review and evaluation of marital and family therapies for affective disorders. *J Marital Fam Ther*. 1995;21:377–401.
40. Jacobson NS, Dobson K, Fruzzetti AE, Schmaling KB, Salusky S. Marital therapy as a treatment for depression. *J Consult Clin Psychol*. 1991;52:547–557.
41. Jacobson NS, Fruzzetti A, Dobson K, Whisman M, Hops H. Couple therapy as a treatment for depression; II. The effects of relationship, quality and therapy on depressive relapse. *J Consult Clin Psychol*. 1993;61:516–519.
42. Dessaulles A, Johnson SM, Denton WH. Emotion-focused therapy for couples in the treatment of depression: a pilot study. *Am J Fam Ther*. 2003;31:345–353.
43. Keitner GI, Ryan CE, Miller IW, Kohn R, Bishop DS, Epstein NB. Role of the family in recovery and major depression. *Am J Psychiatry*. 1995;152:1002–1008.
44. Brent DA, Holder D, Kolko D, et al. A clinical psychotherapy trial for adolescent depression comparing cognitive, family, and supportive therapy. *Arch Gen Psychiatry*. 1997;54:877–885.
45. Amad A, Ramoz N, Thomas P, Jardri R, Gorwood P. Genetics of borderline personality disorder: systematic review and proposal of an integrative model. *Neurosci Biobehav Rev*. 2014;40:6–19.
46. Hooley JH, Hoffman PD. Expressed emotion and clinical outcome in borderline personality disorder. *Am J Psychiatry*. 1999;196:1557–1562.
47. Magnavita JJ, MacFarlane MM. Family treatment of personality disorders: Historical overview and current perspectives. *Family Treatment of Personality Disorders: Advances in Clinical Practice*. Haworth Clinical Practice Press; 2004:3–39.
48. Hoffman PD, Fruzzetti AE, Buteau E. Understanding and engaging families: an education, skills and support program for relatives impacted by borderline personality disorder. *J Ment Health*. 2007;16:69–82.
49. American Psychiatric Association. *Diagnostic and Statistical Manual of Mental Disorder*. 5th ed. American Psychiatric Publishing; 2013.
50. Cobb JP, Mathews AM, Childs-Clarke A, Blowers CM. The spouse as co-therapist in the treatment of agoraphobia. *Br J Psychiatry*. 1984;144:282–287.
51. Hafner RJ. Agoraphobic women married to abnormally jealous men. *Br J Med Psychol*. 1979;52:99–104.
52. Hafner RJ. Predicting the effects on husbands of behavior therapy for wives' agoraphobia. *Behav Res Ther*. 1984;22:217–226.
53. Munby M, Johnston DW. Agoraphobia: the long-term follow-up of behavioral treatment. *Br J Psychiatry*. 1980;137:418–427.
54. Treichel J. Familial OCD: Environment, genes both play role. Psychiatry News. 2013.
55. Calvocoressi L, Lewis B, Harris M, et al. Family accommodation in obsessive-compulsive disorder. *Am J Psychiatry*. 1995;152:441–443.
56. Bisson JI, Ehlers A, Matthews R, Pilling S, Richards D, Turner S. Psychological treatments for chronic post-traumatic stress disorder. Systematic review and meta-analysis. *Br J Psychiatry*. 2007;190(2):97–104.
57. Lock J, Le Grange D, Agras WS, Moye A, Bryson SW, Jo B. A randomized clinical trial comparing family based treatment to adolescent-focused individual therapy for adolescents with anorexia nervosa. *Arch Gen Psychiatry*. 2010;67:1025–1032.
58. Russell GF, Szmukler GI, Dare C, Eisler I. An evaluation of family therapy in anorexia nervosa and bulimia nervosa. *Arch Gen Psychiatry*. 1987;44:1047–1056.
59. Schwartz RC, Barrett MJ, Saba G. Family therapy for bulimia. In: Garner DM, Garfinkel PE, eds. *Handbook of Psychotherapy for Anorexia Nervosa and Bulimia*. Guilford; 1985:280–307.
60. Malenbaum R, Herzog D, Eisenthal S, Wyshak G. Overeaters anonymous: impact on bulimia. *Int J Eat Disord*. 1989;7:139–144.
61. Pope HG Jr, Hudson JI, Jonas JM, Yurgelun-Todd D. Bulimia treated with imipramine; a placebo-controlled, double-blind study. *Am J Psychiatry*. 1983;140:554–558.
62. Vandereycken W. The addiction model in eating disorders: some critical remarks and a selected bibliography. *Int J Eat Disord*. 1990;9:95–102.
63. Koob GF. The neurobiology of addiction: a neuroadaptational view relevant for diagnosis. *Addiction*. 2006; 101(Suppl 1):23–30.
64. Mayfield DG, McLeod G, Hall P: The CAGE questionnaire: validation of a new alcoholism screening instrument. *Am J Psychiatry*. 1974;131:1121–1123.
65. Selzer ML, Vinokur A, Van Rooijen L. A self-administered Short Michigan Alcoholism Screening Test (SMAST). *J Stud Alcohol*. 1975;36:117–126.
66. Saunders JB, Aasland OG, Babor TF, de la Fuente JR, Grant M. Development of the alcohol use disorders identification test (AUDIT): WHO collaborative project on early detection of persons with harmful alcohol consumption–II. *Addiction*. 1993;88:791–804.
67. McLellan AT, Luborsky L, Woody GA, O'Brien CP. An improved diagnostic evaluation instrument for substance abuse patients. The Addiction Severity Index. *J Nerv Ment Dis*. 1983;168:26–33.

68. Marlatt GA, Tucker JA, Donovan DM, Vuchinich RE. Help-seeking by substance abusers: the role of harm reduction and behavioral-economic approaches to facilitate treatment entry and retention. *NIDA Res Monogr*. 1997;165:44–84.
69. Romijn HJ, Hofman MA, Gramsbergen A. At what age is the developing cerebral cortex of the rat comparable to that of the full-term newborn human baby? *Early Hum Dev*. 1991;26(1):61–67.
70. Barnard M. Drugs in the family: The impact on parents and siblings. Joseph Rowntree Foundation; 2005.
71. Roozen HG, De Waart R, Van Der Kroft P. Community reinforcement and family training: an effective option to engage treatment-resistant substance-abusing individuals in treatment." *Addiction*. 2010;105: 1729–1738.
72. Steinglass P. Systemic motivational therapy for substance abuse disorders: an integrative model. *J Fam Ther*. 2009;31(2):155–174.
73. Adams M. Social aspects of the medical care for the mentally retarded. *N Engl J Med*. 1972;286:635–638.
74. American Academy of Child and Adolescent Psychiatry. AACAP practice parameters for the assessment and treatment of attention-deficit hyperactivity disorder. *J Am Acad Child Adolesc Psychiatry*. 1991;30:1–3.
75. Satel S, Southwick S. Consequences for the family of abrupt reduction of chronic symptoms (letter). *Am J Psychiatry*. 1987;144:1362.
76. Chamberlain P, Rosicky JG. The effectiveness of family therapy in the treatment of adolescents with conduct disorders and delinquency. (Special Issue: The Effectiveness of Marital and Family Therapy). *J Marital Fam Ther*. 1995;21:441–459.
77. Rueter MA, Scaramella L, Wallace LE, Conger RD. First onset of depressive or anxiety disorders predicted by the longitudinal course of internalizing symptoms and parent–adolescent disagreements. *Arch Gen Psychiatry*. 1999;56:726–732.
78. Kitzmann KM, Beech BM. Family-based interventions for pediatric obesity: methodological and conceptual challenges from family psychology. *J Fam Psychol*. 2006;20(2):175–89.

19 Family Treatment in the Context of Other Special Problems—Violence to Self and Others

OBJECTIVES FOR THE READER

- To be able to use the family model in the context of family issues such as violence, incest, and suicidal behavior.

For easier reading, we emphasize that the descriptors "couples" or "marital" are used nearly interchangeably in this chapter.

Your parents were fighting machines and self-pitying machines. Your mother was programmed to bawl out your father for being a defective money-making machine, and your father was programmed to bawl her out for being a defective housekeeping machine. They were programmed to bawl each other out for being defective loving machines. Then your father was programmed to stomp out of the house and slam the door. This automatically turned your mother into a weeping machine. And your father would go down to a tavern where he would get drunk with some other drinking machines. Then all the drinking machines would go to a whorehouse and rent fucking machines. And then your father would drag himself home to become an apologizing machine. And your mother would become a very slow forgiving machine.

—Kurt Vonnegut Jr., *Breakfast of Champions*

INTRODUCTION

In the previous chapter, we described the family model in situations in which the family has a member with a diagnosable psychiatric disorder. In other situations, a family member may engage in violent behaviors to self or others that disrupt family functioning such as suicide attempts, verbal or physical abuse, or sexual abuse (i.e., incest). We have grouped these problems for discussion because they so clearly involve the whole family and because such behaviors cut across traditional diagnostic lines. In addition, they require very specific and aggressive treatment by the family therapist and other health care providers.

From both an individual and a family perspective, these behaviors serve multiple functions. A suicide attempt, for example, might be an effort to coerce or control another, an expression of despair, an attempt to get love and support, an expression of anger, or all of the above. The attempt may mobilize a family to change or may be part of the family's usual homeostasis (e.g., every time the father threatens to leave, the adolescent daughter attempts suicide). Violence, although highly coercive, may arise from a calculated attempt at control or may be an expression of internal feelings of helplessness, and it may be part of a familiar violence cycle or a single event of sudden rage. For example, sometimes the only way one spouse knows how to handle intimacy or difficult discussions is to explode or to threaten suicide or homicide.

THE FAMILY MODEL AND VIOLENCE
Description of the Problem
Definition of Family Violence
Shame
Trauma Repetition and Trauma Bonding
Causes of Violence in Families
Relationship between Family Violence and Alcohol or Drug Abuse
How Violent Acts Occur: The Cycle of Violence
Assessment of Individual and Family Systems Issues
Physical and Psychological Consequences of Violence
How to Assess the Degree of Danger
Treatment
Mandatory Reporting Laws
Clinical Issues for Therapists
INTRAFAMILIAL CHILD SEXUAL ABUSE
Individual Issues
Family Issues
Larger System Issues
Assessment
Treatment
THE FAMILY MODEL AND CHILD ABUSE
Incestuous Trauma
THE SUICIDAL PATIENT AND THE FAMILY
Acute Management
Evaluating the Family
Involving the Family
Treating the Family
Discharging the Hospitalized Patient
CLINICAL PRACTICE IMPLICATIONS

THE FAMILY MODEL AND VIOLENCE

Description of the Problem

Definition of Family Violence

Since the early 1990s, there has been an increasing awareness of the prevalence and consequences of family violence in the United States. Family violence is a widespread problem that affects people from all racial, ethnic, religious, geographic, educational, economic, and social backgrounds. Family violence is more than just a family problem; it is associated with social, financial, and legal sequelae that extend to the society.

Economic costs related to family violence include the increased need for police, courts, correctional facilities, and mental health resources.[1] Violence in a family is an umbrella phrase that may refer to physical, verbal, or sexual abuse against an intimate partner, child, or elder. *Physical violence* is an act that in some way directly threatens a family member's safety (e.g., hitting, throwing an object, threatening with a weapon). *Verbal* or *emotional abuse* consists of behaviors that symbolically threaten family members (e.g., threatening to abandon a family member, verbally derogating a family member, destroying property, abusing pets to hurt a family member). *Sexual abuse* refers to acts that are sexually aggressive, coercive, or exploitative (e.g., rape, incest). In violent relationships, violent episodes often involve a combination of assaultive acts, verbal abuse, sexual aggression, and threats.[2]

Once assaultive behavior occurs in a relationship, it usually develops into a stable pattern over time.[3] Assaultive behavior may (and often does) become worse with time and can end in murder. In considering the violent family, it is important to understand whether the pattern is mutual physical violence, verbal aggression on the part of the woman combined with physical aggression on the part of the man, or a completely controlling husband with a severely victimized and silenced wife. Although violence perpetrated by a woman against a nonviolent man does occur, it is a much less common pattern.

Additionally, it is important to first identify the type of family violence that is present and having an understanding of the categorizations of violence:

Domestic violence is defined as a pattern of behaviors used to gain or maintain power and control. Broadly speaking, domestic violence includes elder abuse, sibling abuse, child abuse, intimate partner abuse, parent abuse, and can also include people who don't necessarily live together but who have an intimate relationship. Domestic violence centers use the Power and Control Wheel developed by the Domestic Abuse Intervention Project in Duluth, MN to describe how domestic violence occurs. Domestic violence includes both physical and sexual violence including intimidation, emotional abuse, isolation, maximizing, denying and blaming, using children as in threatening to take them away, using privilege like treating partner as a servant, economic abuse and most important using coercion and threats.

Intimate partner violence is more specific, referring to violence that happens between people in an ongoing or former intimate or romantic relationship, and is a subcategory of domestic violence.

Coercive control is the use of power for control and compliance. It is a dynamic and systematic process described in the top left corner of Power and Control Wheel as, "Making and/or carrying out threats to do something to hurt a partner, threating to leave them, to commit suicide, to report them to welfare, making them drop charges, making them do illegal things." Overt control occurs with the implication that "if you don't follow the rules, I'll kill you." More subtle control is when obedience is forced through monopolizing resources, dictating preferred choices, microregulating a partner's behavior, and deprivation of supports needed to exercise independent judgment. All interpersonal relationships have elements of persuasion and influence, however, the goal of coercive relationships is to maintain power and control. It is a dynamic of the relationship. Coercive control emphasizes the systematic, organized, multifaceted patterned nature of this interpersonal dynamic and can be considered to its origin in the patriarchal dynamic where men control women. Most professionals who work in this interdisciplinary area now refer to domestic violence as coercive control. Victimizers target partners whom they sense they can control to get their own needs met. They are disinclined to invest in relationships with partners who stress their own points of view, who do not readily accept blame when there is a disagreement, and who offer nurturing only when it is reciprocated.

If coercion is present in the interpersonal family dynamics, it is useful to share this control wheel with the patients. Good education is of course our responsibility, though despite adequate psychoeducation, there are those individuals who choose to continue to participate in unhealthy relationships. In either case, the most important first step is to assess safety. Are they afraid of increased violence if they challenge their partner? Restraining orders or other legal deterrents may not offer solace as many people are clear that their spouse will come after them, if not tomorrow, then next week, or even next month. They are sure that they will not be safe. In these cases, it is important to review safety steps with the patient so that if they decide to leave, they will be prepared. The following are key safety points to share with your patients to follow:

- Memorize important phone numbers of people to call in an emergency.
- If your children are old enough, teach them important phone numbers, including when to dial 911.
- If you can, open your own bank account.
- Stay in touch with friends. Get to know your neighbors. Don't cut yourself off from people, even if you feel like you want to be alone.
- Rehearse your escape plan until you know it by heart.
- Leave a set of car keys, extra money, change of clothes, and copies of important documents with a trusted friend or relative: your own and your children's birth certificates, children's school and medical records, bank books, welfare identification, passport/green card, immigration papers, social security card, lease agreements or mortgage payment books, insurance papers, important addresses, and telephone numbers.
- Keep information about domestic violence in a safe place, where your abuser won't find it.

Some women may acknowledge that the risk of physical violence is not the determining factor in their decision to stay, and have difficulty explaining why they choose to stay. In these cases, it is recommended to consider the following frames that have their origin in the study of the impact of trauma.

Shame

From this lens, abusive events are humiliating experiences, now represented as shame experiences. Humiliation and shame hide hostile feelings that the patient is not able to acknowledge. "In shame, the self is the failure and others may reject or be critical of this exposed, flawed self" (Dorahy, 2017, p. 143). Women will therefore remain attached to an abuser to avoid the exposure of their defective self.[4]

Action steps: Empathic engagement and acknowledgment of shame and humiliation are key. For someone to overcome shame, they must face their sense of their defective self and have strategies to manage these feelings. The development of such strategies is a crucial next step in their development.

Trauma Repetition and Trauma Bonding

Women subjected to domestic violence often respond with incapacitating traumatic syndromes. The concept of "trauma repetition" is suggested as a cause of vulnerability to repeated abuse, and "trauma bonding" is the term for the intense and tenacious bond that can form between abusers and victims.[5] Trauma bonding implies that a sense of safety and closeness and secure attachment can only be reached through highly abusive engagement; anything else is experienced as superficial, cold, or irrelevant" (Sach, 2017, p. 85). Trauma bonding may have its origins in emotional neglect, according to self-reports of 116 women.[6]

Action Steps: The literature on trauma is growing and many patients will benefit from good curated sources. Having a good list of books and websites on hand is important. Discussion and exploration of the impact of trauma will be needed, and can be provided by someone who is available on a consistent and frequent basis. Of note, this work may be time consuming and difficult.

Asides:

1. Some psychiatrists offer the explanation that these women must be masochistic. The misogynistic concept of masochism still haunts the halls of psychiatry. It is usually offered as a way to dismiss these women's concerns.
2. One of the obstacles to recognizing chronic mistreatment in relationships is that most abusive men simply "do not seem like abusers." They have many good qualities, including times of kindness, warmth, and humor, especially in the initial period of a relationship. An abuser's friends may think the world of him. He may have a successful work life and have no problems with drugs or alcohol. He may simply not fit anyone's image of a cruel or intimidating person. So, when a woman feels her relationship spinning out of control, it may not occur to her that her partner is an abuser. Even if she does consider her partner to be overly controlling, others may question her perception.
3. Neutrality in family courts is systemic sexism/misogyny. When it comes to domestic violence, family courts tend to split the difference. Dr. S. Brandt notes that even after decades, mental health professionals often have an extremely superficial and outdated view of what comprises domestic violence. The assumption that it is violence alone that matters, has formed the basis of much clinical and legal confusion.[7] As an analyst, she has gone against the grain of a favored neutrality and became active in the courts, noting the secondary victimization that occurs when a woman enters the legal system.

In summary, psychiatrists must reclaim our expertise in systemic dynamics and point out the role of systemic misogyny. Justices and other court officials need education. Ideally, justice should be based on the equality of men and women in a society free of systemic misogyny. Unfortunately, our society has not yet reached this position. In the meanwhile, we must think systematically about interpersonal dynamics. This is our lane. This should not be controversial.

Causes of Violence in Families

Family violence has multiple causes. The strongest predictor of spousal abuse is having witnessed spousal violence in one's family of origin. Similarly, having a history of being maltreated as a child is a major vulnerability factor for committing child abuse. Other factors believed to be important in the genesis of family violence include sociocultural values and norms, sex role socialization, and social isolation. The culture of masculinity in the United States encourages the devaluation of women and, in some subcultures, the idea that violence is a good way to keep women in line. In addition, many men believe they are valued less for their verbal skills than for their ability to fight, drink, and be tough—this pattern encourages men to use anger as an all-purpose emotion with which to replace fear, hurt, or helplessness. The role that individual psychopathology may play in the etiology of family violence is unclear. Studies linking psychiatric diagnoses (e.g., antisocial personality disorder, depression) with spousal abuse have generally been flawed methodologically; however, the amassed evidence suggests that higher rates of psychopathology are found among batterers than among nonbatterers.[8]

Relationship between Family Violence and Alcohol or Drug Abuse

With few exceptions,[9] the bulk of the evidence indicates that domestic violence and alcohol or substance abuse are associated strongly.[10,11] National survey data indicate that 70% of the husbands who reported severely assaulting their wives reported being drunk one or more times during the survey year, as compared with 50% of the husbands who had moderately assaulted their wives and 31% who did not assault their wives.[12] Perpetrators of domestic violence are also more likely to have alcohol problems,[13] binge drink, and have an earlier onset of alcohol use than nonviolent men.[14] Research indicates that alcohol use interacts with personality variables, such as hostility and aggressive personality styles, to create violence.[15]

As with the relationship between alcohol use and domestic violence in the perpetrator, the temporal relationship between victims' use of alcohol and their experience of violence remains unclear. Several relationships are possible. First, individuals who experience violence may use alcohol to medicate themselves after being victimized. Second, alcohol may disinhibit drinkers who then may unintentionally provoke the abuser. Third, victim alcohol use and experience of violence may be coincidental and may be explained by a third variable such as the abuser's use of alcohol. Walker[2] reported that women who reported heavy drinking patterns tended to be involved with men who also abused alcohol.

Finally, evidence suggests a link between alcoholism and child abuse, although more methodologically rigorous research is necessary to determine the strength of this association. Although multiple studies have demonstrated that approximately 50% of abusive parents abuse alcohol, estimates of the proportion of confirmed child abuse cases associated with some sort of parental substance abuse problem have ranged widely.

How Violent Acts Occur: The Cycle of Violence

Violent acts do not have to be frequent to be frightening. A man who has injured his wife once may only have to threaten her to control her behavior, and she may be unaware of how much of her behavior is based on the need to avoid further violence. Violence against things (e.g., breaking objects in the home, throwing things) may also be frightening, and the entire family's behavior may become completely oriented toward averting the angry spouse's rage. On the other hand, wives' violent behavior is less often seen as frightening by husbands. Violence in the family resulting in child abuse is most likely to occur in a context of alcohol and high stress. The fewer resources the caretaking adult has, and the more emotional intensity the child has, the greater the chance of trouble. For many parents, abuse occurs in the context of a child who cannot stop crying or who is talking back. The line between acceptable discipline and child abuse varies to some extent with culture. For example, in the United States "spare the rod and spoil the child" was a common childrearing belief during much of the nation's history. The question remains of whether spanking is abuse or normal punishment. Beyond that gray area, however, it is usually clear what constitutes unacceptable behavior. Later in this chapter we discuss child abuse from the point of view of the pediatrician.

Assessment of Individual and Family Systems Issues

The first step in the treatment of violence in families consists of a comprehensive assessment of individual and family functioning. The clinician must be flexible and shift their focus between individual and family systems issues. Although the treatment of family violence usually should be approached from a systems perspective, the clinician should be aware that individual factors also may be playing an important role. Psychiatric diagnoses such as affective disorders, anxiety disorders, psychosis, and personality disorders may be at the root of the violence and should be treated appropriately (e.g., medication, individual therapy). It may not be possible to conduct family therapy unless individual psychopathology is stabilized first. Another important issue is the motivation of the violent family member to change their behavior.

Perpetrators of violence must be motivated enough to accurately report the extent of their behavior and to acknowledge their behavior as problematic. These criteria may not be present at the beginning of treatment but may represent a preliminary treatment goal. It is unlikely that significant therapeutic progress can be made without the existence of these basic criteria. Identifying potential motivating factors for the participation of a violent family member in treatment (e.g., avoiding jail, preserving the relationship) is an important task to complete during the initial assessment.

If after a careful assessment the therapist believes that the perpetrator is not motivated to stop violent behavior or if the violent behavior cannot be brought under control, family treatment is not an appropriate treatment strategy. Instead, referrals should be made for individual treatment for both the perpetrator (e.g., an anger management group) and the victim (e.g., individual treatment aimed at empowering the victim, women's group). Under these circumstances, the therapist should advocate actively for the abused partner to leave the relationship. While taking the initial history of a family with violence, the clinician should use not only interview skills but also observational skills. In observing the family, the clinician should note whether any family members exhibit apparent injuries. If the family's explanation of an injury is suspect, the clinician's suspicions regarding potential family violence should be heightened. Other behavioral signs that may suggest family violence include clingy and fearful behaviors such as hypervigilance and a strong hesitancy to speak. Any thorough assessment of a family or couple should include questions designed to assess the presence of family violence. The clinician must be sensitive when inquiring about this issue because a good deal of stigma and secretiveness are associated with the problem. By using empathic statements about how difficult it can be to cope with feelings of frustration, hopelessness, and anger, the clinician can help to create a nonjudgmental atmosphere. The clinician should be aware that the victim of violence may be unable to acknowledge the violence in the presence of the perpetrator. If the clinician suspects this is the case, they should conduct individual interviews to assess for violence. If an individual family member reveals in the individual interview that family violence occurs, the clinician should work with that family member to determine whether they feel safe discussing the problem in a conjoint meeting.

When assessing violence between intimate partners, it is helpful to ask questions such as the following: What does a typical fight look like? How are disagreements resolved? Do things ever get out of hand (out of control) when you fight? Do either of you have a short fuse or lose your temper easily? How do each of you express anger? These questions should be followed by more specific questions about the occurrence of violent behaviors (e.g., did you ever hit your partner?). Questions should also assess the severity of injury sustained by the victim (e.g., what is the worst you have ever been injured by your partner? Have you ever sought medical attention for an injury inflicted by your partner?). It is also important that the couple should be questioned about the presence of guns in the home.

When inquiring about child abuse, it may be helpful to begin asking the parents how they discipline their children, whether they have ever felt out of control with their children, and whether they have ever been so frustrated that they felt they might hurt their children. Again, specific questions about violent behaviors should be asked (e.g., have you ever touched or caressed your child in what others would call a "sexual" manner? Have you ever hit your child with an object other than your hand? Have you ever left marks or bruises on your child?). The therapist can sometimes identify abuse by asking about or observing child behavioral indicators such as aggressive behavior, agitation, temper tantrums, withdrawal, hyperactivity, blunt affect, a wariness of adult contact, fearfulness, self-blaming statements, sleep disturbance, or regression from age-appropriate behaviors (e.g., becoming enuretic or encopretic).[16] Obviously, these symptoms are most often related to issues other than abuse, but a reasonable amount of suspicion is warranted.

Physical and Psychological Consequences of Violence

Although both men and women can be verbally and physically abusive, women are much more likely to suffer injuries as victims of physical violence. Victims of family violence may demonstrate emotional and behavioral symptoms of trauma. These symptoms may include a startle response, hypervigilance, psychic numbing, memory loss, denial of the traumatic event, depression, and anger. The clinician should be careful to observe all family members for these symptoms. Abused individuals also frequently present with problems of anxiety, depression, and somatic complaints. Abused children frequently present with both internalizing and externalizing behavior problems, including aggression, anxiety, impulse-control problems, self-destructive behavior, and antisocial behavior.

How to Assess the Degree of Danger

If the clinician has evidence that some form of violence has occurred in the home, it is important to assess the perpetrator's danger to self and others. This assessment should include questions regarding risk for suicide and homicide. Steps must be taken to ensure immediate safety in the home. In order to assess the degree of danger, the clinician should inquire about the severity, nature, and frequency of the violence.

The clinician should also note the degree to which the perpetrator is capable of controlling their hostile or aggressive tendencies and the extent to which they acknowledge the behavior as problematic. Finally, the clinician should determine what weapons are available. Research indicates that a gun in the home adds substantially to the risk of family violence. An individual living in a home with a gun (roughly 50% of the homes in the United States) is eight times more likely to kill or be killed by a family member or intimate acquaintance than is an individual in a home without guns.[1]

During this information-gathering process, the clinician should note the behaviors of family members. If a family's argument begins to escalate during the interview and the family is unresponsive to the clinician's interventions, the clinician may need to conduct separate interviews. The clinician should take a proactive role when dealing with a violent family and not allow arguments to escalate. Through careful observation and questioning, the clinician determines the relative risk for physical harm. If the risk is low, creating a no-violence contract with the family members may be helpful. If the risk is high, the clinician should consider working with the family members to help them establish separate living arrangements until the risk becomes lower.

Treatment

Mandatory Reporting Laws

The clinician should be aware of the mandatory and optional reporting laws for spousal, child, and elder abuse in the state in which they practice. In addition, the clinician should inform patients of the limitations of confidentiality prior to beginning therapy. It is often helpful to do this in an office information form that describes the policies and procedures of the clinician's practice. This ensures that patients will not have grounds to be surprised if the clinician informs them that a mandated report will be made. If the clinician believes that a mandated report is required, they must never be persuaded by the family not to make the report.

Making a mandated report of abuse raises significant clinical issues that must be addressed. A family may react to the clinician in a hostile manner and refuse to take responsibility for the problem. In cases in which the therapeutic relationship is damaged significantly by breaking confidentiality, the clinician may need to refer the family to another clinician for continued treatment. It is sometimes possible to use the mandated reporting process as a means to strengthen therapeutic leverage. For example, the clinician might enlist family members' cooperation by informing them that it would be most beneficial for them to remain in family therapy and that the clinician could act as their advocate with the adult or child protective agency if they complied with the treatment recommendations. This may be facilitated by the clinician allowing the family to be present in the room when they make the report by phone or by having a family member make the report themselves while the clinician provides support. Making a report of family violence can be an empowering act that helps family members begin to take control of their lives. It may also be helpful for victims of violence to watch others taking a stance against violent behavior by reporting it to authorities.

Safety as a first step. The primary goal of the family assessment and subsequent therapy is to stop the violence. Even if the clinician determines that the family does not need to be separated physically, they should initiate a discussion of separation as an option if the violence increases. Getting family members to discuss what they imagine a worst-case scenario might look like may help to empower the family to work toward change. The development of an escape plan for the victim to use if conflict escalates is recommended to reduce stress and ensure physical safety. This plan should be accomplished individually with the victim of the violence and may include calling 911; having car keys, money, and important documents accessible; alerting friends or neighbors to the violence; setting up places to stay; and getting out of the house if the perpetrator is under the influence of alcohol or drugs. The therapist should also provide the victim with a phone number for a domestic violence hotline and a list of domestic violence shelters. Legal options (e.g., restraining orders) should also be discussed.

The clinician must insist that violent behaviors and threats of physical violence not occur during and after the family therapy. The therapist must take a clear stance against violent behavior, even if that means potentially alienating the perpetrator of the violence. If lethal weapons are readily available, the clinician should contract with the family to immediately remove these from the home to an inaccessible location. Asking the family members to describe the ways in which the no-violence contract might fail will help them both to take responsibility for the problem and to identify ways in which they are prone to sabotage themselves. The no-violence contract should be signed by both spouses and the therapist. It should state that one consequence of violence is that the couple will separate in order for the therapist to continue conducting therapy. Regularly checking in with the family to assess the usefulness and clarity of the contract is important. For example, the clinician might begin each session by asking whether the family was able to abide by the contract.

The clinician must understand the sequence of events leading up to the violence and identify the critical points of escalation. If alcohol or substances are involved as precipitants to violence, the clinician must be clear with the family that the substance user must agree to abstain from alcohol or substances in order for family therapy to be successful. This may require a referral to a self-help group (e.g., Alcoholics Anonymous, Rational Recovery) or to an alcohol or drug treatment facility.

The clinician's basic stance in working with violent families should be one of supportive confrontation. Violent families need help in setting limits and gaining control over their lives. Violent family members may be struggling with low self-esteem and profound feelings of powerlessness. If this is the case, an important goal of family therapy would be to increase feelings of self-esteem and mastery while rejecting the violent behavior. The clinician should reinforce the distinction between rejecting the violent behavior and rejecting the person who exhibits the behavior. They may need to transmit this perspective through repeated and clear verbal and nonverbal communications. Another crucial initial goal of family therapy is the reduction of family isolation. Violent families are often closed systems that promote secrecy, mistrust of outsiders, and strong family loyalty. These factors perpetuate the violence by isolating family members from help and support. The clinician should attempt to create a more open family system by referring family members to appropriate community resources, which may include support or therapy groups (e.g., assertiveness training, codependency groups, groups for perpetrators of violence). Family members may demonstrate resistance to following through on referrals, in which case the clinician should help the family to examine the underlying sources of its resistance and work toward change.

Therapy approaches. Cognitive-behavioral models of family violence view violent behavior as a learned behavior and a skills deficit. Violence is learned through direct and indirect modeling of behavior. Once learned, violence continues to be used because it is functional for the perpetrator. These models also assume that perpetrators of violence have difficulty controlling their anger and have deficits in interpersonal and communication skills. Therefore, treatment focuses on helping the perpetrator to manage anger effectively and on teaching nonviolent alternative behaviors.

Ways to reduce violent behavior include mandating the use of time-outs (described below), coaching the family to anticipate stress, identifying conflicts, and teaching negotiating or "fair fighting" skills. Improving communication skills will be an essential goal to help family members express anger, fear, hopelessness, and other feelings without verbal or physical abuse. The family must learn new techniques for the expression of anger and the resolution of conflict. In conducting this work, the clinician should be active and directive, pacing the therapy so that it challenges but does not overwhelm the family.

The time-out procedure begins with teaching the family to identify physiologic, behavioral, and cognitive cues that signal impending violence. Cue recognition can be facilitated by having family members self-monitor their feelings, thoughts, and behaviors during times when they feel angry. In this way, high-risk situations can be identified and time-out procedures are taught to help the perpetrator or victim leave an escalating conflict before violence occurs. The family is coached to return to the discussion after all family members have calmed down. A common problem that occurs is that when the perpetrator states the need for a time-out, the victim may try to prevent the perpetrator from leaving so that the conflict may be resolved. The therapist may deal with this problem by reminding the victim that the function of the time-out is not to leave an argument unresolved but to protect the victim from violence.

Once the time-out procedure is provided, families are taught new communication and conflict-resolution skills. These skills include the use of "I" statements and assertive statements, expression of feelings, active listening, validation, and problem solving. Families are taught to use these skills in conjunction with the timeout procedure to avoid escalation of conflict into violence.

Exploring family dynamics. Once the violence is under control and a sufficient sense of safety is established, more intensive work focusing on dysfunctional family dynamics can take place. Family systems, intergenerational, and structural family therapies are clinically useful in guiding this work. Enhancing deficient communication skills is often one of the first steps in the treatment of family violence. Examining the intergenerational aspects of violence and other salient family dynamics can help the family view its patterns of interacting in a broader context. This process may ease questions of blame and vilification as family members take responsibility for their behavior while recognizing that their patterns of behaving may have been formed in a context in which they had little control. It can be particularly helpful to use genogram work to elucidate these intergenerational patterns by creating a detailed family history and providing a visual representation of the family system. Structural family therapy can be helpful in identifying important family subgroups, coalitions, triangles, power dynamics, and boundaries. As we said earlier in this chapter, many families in which violence occurs are closed systems. Increasing support resources for these families is an important goal of the therapy. Family members should be referred to appropriate support resources, such as assertiveness training groups,

groups for batterers or victims of battering, 12-step groups, and so on. In some closed family systems, family members also may be enmeshed and may experience ambivalent feelings about their dependency on other family members. These family members may use violent behavior as a means of creating distance between family members or as a way of releasing pent-up anger about the unhealthy dependency in the family. The goal in these cases would be to develop support resources outside of the family and healthy differentiation among family members. Violent families need help in creating appropriate boundaries and in reestablishing these boundaries quickly after they have broken down.

Another relevant issue for violence in the family is the extent of any power imbalance in the family. Family violence usually can be conceptualized as a means for one family member to exert control over other members. In such family systems, any direct or indirect threats to the controlling family member's power are met with intimidation and violence. The controlling family member must begin to see that their intimidating behavior accomplishes the opposite of the goal. For example, if the controlling family member fears that his wife will leave him, he must be made to understand that by intimidating her, he will not gain her love or trust but rather her fear and mistrust. The controlling family member must come to understand the difference between overt and covert power and demonstrate a willingness to give up overt power in order to gain more indirect forms of power. Overt power refers to influence gained by intimidation and fear. Covert power refers to influential power gained by behaving in a respectful and caring manner. This message is not likely to be grasped easily by the controlling family member. A review of over 1 million tweets, between April 12 and July 16, 2020, found an increase in calls to hotlines and increased reports of a variety of types of family violence. There were also more inquiries about social services for family violence, an increased presence from social movements, and more domestic violence-related news.[17] It may take considerable time before family members are comfortable enough to openly share their feelings about the controlling behavior and thus confront the abuser with the negative effect of their behavior on the relationship.

When working with families in which child abuse is involved, clinicians will likely incorporate parenting training as an essential component of family therapy. Educating parents about developmentally appropriate behavior for children can help to eliminate unrealistic expectations. Parents should be taught to be aware of feelings of anger and frustration and to identify cues that indicate behavioral escalation to violence. Parents should be taught to take their own time-outs and to use rational self-talk to calm themselves down. Stress reduction and relaxation exercises may be used to decrease physiologic arousal. Parents should also be taught alternative methods of discipline. These methods include using time-outs with their children, using new communication skills, setting limits with their children, and applying consequences consistently. Clinician modeling of appropriate behavior and behavioral rehearsal are helpful to enhance skills and confidence. Referrals to parent-training courses in the community can reduce isolation and reinforce new knowledge and skills.

Additionally, the strains of the COVID-19 pandemic have also had a profound effect on family dynamics. Despite the ability of some couples to pull together and manage through the pandemic, some couples and families fail to thrive. Increasing divorce rates have been noted nationwide with many disagreements being specifically about COVID-19.[18]

Clinical Issues for Therapists

Although the therapeutic alliance is always an issue when working with families, maintaining alliances may be particularly problematic when working with violence in the family.[19] Alliance problems are set up initially as the therapist focuses on stopping the violent behavior of the perpetrator and ensuring the safety of the victim. The therapist must be able to ally with the perpetrator. One way to accomplish this is to accept the perpetrator without accepting the violent behavior. Because perpetrators of violence often expect to be rejected or judged by the therapist, the therapist needs to convey that the behavior is unacceptable without condemning the abuser as a person. Finally, while recognizing that the perpetrator is responsible for the violent behavior, the therapist must view the family dysfunction and discord as a systems issue.

That is, the therapist should acknowledge and validate the provocation described by the perpetrator while emphasizing that provocation never equals justification for violent behavior.

Because perpetrators of violence often feel out of control, it is important for them to believe that the therapist can deal with them and the violence.[19] The therapist needs to set limits about violence. When the perpetrator tests these limits, the therapist should not show fear but should lay out the consequences for such behavior. This may be difficult for some therapists, particularly for those who are afraid for their own safety. Therapists must be concerned with their own safety when working with violent families. For example, therapists should not work with violent people when they are the only ones in the building, at the end of the work day when everyone else has gone home. If guns have been involved in the violence, it must be clear that guns may not be brought into the building where therapy takes place. (This seems obvious, but therapists are often afraid to bring it up.) For example, the therapist could say, "I can't work if there is a gun around because guns make me nervous." The therapist must have a plan if violence erupts in the office. Most importantly, the therapist must learn to monitor the session so that escalation points are not reached.

Working with violence in the family presents multiple challenges for clinicians. Therapeutic progress may be slow and gradual. Clinicians must track their countertransference reactions so that they do not impart feelings of hopelessness or negativity to their patients. Just as families where there is violence should be encouraged to seek support resources, so should clinicians readily seek support for themselves in the form of consultation or the enlistment of a cotherapist as they feel the need.

INTRAFAMILIAL CHILD SEXUAL ABUSE

Incest is a nonconsensual sexual act between family members in which one person's abuse of power violates and victimizes others whose access to power is not comparable.[20] In addition to the serious damage done to the abused child, the family as a whole is damaged by the boundary violations, the secret keeping, and the knowledge of destructive and violent behavior by one of its members.

Intrafamily child sexual abuse encompasses any form of sexual activity between a child and a family or extended family member, including adults in surrogate parent roles such as a live-in boyfriend. This activity is by definition exploitative and nonconsensual, as it is imposed on children who lack the emotional, physical, and cognitive ability to protect themselves. A child may appear to acquiesce to a particular sexual act for the purpose of gaining love or attention, avoiding violence, or protecting another. In some cases, incest may occur between an adult child and a parent or adult sibling. This situation is rare and tends to occur after a history of childhood incest. Individual, family, and larger system dynamics interact to create a climate in which incest is possible, and it is impossible to examine incest within the family without examining all three systems.

Intrafamily child sexual abuse encompasses any form of sexual activity between a child and a family or extended family member, including adults in surrogate parent roles such as a live-in boyfriend.

Sexual contact between siblings is the most common form of incest, although father–daughter incest is more commonly reported to the authorities than are other forms. Male siblings are overwhelmingly the perpetrators. Sibling incest in some cases is experienced as less traumatic, especially when the siblings are close in age. Studies indicate that most sibling contact occurs before age 12 years and is associated with parental absence or overly stimulating sexual behaviors. Father–daughter incest is by far the next most common type. Men constitute about 95% of the perpetrators in abuse of girls and 80% in abuse of boys. Father–son incest and mother–child incest are, to our knowledge, far less common, although underreporting has probably seriously skewed these statistics. Mothers implicated in incestuous relationships are more likely to have obvious and severe psychiatric disorders than are fathers.

Individual Issues

Key individual issues are a history of abuse in the lives of the parents and alcoholism, psychosis, violence, or pedophilia in the perpetrator. Sibling perpetrators may be violent, angry, confused, and sexually immature, using their siblings to shore up their sense of power and meet their sexual needs. Once the abuse begins, the abused child will often exhibit symptoms of depression, withdrawal, or sexual precocity. Older children may begin acting out sexually, believing that they have been damaged or that they are so worthless that sex is the only thing good about them. Many victims begin to split off parts of themselves and can go on to experience severe dissociative symptoms.

Family Issues

Families in which abuse occurs are frequently disorganized, rigid, and socially isolated. The parents themselves, more often than not, have histories of neglect and abuse. This means they are unlikely to know how to get their own dependency needs met and are unlikely to be able to give much to dependent children. As the marriage progresses and the marital relationship becomes more difficult, fathers (and occasionally mothers) may turn to their dependent children for sex and affection. Two major patterns of interacting have been described with father–daughter incest. In one pattern, a rigid family is led by a domineering father who uses force and coercion to maintain his role. In the other pattern, the mother is dominant and the father develops incestuous relations to secure feelings of power and self-worth in the family. Both patterns involve closed and avoidant family systems and feelings of powerlessness in the man, although the feelings are managed in opposing ways. If the parent is a pedophile, is disinhibited by substance abuse, is a victim of abuse himself, or is under severe stress, he is vulnerable to progress to more and more explicit sexual contact with the most vulnerable people in the family, the children. Because children do not want to admit that a person who loves them could betray them, and because the cost of reporting the abuse is so high (e.g., loss of the parent, loss of family income, loss of trust, public shame), the victim is less likely to tell anyone of the abuse, and family members are likely to deny and minimize the problem. Many victims are told that they, other family members, or their pets will be killed if they tell. For the mother, the cost of not believing the abuse is to betray her child, but the cost of believing it means she may lose her spouse, break up the family, and perhaps descend into poverty. The ensuing denial creates secrecy, isolation, and shame within family members. Sibling abuse is easier to report in some ways, but this involves enormous shame and the fear of retaliation from the perpetrator. Abuse by the mother is perhaps the hardest to report; virtually all children abused by their mothers do not report the abuse at the time.

Larger System Issues

Incest takes place more commonly in any society that gives males power over females and condones many types of exploitation. The assumption that a man has a right to the women in his family allowed such a society (until recently) to deny the possibility of incest or marital rape.

For many men, any affection has sexual overtones, so that a woman or a child being affectionate must be "asking for it." Because men are often encouraged not to act feminine, or dependent, and are encouraged to be dominant, strong, and invulnerable, the only way for some men to meet their dependency needs is through sex. Such men are not taught to be empathic or sensitive to the needs of those around them but rather to control and be taken care of by women. When the man is a live-in boyfriend or stepfather, the lack of genetic connection may be taken as a license to abuse. Because most women are considered the gatekeepers for the family's emotional life, when incest does occur, society is more likely to blame the woman for not protecting the children than the man for the abuse, even though the woman may have no power in the relationship and no ability to make her husband do what she wants.

Assessment

Abuse must be considered when alcohol and drug use are present, when the family is secretive and depressed, when a small child begins speaking knowledgeably about sexual material with which they should not be familiar, when a major personality change occurs in a child who was previously functioning well, or when the child reports abuse. Although false allegations of incest are uncommon, when it occurs, it usually is in the context of a custody or other divorce proceeding, or in a chaotic home with an adolescent girl who is angry at her father or stepfather. The clinician should be alert for this possibility but should also err on the side of protecting potential victims. Evaluation of the family in which incest occurs involves several stages. The key first stage involves identifying the degree of incest and the need for protection of family members from ongoing abuse. This may involve child protective services intervention and other legal decisions depending on the local reporting laws. The next stage takes place after the safety of family members has been established; the therapist's job is to evaluate the family as a system and each individual member. They must consider whether alcohol or drug abuse, violence, psychosis, or pedophilia are present. Finally, it is particularly critical to allow abused children to talk about their feelings (good and bad), about the abuser, and about themselves. If one child has been abused, the siblings likely know about it and have likely been abused as well.

Treatment

Treatment must be organized around stopping the individual and systemic dynamics that maintain the incest and understanding the crucial distinctions between incest and other dysfunctional dynamics. In addition, treatment must be dedicated to stopping not only the physical aspects of the abuse but also the other exploitative and intimidating behaviors in the perpetrator and the family. The therapist must be prepared to deal with a perpetrator mourning the loss of their abusive power and the family mourning a major, unexpected, and unwanted loss of its self-image and of family members. The family may be facing the mandated loss of either the abuser, who has been separated from the family, or the abused child to foster care. Legal, social work, and other uninvited health professionals have suddenly invaded their lives. Treatment will likely be mandated rather than chosen freely; therefore, these families often respond with shock, anger, and denial. The family therapist must find a way to work with many members of the helping community who may disagree about how to help or who should be punished. The legal system will often encourage the perpetrator to deny the offense and avoid entering treatment until litigation is completed, which may take months. The therapist must attend to these dynamics while dealing with the family. In abusive families, the initial impulse is to deny the facts, deny responsibility (e.g., it was my wife's fault for not stopping me), or deny the effect (e.g., it was only once and didn't matter). This may be very frustrating to the therapist who does not understand the needs that prompt this denial. The therapist must be clear and explicit about the negative consequences of the abuse while supporting the family's wish for connection and whatever strengths are available. The perpetrator is often sent to a group for perpetrators that can challenge them directly. The family is encouraged not to blame the nonprotective parent (usually the mother) more than the perpetrator and to understand the nonprotective parent's own powerlessness and fear. Efforts must be made to support that parent's growth and their ability to parent. The abused child needs adequate individual support to deal with dissociative phenomena or other symptoms (e.g., posttraumatic stress disorder) that have already occurred and to find a way to deal with the loss and shame. The complexity of treatment demands patience and willingness to work in complex systems.

Countertransference feelings of anger, disgust, and wishes to rescue the victim and family from the perpetrator are common responses in the family therapist. The therapist must be self-aware and resolve these feelings if they are to be effective with these families. It is often helpful to work in a team or to have an outside therapist review these cases.

THE FAMILY MODEL AND CHILD ABUSE

Child abuse is a major clinical problem throughout childhood. Child maltreatment occurs in families from all social classes and ethnic groups. Child neglect is the most frequently reported form of abuse but can also be linked to the family's capacity to provide basic needs such as shelter, food, and health care. In the view of some clinicians, maternal substance abuse and domestic violence directed at the pregnant mother may constitute the earliest forms of child abuse.

Diagnosing accidental versus abusive forms of injury during early childhood requires evaluating the age and developmental ability of the child and the seriousness and likely mechanism for the injury. In addition, a careful history is needed to detect inconsistencies. Infants are especially likely to sustain intracranial bleeding from severe intentional shaking because of muscle weakness and their relatively large head size, which creates sufficient force momentum to tear vessels and cerebral matter.

Blunt trauma to the chest and abdomen from a kick or punch can result in serious or fatal heart, liver, intestinal, or pancreatic injury. Skeletal trauma is also age related: 80% of fractures associated with abuse occur in infants younger than 18 months, and joint fractures are strong clues to nonaccidental injury.[21] Toddlers and school-age children often present with suspicious bruises, burns, or human bite marks. Because common pediatric infections (e.g., ringworm, impetigo) or birthmarks have been mistaken for cigarette burns or other surface signs of abuse, a careful evaluation of each child is important to avoid false reports of abuse.[22] Bruises on the face, ears, neck, trunk, or buttocks are less likely to be accidental, and pattern bruises resembling a hand, belt, extension cord, or other object should be noted carefully and documented photographically, if possible.[23] Less common forms of child abuse include Munchausen syndrome by proxy, in which the parent (usually the mother) fabricates a history and secretly induces a host of factitious symptoms in the child (e.g., fever, bleeding, vomiting, diarrhea, electrolyte imbalance) to gain entrance to the hospital, ostensibly for care of the child but also to participate in the medical care system as a dedicated and devoted parent attending to a child with an illness that medical science seems unable to diagnose and cure. A team approach to uncovering this syndrome is mandatory if the child is to be protected from harm.[24]

The consequences of child abuse are both immediate and long term. For the child who remains in an abusive environment, recurrent physical injury and the accompanying emotional abuse occur. A physically dangerous and threatening family environment focuses the child's energies on survival strategies and may leave little margin for normal emotional and psychological development. Recent studies of such children emphasize the potential for neurologic impairment of the brain structure and function owing to abuse. This impairment is described as a posttrauma experience with persistence of the freeze, flight, or fight stress response that may show up later as negative personality and behavioral traits such as poor self-esteem, fear of failure, indiscriminate and shallow relationships with peers and adults, and use of aggression and violence to solve problems.[25] School-age children may show behavioral and learning problems that reflect past or present abuse.

Perpetrators of child sexual abuse are often known to the child as family, friend, or caretaker. Adolescents are often victimized by peers. The sexual contact may go on over time and become progressive but is usually concealed from others. Stranger assault is less common but usually more violent and acute than is assault by a perpetrator known to the child. The child may disclose some or all of the abuse to a family member, friend, or teacher. Health-care providers may encounter masked presentations such as psychosomatic symptoms, unusual or vague physical complaints, encopresis or enuresis, behavior disorders, school truancy, and adolescent pregnancy. Although not common, the diagnosis of a sexually transmitted disease in a prepubertal child is a strong indicator of abuse and requires investigation.

Current procedures involve reporting suspected child sexual abuse to protective services or law enforcement authorities who conduct an initial intake investigation and may then bring the child to a specialized child protection center for a forensic interview and medical examination by trained examiners. Physical evidence of abuse of the prepubertal child may be revealed with the aid of photo or video colposcopy (external magnification and good light source), a useful tool in child sexual abuse cases that has been of great help in expanding the knowledge of normal versus abnormal findings.[26] Therapy for the victim and the family is crucial in most cases of child sexual abuse. Children need to hear the message that despite what happened to them they are still normal with intact bodies and that friends cannot tell they were abused simply by looking at them. Parents also need reassurance that although physical signs of trauma may be (but more often are not) found on examination, their children are not damaged goods. Some children require out-of-home placement for protection from repeated abuse if the caretaking parent is unsupportive of the child. Knutson and Schartz[27] have reviewed in detail the physical abuse and neglect of children.

Incestuous Trauma

Incestuous trauma of whatever type is not limited to the victim. Studies of sexual trauma indicate that members of the entire family are at risk for ongoing difficulties, including somatic complaints, posttraumatic stress disorder, mistrust, poor self-esteem, depression, suicidal behavior, increased aggression, impaired peer relationships, poor school performance, substance abuse, and disturbance of sexual behaviors. Families that receive appropriate early and continued assistance as they recover from the trauma of incest are likely to have the best outcomes and thereby mitigate the development of some of these problems. Kaplan and Pelcovitz[28] have reviewed extensively the area of incest as it relates to the family.

THE SUICIDAL PATIENT AND THE FAMILY

The suicidal patient poses a major unresolved public health problem. Whether the suicidal act is viewed as a maladaptive response to an acute family crisis (e.g., from the perspective of a family model, in which one identifies a family problem and interprets the suicidal behavior as an attempt to resolve the family crisis) or a maladaptive coping response to other stressors, engagement of the family in the treatment of the suicidal patient is an important adjunct to treatment. This is true when monitoring suicide risk and when intervening to manage the risk for suicidal behavior. Suicide is the end result of a variety of mental disorders; it also occurs when no major psychiatric disorder is present.

In this section, we present a step-by-step management plan for the assessment and treatment of those patients who, with their families, present at a time of threatened or actual suicidal behavior. Such families most often present to the family therapist in crisis, and we begin at that point.

Acute Management

Recognizing that the truly accurate prediction of suicide risk is virtually impossible, the clinician must nevertheless make an immediate judgment of risk, as a first step in the management of an acute clinical condition. We dichotomize patients into the seemingly simplistic categories of "probably will try" and "probably will not try." In our experience, the best (although not exclusive) predictor of suicide attempts is a history of a life-threatening suicidal act (e.g., one that required hospitalization in an intensive care unit). Other indicators include a history of a medically damaging suicidal act that required medical intervention, the suicide of a close family member, or the recent acquisition of the means to commit suicide (e.g., purchasing a gun).

We believe that patients in the "probably will try" category should be managed with one-to-one, round-the-clock, family observation or hospitalization, pending collection of further information from other family members. Patients in the "probably will not try" category are thought to be less likely to require such observation. In all cases, a more extensive psychiatric evaluation and mental status examination is indicated.

The baseline evaluation of acute suicide risk should focus on current and past suicidal ideation, planning behaviors, and indicators of suicide intent (e.g., availability of a method and means, attempts to avoid detection, attempts to communicate intent). Knowledge of circumstances, events, and clinical conditions associated with current and previous attempt behavior can help in terms of identifying specific risk indicators for extended monitoring of suicide risk and determining appropriate conditions and treatment parameters for managing acute suicide risk.

Evaluating the Family

Once the decision has been made about whether to use maximal suicidal precautions by hospitalizing the patient, the next step is to obtain a family history, assessing the history of family functioning, key events of past and current stages of the family developmental cycle, and current patterns of family adaptation to problems. At this point, some families ask, "Why should we be involved?" At our hospital, we explain that our routine practice is to require that families be involved in inpatient treatment (if indicated) in order to achieve treatment efficacy. By establishing family involvement as one of the preconditions of inpatient treatment, the aim is to induce the patient and the family to pursue treatment and to minimize the risk of premature dropout from treatment and suicidal behavior. If the family does not participate, we explain that we will consider discharging the identified patient to their family. If the patient is not hospitalized, they should receive supportive care and monitoring.

The next step is to evaluate the role of suicidal behavior and the identified patient in relation to the family. Although the suicidal act is often unrelated to a family crisis or problem, in many situations suicide attempts are premeditated acts that are attempts to resolve mounting family conflict. The focus is on the evaluation of the historical and developmental aspects of the family context in which the presenting problem has evolved.

A final step in the evaluation involves determining whether the identified patient has a current psychiatric disorder or a history of one. Dealing with family dynamics alone will seldom completely alter the course of these illnesses. Considering the known epidemiology of suicide and suicidal behavior, we are particularly concerned with determining the presence of a history of mood disorder, schizophrenia, and alcohol or other substance use disorders. For example, therapists have had the experience of seemingly restructuring and restabilizing a family after a suicide attempt only to discover (several years later) that the identified patient had a recurrent depressive disorder with associated suicidal ideation largely unrelated to family problems. It later emerged that the presence of severe depression was a consistent and probably causal factor in the recurrence of suicidal behavior.

Involving the Family

The next step is to involve the family in the treatment. The family often attempts to dump the patient on the hospital's (or family therapist's) doorstep as a solution to a family crisis. At this point, the therapist has increased leverage. As we mentioned earlier, we choose this point to inform the family that the patient cannot be treated without its involvement. The family is told that if it doesn't agree to participate in treatment, treatment cannot take place (i.e., start). This statement is used as a tactic to involve the family rather than (as the family may view it) as a consequence of ignoring the patient. We believe that effectiveness of treatment for the identified patient and the family is impaired seriously by lack of family involvement. Furthermore, if we collude with the family to allow uninvolvement, we tend to find that acutely suicidal patients are readmitted to the hospital over and over again (as indicated in follow-up studies).

After the family agrees to participate in the treatment, the next step is joining the family. This is a tactic by which we convey to the family that we're on its side—a tactic that facilitates the development of a treatment alliance with the therapist. If the patient is not hospitalized, the family should be given the therapist's telephone number, and intensive therapy should be started.

If the suicide attempt has been a response to a threat of divorce, it is critical to involve other family members such as siblings or parents when possible in order to form an alternative support system. If the partner has decided definitely to leave the relationship, they will not be much help in supporting the suicidal family member. Although suicide attempts are not an effective way of keeping a partner in a relationship if they do not want to be there, sometimes a suicide attempt will trigger a renewed attempt to improve a marriage. In such cases, a trial of marital therapy is often useful. Suicide attempts may trigger a great deal of anxiety in a beginning therapist or in one who does not see such cases frequently. The therapist must be clear that, just as with family members, their care and concern alone cannot prevent a determined person from committing suicide. Because most people who attempt suicide are ambivalent, the therapist often has a good deal of leverage but not omnipotence. Because of legal concerns and therapist worries, it is particularly helpful to treat these cases with the supervision of an experienced psychiatrist.

> The therapist must understand that, just as with family members, providing care and concern alone cannot prevent a determined person from suicide.

Treating the Family

It has been our experience that the suicidal ideation gradually decreases as the family problem is addressed. At the stage of acute symptom remission, the task is to treat the family problem rather than to focus exclusively on to the patient with suicidal ideation. For example, in many cases, the suicidal act may serve as a way to wake up the family. In such cases, the act represents an attempt to find a new option or solution to the family problem. Throughout this stage of treatment, the therapist emphasizes that although the focus of treatment began with the suicidal act, the act is essentially a symptom of a larger problem. Thus the message is conveyed that dealing with the other family problems is the most effective way to change the problem in the long run.

What often becomes evident at this stage is a continuing struggle between the family's need to keep the identified patient in the present role versus the family's feelings of wanting to help the patient (and to thereby move them out of that role). In our experience—especially with the families of hospitalized patients—family forces may be extremely powerful in maintaining the patient in the depressed, acting out, or suicidal role as an adaptation to the family conflict. Family members often feel guilty and in part want to help, but they are at a loss to find a new solution to the problem. This is the crucial stage of the therapy—a pivotal point at which the family is most amenable to working on reframing and redefining the family problem.

Discharging the Hospitalized Patient

After the family has reached a new equilibrium in which the family problem has been reframed and redefined, the patient can be discharged to the family for continued family therapy in the community using the more traditional family therapy techniques.

CLINICAL PRACTICE IMPLICATIONS

Although violence, incest, and suicidal behavior are not DSM disorders, the frequency of these behaviors, the damage to individual and family life they cause, and the difficulty in detecting and treating them is considerable. As such, the clinician must understand the material in this chapter in order to provide thoughtful diagnostic and treatment intervention.

SUGGESTED READING

Heru AM, Stuart GL, Rainey S, Eyre J, Recupero PR. Prevalence and severity of intimate partner violence and associations with family functioning and alcohol abuse in psychiatric inpatients with suicidal intent. *J Clin Psychiatry*. 2006;67(1):23–29.

REFERENCES

1. Seppa N. *APA releases study on family violence*. American Psychological Association Monitor; 1996.
2. Walker LEA. *The Battered Woman Syndrome*. Springer; 1984.
3. O'Leary KD, Barling J, Arias I, Rosenbaum A, Malone J, Tyree A. Prevalence and stability of spousal aggression between spouses: a longitudinal analysis. *J Consult Clin Psychol*. 1989;57:263–268.
4. Dorahy MJ. Shame as a compromise for humiliation and rage in the internal representation of abuse by loved ones: Processes, motivations, and the role of dissociation. *J Trauma Dissociation*. 2017;18(3):383–396.
5. Dutton DG, Painter SL. Traumatic bonding: The development of emotional attachments in battered women and other relationships of intermittent abuse. *Victimology*. 1981; 6(1):139–155.
6. Krüger C, Fletcher L. Predicting a dissociative disorder from type of childhood maltreatment and abuser-abused relational tie. *J Trauma Dissociation*. 2017;18(3):356–372.
7. Brandt S, Rudden M. A psychoanalytic perspective on victims of domestic violence and coercive control. *Int J Appl Psychoanal Studies*. 2020;17:215–231.
8. Hamberger LK, Hastings J. Characteristics of male spouse abusers consistent with personality disorders. *Hosp Community Psychiatry*. 1988;39:763–770.
9. Barnett OW, Fagan RW. Alcohol use in male spouse abusers and their female partners. *J Fam Violence*. 1993;8:1–25.
10. Flanzer JP. Alcohol and other drugs are key causal agents of violence. In: Gelles RJ, Loseke DR, eds. *Current Controversies on Family Violence*. Sage; 1993:171–181.
11. Kyriacau DN, Anglin D, Taliaferro E, et al. Risk factors for injury to women from domestic violence. *N Engl J Med*. 1999;341:1892–1898.
12. Kantor GK, Straus MA. The drunken bum theory of wife-beating. *Soc Probl*. 1987;34:213–229.
13. Pan HS, Neidig PH, O'Leary KD. Male-female and aggressor-victim differences in the factor structure of the modified Conflict Tactics Scale. *J Interpers Violence*. 1994;9:366–382.
14. Murphy CM, O'Farrell TJ. Factors associated with marital aggression in male alcoholics. *J Fam Psychol*. 1994;8:321–335.
15. Heyman RE, O'Leary KD, Jouriles EN. Alcohol and aggressive personality styles: potentiators of serious physical aggression against wives? *J Fam Psychol*. 1995;9:44–57.
16. Veltkamp LJ, Miller TW. *Clinical Handbook of Child Abuse and Neglect*. International Universities Press; 1994.
17. Xue J, Chen J, Chen C, Hu R, Zhu T. The hidden pandemic of family violence during COVID-19: unsupervised learning of tweets. *J Med Internet Res*. 2020;22(11):e24361.
18. Ellyatt H. *Arguing with your partner over Covid? You're not alone, with the pandemic straining many relationships*. CNBC; 2022.
19. Rosenbaum A, O'Leary KD. The treatment of marital violence, In: Jacobson NS, Gurman AS, eds. *Clinical Handbook of Marital Therapy*. Guilford; 1986:385–405.
20. Erickson MT. Rethinking Oedipus: an evolutionary perspective of incest avoidance. *Am J Psychiatry*. 1993; 150:411–416.
21. Leventhal JM, Thomas SA, Rosenfield NS, Markowitz RI. Fractures in young children; distinguishing child abuse from unintentional injuries. *Am J Dis Child*. 1993;147:87–92.
22. Reece RM. *Child Abuse: Medical Diagnosis and Management*. Lea & Febiger; 1994.

23. Reece RM. Unusual manifestations of child abuse. *Pediatr Clin North Am*. 1990;37:905–921.
24. Light MJ, Sheridan MS. Munchausen syndrome by proxy and apnea (MBPA). A survey of apnea programs. *Clin Pediatr (Phila)*. 1990;29:162–168.
25. Perry BD. Neurodevelopment and the neurophysiology of trauma II. *The APSAC Advisor*. 1993;6:1–14.
26. McCann J. Use of the colposcope in childhood sexual abuse examinations. *Pediatr Clin North Am*. 1990; 37:863–880.
27. Knutson JF, Schartz HA. Physical abuse and neglect of children. In: Widiger TA, Frances AJ, Pincus HA, First M, Davis W, eds. *DSM-IV Sourcebook*, Vol 3. American Psychiatric Association; 1997:713–804.
28. Kaplan S, Pelcovitz D. Incest. In: Widiger TA, Frances AJ, Pincus HA, First M, Davis W, eds. *DSM-IV Sourcebook*. Vol 3. American Psychiatric Press; 1997:805–860.

20 The Family and Treatment of Acute and Chronic Psychiatric Illness

OBJECTIVES FOR THE READER

- To understand the role of the family in the acute and chronic treatment of one of its members
- To be able to treat such a family with the goal of preventing rehospitalization and of reaching the highest functional level and quality of life for the identified patient and family
- To become aware of family approaches and alternatives to hospitalization as most psychiatric care is delivered in outpatient settings

For easier reading, we emphasize that the descriptors "couples" or "marital" are used nearly interchangeably in this chapter.

INTRODUCTION

Now that we have examined the role of the family in individual psychiatric disorders and problems, it is necessary to address the issue of how the family model is used in acute and chronic care settings. Inpatient units are no longer the solitary sites for acute care. Crisis units now receive and evaluate the acutely ill or those in crisis. Some patients are hospitalized and some are held briefly, stabilized, and discharged to intensive (though not inpatient) levels of care. These include 24-hour residential programs, partial hospital services, and intensive outpatient treatment and home care. For patients who begin in a hospital, their stays are typically brief and they are later "stepped down" to less intensive, less costly services. For chronically ill patients, multiple treatment sites are available, from chronic inpatient units to board and care homes to community health centers, and so on.

In this context, we must point out that the nature and quality of work with the family has varied enormously throughout the history of the treatment of psychiatric illness. The regard and help given to families have generally reflected prevailing theories of individual patient psychopathology and a tendency for clinicians to temporarily "adopt" patients from their families. Shorter lengths of hospital stays and a now developed literature on family theory and practice have combined to inform us of the limits of hospital practice and the importance of including, allying, and relying on families for the effective short- and long-term care of the psychiatric patient.[1,2] The family involvement in the discharge planning process is key for increase involvement in follow-up care postdischarge.

In this chapter, we focus on a new model for the evaluation and treatment of families. The model is empirically rather than theoretically based (where data exist). We provide general guidelines for family work and detailed approaches for specific disorders.

Now in the year 2024, hospitalizations are very brief and often less than 1 week. As such, the crucial issue to change posthospital trajectory of the illness is for the family therapist to be proactive in contacting the family at the time, or before admission. The involvement of family members if in touch with the patient's family should be a required piece of the discharge process. Neighbors and friends may also want to be involved and be key supports.

BACKGROUND
ACUTE TREATMENT
The Function of the Acute Team for the Family
Family Responses to Mental Illness of a Family Member
Families of the Acutely Ill
The Family Burden in Psychotic Illness
Rationale for Acute Treatment of Families
Process of Family Treatment in Acute Care
Allying with the Family
Evaluating the Family
Setting Goals
Common Goals of Acute Family Intervention
Goal 1: Accepting the Reality of the Illness and Understanding the Current Episode
Goal 2: Identifying Current Episode Stressors
Goal 3: Identifying Potential Future Stressors, within and Outside the Family
Goal 4: Elucidating Stressful Family Interactions
Goal 5: Planning Strategies for Managing or Minimizing Future Stressors
Goal 6: Accepting the Need for Continued Treatment
Particular Decisions in Acute Care and Family Intervention
Timing
Staffing
Family Techniques
A Working Model of Acute Family Intervention
Guidelines for Recommending Family Intervention in an Acute Care Setting
Empirical Studies
FAMILIES OF THE CHRONICALLY ILL
Expressed Emotion
COMMUNITY-BASED SUPPORT GROUPS
CONTROVERSIES IN THE TREATMENT OF ACUTE AND CHRONIC PSYCHIATRIC ILLNESS
CLINICAL PRACTICE IMPLICATIONS

BACKGROUND

In many cultures (other than Western), families typically have a vital role in the psychiatric care of their members.[3] Because of the scarcity of trained professionals in these cultures, families must provide for the needs of the identified patient. Family members often stay with the patient in or near the hospital. The assumption is that the patient is an integral part of their family, and it is unthinkable that the patient would return anywhere but to the family.[4]

In an article published in 1977, Anderson outlined some of the difficulties of working in acute settings, many of which still remain to some degree.

Regrettably, however, the family therapy literature is not particularly helpful to those working on inpatient units; such concepts as "defining the family as the patient" tend to alienate the medical staff of an institution and the already overwhelmingly guilt-ridden families. The polarized approaches of family therapists, who generally operate on a "system" model, which overemphasizes interactional variables, and of psychiatrists, who generally operate on a "medical" model, which overemphasizes individual variables, disregard the complex and complementary interplay of biologic, psychodynamic, and interactional factors.

Anderson's[5] comments highlight the problem of integrating theories of etiology and pathogenesis, a problem shared by patients, families, and hospital staff. To be sure, advances have been made since 1977. For example, research on expressed emotion (EE) in the family environments of patients with schizophrenia has demonstrated the interplay between biology and environment, thereby focusing treatment.[6] The degree of family warmth is an additional research finding that supports better patient outcomes, across different cultural settings.[7] In addition, research designs that include pharmacotherapy in various doses combined with family intervention[8,9] recognize and provide data on the importance of attacking biologic and social factors simultaneously. During the 1990s, families came to be seen as "colleagues" on the treatment team. Accordingly, our prescription for acute help for families has undergone major changes. People with severe mental illness typically experience social impairment, low levels of employment, and increased isolation. Not only does the literature support that family involvement leads to better discharge outcomes, but it also has been found to decrease rehospitalization and relapse rates.[10]

ACUTE TREATMENT

The Function of the Acute Team for the Family

Brief acute psychiatric intervention (through hospitalization and other acute residential services), which is the norm in the United States, provides a safe and controlled environment in which to treat acute symptoms of depression, mania, suicidal ideation, substance intoxication and withdrawal, severe personality disorders, and psychosis. In addition, acute care with residential support serves major functions for the patient's family. The identified patient is removed temporarily from an overwhelmed family environment. In an acute family crisis, removal from home can decrease behavioral eruptions and offer substantial relief to a desperate family. During this separation, a critical goal is to evaluate the family's patterns of interaction and change maladaptive ones.

Acute residential care also can provide a setting in which the problems of the patient and their family surface, allowing for resolution of these problems. Psychiatric intervention can disrupt a rigidly pathologic pattern of family interaction, throw the family temporarily into turmoil, and create an opportunity for change that can be more rapid and substantial than without separation. Moreover, 24-hour care permits observation, evaluation, and discussion of family interaction patterns, which can motivate the family to seek marital or family treatment after discharge. Acute care also may set the stage for overt (as opposed to previously covert) consideration of separation in deadlocked marital or parent–child interactions. In our opinion, the clinician should consider four family-relevant functions when a patient with a serious mental illness presents for treatment.[11]

1. **Treat the patient.**
2. **Evaluate the family. Identify families with specific difficulties who need immediate or intense support.**
3. **Develop a therapeutic alliance with the family, which can later be shifted to community-based care.**
4. **Begin psychoeducation with the family.**

In performing these functions, especially when evaluating the family, the clinician should identify the family's patterns of coping with the patient's mental illness and intrafamilial differences in coping that evoke conflict (e.g., when one parent sees the patient as bad and the other sees the patient as sick). It's important to keep in mind that the family response always must be understood in its cultural context. Finally, a good clinician needs to recognize how families cope can change over time.

Family Responses to Mental Illness of a Family Member

Families of the Acutely Ill

Families experience a patterned sequence of responses to the occurrence of mental illness in a family member (i.e., the identified patient). These stages are as follows:

1. Beginning uneasiness: the family does not know what to expect.
2. Need for reassurance: the family hopes that everything will be all right.
3. Denial and minimizing: the family denies that anything is wrong and minimizes the patient's difficulties.
4. Anger and blame: the family begins to see the extent of the problem, and each member lays blame on the others or on the hospital staff.
5. Guilt, shame, and grief: each member perceives their role and feels guilt and shame.
6. Confusion in the changed family: the family adopts new roles with resultant confusion.
7. Acceptance of reality: the family adapts to a new homeostasis.

In treating families in which the identified patient has a psychiatric illness, the therapist needs to be aware of these stages in order to make effective treatment plans. For example, to ensure that the identified patient with a bipolar illness takes their lithium medication as regularly as an individual with diabetes mellitus takes insulin, the therapist needs to know how the family feels about the illness and its treatment. Later in this chapter, we translate these functions into goals.

The Family Burden in Psychotic Illness

Researchers on family factors in the major psychiatric disorders have identified several types of stressors confronted by families attempting to cope with mental illness—for example:

- The objective and subjective burdens imposed on family life by salient aspects of the illness and by the need to provide caretaking
- Family members' tendencies to respond to the patient with criticism or emotional overinvolvement (EOI) (i.e., high EE), which is hypothesized to increase the stress climate for the patient[12]
- Additional stress associated with psychiatric disorders in the patient's spouse, as a consequence of assortative mating

Except for a handful of studies cited later in this chapter, management of these stressors has been fruitful with patients suffering from schizophrenia but has not been included in investigations of mood disorders in general and bipolar disorder in particular. More recently, a study has been published on improving the treatment process of families with whom a member suffers from bipolar disorder.[13] Commonly, families are excluded from treatment due to desire to protect confidentiality. Additionally, many mental health care providers lack training in how to communicate and how to include a patient's family in the treatment care plan. Below we will discuss the roadblocks that affect family integration in the discharge planning process. *Objective burden* refers to the effects of mental illness on the family's finances, use of time, living conditions, and relationships with others. *Subjective burden* refers to the emotional stresses that the illness imposes on the family. Research on both types of family burden has demonstrated that families of patients with both psychotic and mood disorders experience considerable emotional distress and social and financial problems in relation to their relatives' illness. Caretakers of patients with chronic schizophrenia face psychological problems much greater than those of the general population in the care of these patients. These burdens significantly affect the lives of families of the mentally ill and may be particularly prominent among the families of patients with bipolar (as compared with unipolar) disorder. Higher levels of burden are experienced in lower-class families and in families of patients who are male, have negative symptoms, and who have been ill for a relatively long period before hospitalization. Symptom severity and illness chronicity have been associated with increased levels of family burden. Falloon et al.[14] assessed levels of family burden before and after a psychoeducational intervention; this study found significant decreases in burden in the psychoeducational but not the control condition.

Rationale for Acute Treatment of Families

Although it is our belief that most family interactions are not a major or sole cause of serious individual symptoms, it seems clear that acute intervention with family members can produce both helpful and maladaptive changes for a family system. Consider the following situations:

1. The family is in crisis and uses acute care to adaptively resolve the crisis. For example, some dysfunctional couples have described the process of coping with a psychotic episode in one partner as a strongly positive experience for both partners.
2. The family extrudes an identified patient from the family by hospitalization in an attempt to solve a crisis. Consider the following case example:

   The A family consisted of a mother, Ms. A, her boyfriend, and her two teenage daughters. The older daughter had anorexia nervosa, but the younger daughter was functioning well. Ms. A had long-standing paranoid schizophrenia and was extremely dependent on her own mother. She had been divorced about 10 years previously but had recently become involved with a boyfriend. After Ms. A became very involved in this relationship and was considering marriage, she began to argue frequently with her older daughter. When this daughter began eating less and became paranoid, Ms. A contacted a pediatrician, stating that her daughter was seriously ill and needed hospitalization. Ms. A confided to the family therapist that she was unable to take care of her daughter because caring for her daughter would prevent her from spending time with her boyfriend and thereby would threaten the relationship. Instead of a family intervention, the pediatrician (unknowingly) hospitalized the daughter.

   The preceding case example illustrates how one family member can change the life of another in the service of individual needs. In order to prevent the loss of her boyfriend, the mother restructured the family by having her daughter (i.e., the identified patient) hospitalized.

3. The family uses the care system to obtain treatment for a member other than the identified patient. The identified patient is not necessarily the only sick one (nor even the sickest one) in the family.[15] For example, the mother may be hospitalized for depression, which ignores the father's alcoholism. A family approach allows the therapist to observe and evaluate all family members and advocate for appropriate treatment (including medication) for whoever may require it. Therapists who concentrate on one individual may overlook or not have access to psychological disturbances in a close relative.
4. The family uses the care system as a means to regain a lost member. For example, an alcoholic father who is never home may finally be convinced to enter treatment. In this case, the family's motivation is to regain a functioning father and spouse.
5. For an identified patient with a chronic or deteriorating condition (e.g., childhood or adult schizophrenia), the family can turn to an acute care system as a necessary respite from family burdens.

These situations illustrate that the treatment program is inadequate unless it includes the family. Acute care psychiatry will not fulfill its responsibility to provide effective and efficient care unless treatment includes a focus on the family.

Process of Family Treatment in Acute Care

The process of family intervention involves allying with the family, evaluating the family, defining the problem, setting goals, starting treatment (in some cases), and referring the family for continued care after discharge. Intensive psychoeducation about a specific illness and a specific treatment for that illness is an essential service. Particular attention should be paid to single-parent families and remarried families that have to cope with serious long-term mental illness. The National Alliance on Mental Illness (NAMI) has found that a high proportion of its members are single parents who often express the opinion that mental illness in a child caused the marital breakup.

Allying with the Family

Contact with the family should start as early as possible. If the patient is hospitalized, contact should start preferably before hospitalization, when the family is trying to arrange admission or certainly by the time of admission. A principal focus with the family should be discharge planning. The family must be helped to understand that hospital treatment of the identified patient involves (or requires) education, support, and involvement of all family members. This may be made a condition of all acute care. A family representative should be appointed as the accountable communicating link with the primary clinician outside of formal treatment sessions.

A more relevant question is whether to treat family members using psychoeducation or a consultative approach and in which order. Grunebaum and Friedman[16] suggest that the first encounter should be psychoeducational rather than consultative. Therapists need the family "in order to learn about the history of the patient's illness and the family's story. Families need us to help explain to them about what they are facing, often for the first time." Consultation is more appropriate later in treatment.

Evaluating the Family

Evaluation of the family should involve the identified patient unless they are too psychotic or cognitively impaired to be present. The evaluation follows the customary outline for acute work and begins with the construction of a family genogram. In addition, the therapist examines immediate events, especially notable family events and changes that led to the contact. The evaluation should help the therapist to determine whether family intervention is needed and, if so, with what focus. A necessary goal of the family evaluation is to move the family from a frightened, defensive stance (in which family members presume they will be blamed) to a position of early trust and collaboration with the treatment team. The therapist also seeks to enable the family to find the best possible coping mechanisms for the patient's symptoms. Coping mechanisms must be understood by the therapist and the family as the best of difficult alternatives. Adaptation to illness is a process of building adaptive responses.

Setting Goals

Keeping in mind that acute treatment is brief, the therapist must immediately focus on the general goals of family intervention and on the goals specific to the individual family. Negotiating these goals with the family should be accomplished by the end of one or two evaluation sessions. Negotiation must be done with confidence, delicacy, firmness, and empathy. Family members are upset about the patient's condition; they may see no need for their participation in therapy or may be hostile to the treatment team for not quickly curing the ill family member. In the worst-case scenario, the family consciously or unconsciously seeks to push out the patient. These varied responses often occur because of the burden of dealing with illness. Education about the illness from all therapeutic staff members (e.g., doctors, nurses, social workers) helps to reduce family guilt. Information about the type and length of treatment, and about what can realistically change, will reduce anxiety and allow for focus. Realistic expectations can diminish subsequent disappointment and devaluation of the treatment and staff. Education about needed family assistance will help in discharge planning and treatment compliance. Family sessions can vary in length from 30 minutes to 1 hour and may be scheduled on a daily, biweekly, or weekly basis, depending on needs, goals, or anticipated discharge date.

Psychoeducation rarely proceeds as smoothly as its description might imply. Families frequently resist participating in treatment, deny the patient's illness, or magnify its severity and intractability. The family sometimes is more accurate than the therapist, especially one who is too optimistic or who appears to give up. The therapist must take family concerns seriously and not assume that they are right, especially on first contact. These are the complexities and challenges of family intervention. The family intervention must then switch from an educational focus to an interpretive one in order to overcome or circumvent family resistance to treatment.

We discuss the other parts of this process—that is, starting treatment and referring the family for continued care—elsewhere in this chapter. For example, the issue of treatment is addressed in several sections, starting with "Particular Decisions in Acute Care and Family Intervention," and continued care is addressed to an extent in the section on community-based support groups at the end of the chapter.

Common Goals of Acute Family Intervention

Six goals dictate the focus and course of acute family intervention (AFI). Although our inpatient family intervention research[17] has focused on two major diagnostic groups (i.e., schizophrenia and mood disorders), these goals generalize to major mental illnesses. Whatever diagnosis the patient receives, the family faces multiple tasks: (1) understanding the patient's illness; (2) appreciating the family's own influence on the illness; (3) allying with treatment staff; (4) acknowledging the course of the illness; (5) adjusting the family's expectations of the ill member; and (6) deciding on a discharge treatment plan, including the optimal living arrangement for the ill family member. Because these are enormous tasks, especially for the first episode of illness, they require considerable focused attention from the therapeutic staff.

The sections that follow describe the six goals and corresponding treatment strategies of AFI that are designed to meet the family's needs. When family needs are met, the family becomes a major asset in the patient's recovery. When family needs are not met, the family will respond with aversion, hostility, and chaos and add to a patient's risk of destabilization.

Goal 1: Accepting the Reality of the Illness and Understanding the Current Episode

The goal of accepting the reality of the illness and understanding the current episode is the cornerstone of all other goals. Unless the family achieves some acceptance and understanding of the illness and the seriousness of the episode, it cannot aid in future treatment. If this is a first episode, the subsequent course of the illness may not be clear to anyone. The therapist must be up-front about this.

The therapist can choose from a number of techniques to accomplish this goal. All techniques require a working alliance, which is accomplished by appreciating and expressing the family's burden. The therapist should ask each family member about their perception and understanding of the illness. Although the therapist may not agree with a family member's view, they can empathize with the family's attempts to cope. In order to reduce inordinate feelings of responsibility for the illness, the therapist can provide the family with facts about the illness and (especially in the case of schizophrenia and major mood disorders) articulate the biologic and genetic causes. When the family members realize that the therapist is not blaming them, the family can begin to trust the therapist. The therapist then may explore the emergence of the current episode in order to identify family stresses and environmental problems. Finally, the family can be educated about the course of the disorder, including early warning signs, progression, relapse, and recurrence.

Goal 2: Identifying Current Episode Stressors

Once the family has tentatively accepted the reality of the illness, the next step is to identify precipitating current episode stressors while they are still fresh in the minds of family members. The abstract notion that stress can influence a psychiatric illness becomes a reality when the link between theory and reality is forged.

The strategies and techniques for achieving this goal are mainly educational, cognitive, and problem-solving oriented. The therapist encourages the family to think about recent stresses, within and outside the family, that may have contributed to the patient's regression. In addition, the family can rank the stresses and assign priorities for brief interventions.

Goal 3: Identifying Potential Future Stressors, within and Outside the Family

Goals 1 and 2 are principally concerned with the immediate and remote past and with a didactic approach to illness. If these goals are accomplished even partly, there is a natural tendency to consider the future. In some cases, a future orientation (e.g., discharge) comes too early. This generally signals defensive denial that must be met with a refocus on Goals 1 and 2.

Family attitudes toward the patient and treatment have an effect on outcome. For example, positive family attitudes about hospital treatment have correlated with patient improvement, whereas resistance to treatment has correlated with discharge against medical advice.[18,19] In addition, Greenman et al.[20] (p. 228) found that certain parental concerns on admission to a hospital affect patient behavior. Interestingly, these concerns were gender-linked: mothers were concerned with limit setting (i.e., preventing impulsive and self-destructive behavior), whereas fathers "had difficulty supporting treatment because they were afraid that taking such a position would anger the patient, leading to a loss of their relationship with the patient." This observation is not surprising because mothers were often home all day with the patient and they already had a deeper relationship with the patient.

Goal 4: Elucidating Stressful Family Interactions

Informing a family that it can stress a patient is both intellectual and vague. However, when a family is shown how its behavior is destabilizing the patient (e.g., causing the patient to become paranoid or disorganized or to smash an object), real learning can occur.

An impressive body of evidence has suggested that families high in EE run an increased risk of patient relapse. EE is a qualitative measure of the criticism, hostility, or EOI that a family member or significant other expresses when speaking about a loved one who suffers from mental illness. Family techniques that lower EE result in better patient outcome.

Although Goals 1 through 3 are mediated by cognitive and educational strategies, techniques that demonstrate how family interactions stress the patient more closely approximate traditional (or systems-oriented) family therapy. The following statement illustrates a systems-clarifying technique: "Every time you criticize him, as you did just now, he puts his head down and murmurs something under his breath that sounds like nonsense." By using this technique, the therapist educates the family about how an interaction does not cause the disorder (thereby reducing guilt) but is likely to trigger current symptoms (thereby focusing controllable and adaptive behavior). The family's frustration and anger toward the patient's behavior, which lead them to criticize the patient, can then be redirected.

Goal 5: Planning Strategies for Managing or Minimizing Future Stressors

By the middle or toward the end of an acute episode of illness, family members may believe that their troubles are over. The next goal of family intervention, therefore, is to help families recognize that planning is needed to ensure that history does not repeat itself. The therapist can initiate discussion of the possible return of symptoms and how the family can cope. Family members also need to be encouraged to discuss their expectations of the patient's future level of functioning. For some families, expectations must be realistically lowered; for others, hope needs to be stimulated. Families also need help anticipating potential stressors related to the patient's reentering the community, including employment, education, and social functioning. If the family members are also experiencing illness or addiction, they should be encouraged to begin treatment.

Goal 6: Accepting the Need for Continued Treatment

This goal, central to preventing relapse, brings the family full circle with Goal 1 (reducing denial of the illness). Families that have experienced repeated episodes of illness have little problem anticipating the possibility of relapse. Because these families are often discouraged and burdened, they need support and encouragement. For families going through a first hospitalization, there is the danger that they will deny future illness and the need for aftercare.

The therapist can use the family technique of visualizing in the future replays of what led to the current illness. How would the patient tell the family (or vice versa) that something is the matter? What are the early signs of illness? Who would the family contact? Additional education about the course of the condition further emphasizes the need for aftercare.

Not every family will need work on all goals. Some families will be so traumatized or limited that the therapist can approach only a few of these goals.

The ultimate goal of family intervention is to extend the gains of acute care into the family. If the family can understand precipitating stressors, modulate high EE, and ensure continued treatment, the transition from intensive treatment to community care will be facilitated greatly. This is especially important in an environment in which hospitals find it advisable to reduce hospitalization in order to limit regression and, especially, to reduce health care costs through brief stays.

Particular Decisions in Acute Care and Family Intervention

Timing

The two key moments of timing are when to make contact and when to start therapy. Contact with the family should start during the decision-making process leading to acute care (e.g., in the emergency room). Family therapists typically disagree about when the patient should be present. Some therapists believe that family intervention with the patient should begin only when the active symptoms have begun to diminish. In our experience, this position rationalizes putting off family intervention and treatment. Many patients, even in a psychotic state, become more coherent during well-planned and focused family sessions.

Staffing

Who should do the family intervention? In our opinion, the primary clinician or therapist is in the best position to work with the family because they have an overall grasp of the case. In the hospital setting, we believe that the individual and family treatments should be done by the same therapist; however, time constraints, or the need for supervision, may make this impossible. Primary clinicians may be of any discipline (e.g., psychology, social work, nursing), but experience with families and family therapy is critical. The key issue is training; that is, whoever does the family therapy must have training in the theory and practice of family therapy and must have experience with the disorders that are prevalent in acute care psychiatry.

The partial hospital or inpatient milieu is especially advantageous for identifying patterns of family interaction. Accurate, on-the-spot observation of a family may reveal how a patient's symptoms may be aggravated. For example, a male adolescent's repeatedly recreating problem family interactions with female staff on the psychiatric unit can present an opportunity to demonstrate to him that this is similar to the way he reacts to his mother.

Family Techniques

A variety of family therapy techniques are needed in the acute setting: individual family intervention, multiple family groups and conjoint couples groups, and family psychoeducational workshops (also known as family survival skills workshops or family support groups).

Clinical family therapy by itself is rarely used today for hospitalized or acute care patients when hospital stays are less than 2 weeks long. For psychotic patients, family intervention complements medication and rehabilitative therapies. For nonpsychotic patients, family intervention is part of a treatment plan consisting of pharmacotherapy and individual therapy. Consider the following case example:

Tom B, a 17-year-old adolescent, was admitted to the hospital after having been extremely agitated and disoriented at home, where he refused to eat or sleep. The working diagnosis was of a schizophrenic disorder. In the hospital, he continued to be very paranoid, eating only with a parent and avoiding other patients. The staff met with the boy and his mother and explained their observations and concerns and discussed how a neuroleptic medication could help. They also discussed side effects and how to evaluate the effectiveness of the medication (e.g., by observing Tom's ability to think more clearly and understand what was going on around him). Tom was told that he could help the staff decide the best dose.

Tom hesitated and his mother, Mrs. B, had questions. But it was she who convinced Tom that he should begin taking medication. Two days later, he reported that he felt better and wanted to stop the medication. The staff spoke again with Tom and his mother and indicated that more time was needed to keep him well. Again Mrs. B persuaded her son to continue. Some days later, he said he felt better but wondered if an increased dose would help him sleep better. In another meeting with Tom and his mother, a new dosage was arranged. The medication discussions provided Tom and his mother with a cooperative, respectful relationship with each other and the staff. Decisions were not made for him; instead, he was included in the decision making. As the hospitalization progressed, Tom more readily questioned his family and the staff, and the answers he received helped to clarify and quiet his psychotic confusion. The neuroleptic medication and the therapy described had worked synergistically.

The acute treatment team must choose a family treatment model: psychoeducational, insight-awareness, or a systemic-strategic approach. All three are useful but at different times in the course of a disorder or with different disorders. Because of the brief duration of acute care and the cognitive impairment of an acutely ill patient, we recommend a psychoeducational approach, reserving insight-awareness and structural approaches for continued care.

A good description of the need for psychoeducation is found in the following communication from a parent of a patient with schizoaffective disorder: when my daughter and son-in-law entered the clinic with their newborn son, diagnosed with spina bifida and hydrocephalus, the chief nurse said, "You will be with this child every hour of the day. We will teach you what to look for, and then you will be able to tell us what is wrong with the baby." When my other daughter accompanied her son to the allergist about the boy's asthma, the doctor gave specific instructions about the dosage of medicine, and the desired response. The doctor told her when to go up and come down with the medication dosage and what to do in an emergency. As a pathologist who has worked closely with my son who has schizoaffective disorder, I believe it is important that a parent or family member be involved equally in the treatment of mental disorders.

The principle is that a patient and his family should be given medical education and training to enable them to carry out the treatment program.

Like any chronic illness, psychiatric illnesses require he care of a mental disorder, like many persistent or unstable illnesses, requires daily attention to symptomatology, stresses, and treatment.

A Working Model of Acute Family Intervention

In current practice on an inpatient psychiatric unit, brief assessment of patients and quick resolution of symptoms is the standard of care. Families, when given the opportunity, will ask basic questions such as "Should we be quiet when she comes home? Does she need to rest? Can she go back to work? What should I do if she gets upset and cries? What do I do if she refuses to get up in the morning? Should she be able to take her medications on her own? Do I need to supervise her taking the medications? Can she be left alone?"

It is important therefore to meet with families to educate them about the illness and how to manage the patient when they come home. Educational material should be available that describes specific illnesses and the typical course of recovery. There is a great deal of information on the internet and families need guidance as to what sites are reliable. If possible, families should be connected with local support groups that meet in person or virtually.

Working with families on the inpatient unit means that all the unit staff are welcoming to the family and that psychiatric residents and other staff are available and willing to meet with families and answer basic questions.

When indicated, family treatment can be started in the acute care setting, although most goals will be accomplished in a continued care setting. One easy intervention that can be done on an inpatient unit is the construction of a family genogram. This might show the family for example, where family support can be accessed, which relatives are supportive, and where family tension exists. A good textbook resource is Heru and Drury, Working with Families of Psychiatric Inpatients, a Guide for Clinicians.[21]

Guidelines for Recommending Family Intervention in an Acute Care Setting

Examples of acute situations that call for family intervention include the following:

- A suicidal and depressed adolescent living in the parental home is hospitalized following a car accident. There is some suspicion that the father is alcoholic and that the parents are not aware of the adolescent's depression or of his daily functioning.
- A 22-year-old college student presents with an acute psychotic episode in the fall of his first year away from home. Family sessions are needed to educate the family about the unexpected illness, to help the parents and the patient evaluate their mutual expectations for his performance, and to encourage follow-up psychiatric care.
- A 39-year-old divorced woman living with her 11- and 13-year-old children is hospitalized following a paranoid psychotic break in which she stabbed herself in the abdomen in the presence of the children. Family sessions with the children are needed to help the mother, now in a denial phase, to explain her illness and to talk about the future. An urgent need also exists for the children to discuss their feelings about witnessing their mother stab herself. The treatment team needs to find more family and community resources for the mother and her children, as well as assessing whether the mother can care for her children adequately.

- A 23-year-old woman who lives with her parents is hospitalized following an exacerbation of schizophrenia occasioned by her younger sister leaving for college. The patient also had stopped taking her medication. The parents have high EE (they are critical of the older daughter, and one parent is with her constantly). Family treatment is started to increase the likelihood of compliance with aftercare (i.e., aftercare includes medication, family therapy, and a partial hospital program).

Indications for family intervention come from the patient, the family, and the observable interactions between the family and the patient's illness. Patient-related criteria include current living conditions (e.g., living with spouse or family of origin) and life cycle issues (e.g., patient is a young adult trying to separate or an older adult living with or dependent on the family). Family criteria include conflict that contributes to the patient's difficulties or psychiatric illness in another family member. Criteria related to the interaction of the family with the patient's illness are family denial or inadequate support of the illness, family resistance to treatment, and danger of harm to the family.

Contraindications include the individual patient who is striving (with a good chance for success) for independence from the parents and parents in severe conflict, in which case marital treatment may be indicated.

Empirical Studies

Glick et al.[22] have reported the only controlled study of family intervention in an inpatient setting. Inpatient family intervention (emphasizing family psychoeducation [FPE]) was compared with hospitalization without family intervention for patients with schizophrenic and mood disorders. The sample included 169 patients and their families for whom family intervention was indicated. The families were randomized into the two treatment conditions. Assessments were made at admission, discharge, and 6 and 18 months post admission, using patient and family measures from the vantage points of patient, family, and independent assessors. Overall, family intervention in the hospital setting was found to be effective but not for everyone.[22–25] For some patients and families, inpatient family intervention appeared not to add anything to standard hospital treatment. The positive effect of inpatient family intervention was principally in female patients with mood disorder and their families, to a lesser extent in schizophrenic patients who had good prehospital functioning, and in patients given other diagnoses. In a follow-up study, the statistical interactions indicated that any therapeutic effect was generally restricted to female patients with schizophrenia or major affective disorder. The effect of family treatment on male patients given these diagnoses was minimal or slightly negative. The effect of inpatient family intervention on schizophrenia did not appear until 18 months post admission, and the most striking effect was observed in the prehospital poorly functioning group. Similarly (in contrast to the discharge results), the follow-up results for patients with mood disorder revealed positive findings favoring the inpatient family intervention but only in the bipolar subgroup. Composite means showed that family treatment was somewhat better for the families of patients (primarily females) with the major psychoses, whereas families of patients given other diagnoses did better without family intervention.

Clinical research on hospital treatments has typically focused on outcomes for patients; the outcomes for families are not known. One hypothesis-generating, three-country study of family outcome after an episode of major affective disorder found that families were less financially well-off (because of hospitalization costs), frequently functioned worse than before the episode, and, without psychoeducation, were unprepared for the next episode.[26]

Our clinical experience suggests that the specific interventions of psychoeducational groups can help the often demoralized family of the chronically ill patient to reestablish itself as a viable unit and lessen family members' burden of shame, guilt, despair, and isolation.[27] As to the effectiveness in outpatient settings, five studies in three countries have found that family intervention coupled with medication significantly lowers the risk of relapse for outpatients with schizophrenia. "Since 1980, twenty-two controlled studies of long-term cognitive-behavioural family interventions integrated with optimal drug and case management have shown substantial additional benefits for people with schizophrenic disorders. These include 14 random-controlled comparisons carried out with sound scientific methods that document the significant clinical, social and economic advantages of these new approaches that include patients, relatives and close friends in the continuing care program.... All recent authoritative reviews of this body of research have reached a consistent conclusion that further delays in implementing these methods in clinical practice can no longer be justified, either on the grounds of insufficient scientific evidence for their effectiveness, or on account of problems with securing additional manpower resources for implementation."[28] As such, one might extrapolate from these studies that family intervention may be mandatory as part of the multimodal prescription for most mental disorders.

FAMILIES OF THE CHRONICALLY ILL

Thirty percent of the patients discharged from psychiatric hospitals are rehospitalized during the first year after discharge. Sixty percent of all admissions to state hospitals are readmissions. For many patients, rehospitalization occurs more than once and indeed becomes a way of life and for many patients the family has become more involved in their long-term outcome.

Expressed Emotion

In 1966, EE was conceived as a measure of the family emotional climate, the premise being that the expression of emotion in families had an impact on the member with psychiatric illness, namely schizophrenia. The Social Psychiatry Unit of the U.K. Medical Research Council created six family measures with construct validity: warmth, number of positive comments, severity of criticism, number of critical remarks, dissatisfaction, and hostility. The final measure consisted of critical comments, hostility, and EOI. These terms were considered normative at the time, but they now sound culturally deaf and outdated. A more culturally appropriate and normative concept/language would be family emotional expressiveness/climate or family cohesion. The measurement of warmth was dropped because of its complex relationship with the other variables; however, the original researchers made several comments about the importance of family warmth.

Using these parameters, patients with schizophrenia in high-EE families had a relapse rate of 58%, compared with 16% for those in low-EE families. The key relative's initial EE score was considered the best single predictor of relapse 9 months postdischarge. EE was the first psychosocial construct that assessed the family emotional climate using a semistructured clinical interview, the Camberwell Family Interview, rather than a checklist of behaviors.

An initial hypothesis was that patients with more symptoms would evoke more family distress, but this was not found to be the case. No consistent relative variables were correlated with high EE, although these relatives were found to be more conventional, less satisfied with themselves, less flexible, less tolerant, lower in empathy, more conscientious, more burdened, more distressed, and caring for a longer period of time.

Low-EE relatives were more fatalistic and less active in managing problems, whereas high-EE relatives were noted to be more active, more critical, disagreed with patients more and showed lower levels of accepting behavior. However, family beliefs about illness show that high-EE relatives believed that patients could and ought to exert more control over their symptoms. This finding led to the development of interventions based on FPE that focus on illness education, resulting in reduced relapse rates.

However, when FPE is applied across cultures, there is no single "universal" successful FPE intervention, and McFarlane notes that the American version of FPE may mesh better with certain cultures than with other cultures. The differences in efficacy may lie in the quality of cultural adaptations, specific aspects of the studies' design, or cultural context.

In African American families with a person with schizophrenia, high EE/high criticalness is associated with better patient outcomes. On qualitative analysis, patients perceived high-EE family comments as "direct and expressive," supportive, and an expression of concern, whereas low-EE family comments were perceived as passive and uncertain. So, interventions to reduce EE will not be helpful for patients in African American families.

In Mexican American families with a person with schizophrenia, high EE/high EOI is associated with relapse, even when sampling (total $n = 224$) differed across time (1980 and 2000), recruitment sites (in-patient versus out-patient), years of illness, illness course and different interviewers/coders.[20] In one sample, a subset of "Anglo-Americans" ($n = 54$) had the same EE scores as Mexican Americans, but the EE score had different internal components: Anglo-Americans had 72% criticism/hostility and 8% EOI, whereas Mexican Americans who had 44% criticism/hostility and 40% EOI. An intervention focused on reducing criticalness will, at best, be irrelevant for families that have high EOI. Interventions for Mexican Americans should therefore focus on reducing EOI. Kopelowitz and colleagues successfully adapted an FPE intervention for Mexican American families. Before the intervention, a systematic assessment of each family enabled the clinical researchers to capture the cultural elements considered important for the adaptation. As a result, family members ($n = 174$) were successfully taught how to support medication adherence. Warmth and moderate EOI emerged as good prognostic factors.

Warmth was an original component in the EE construct but was dropped because of its complex relationships with the other components. The original observers of the importance of family emotional climate predicted that if critical comments and EOI were controlled, then warmth predicted a better outcome. After 40 years, the importance of this research is now reemerging. When family warmth is high, several international studies show that individuals with psychosis have a better outcome. In Mexican American families, the best predictors of good patient outcome were high warmth and moderate EOI.[20] In families from Barcelona ($n = 21$ dyads), high warmth as measured by the Camberwell Family Interview was correlated with fewer patient symptoms. In Puerto Rican children, high parental warmth was found to be protective against psychiatric disorders. In this study, measurement of warmth included assessment of feelings of closeness, trust, and anger towards the child. For further discussion, see ref. 7.

A remarkable change has taken place among the families of the seriously and chronically mentally ill. These families have organized together, shared their common experiences, sought educational information, and destigmatized their views of themselves. As a result, beginning with the American Schizophrenic Association, which stressed orthomolecular therapy, parent groups have formed throughout the country. In 1979, NAMI was formed, which currently has 200 chapters. The groups are remarkably similar, seeking to end the tendency in psychiatry to blame the family, to advocate for themselves, to support one another, to increase research efforts, and to advocate for a more efficient and effective service delivery system.[14,29,30] Families also are concerned that they, who know what has worked and what has not worked, are frequently not consulted by professionals during treatment planning.[31] Families point out that their views are often different from those of their ill relatives. For example, they tend to think that hospitalization and conservatorship are too difficult, discharge is too abrupt, the system is too permissive, and patients are allowed to refuse their medication too easily. It has often been pointed out that one reason that the mentally ill have been placed in community care less successfully than the mentally retarded is because of the stigma felt by their relatives; that is, they often feel a need to hide their love because of the stigma of loving a mentally ill adult.[32]

Families have demonstrated that their willingness to keep mentally ill relatives at home is much greater if certain system changes are made, such as providing fiscal support, respite services, a sound social services program that reduces the family burden, and a true community care system.[33] Although most programs have described their interaction with families in general terms, further work needs to be devoted to identifying the specific coping strategies that work with the chronically ill and the attitudes and behaviors that are most useful.[34]

COMMUNITY-BASED SUPPORT GROUPS

Support groups provide a safe environment for sharing personal experiences, thoughts, feelings, and emotions. A variety of organizations offer group therapy and support groups for psychiatrically ill patients. Whether peer led or led by a mental health professional, these groups can provide a friendly haven for the exchange of information and support.

Mental health professionals should be aware of these community resources and refer patients to websites and organizations like NAMI, the Depression and Bipolar Support Alliance, and the National Education Alliance for Borderline Personality Disorder. These organizations also provide useful handouts and resources. *NAMI Family-to-Family* is a free 12-week course for family caregivers of individuals living with mental illness. Designated as an evidence-based practice in 2013 by SAMHSA, research has found that *Family-to Family* enhances coping and empowerment in loved ones suffering from mental illness.[35] For more information on these groups and other support groups, please visit the Mental Health America website.

Patients also might benefit from local religious communities and programs. Research has found that religion can enhance remission in patients with medical and psychiatric diseases.[36] In addition, many patients with psychiatric disorders frequently use religion to cope with their distress. Regardless of the level of mental illness, the social support, comfort, and meaning that might be found in religious belief can prove powerful.

The Clubhouse Model of Psychosocial Rehabilitation movement continues to grow as a viable alternative to the day treatment program. Clubhouses provide a therapeutic environment for adults with mental health problems to acquire a greater sense of self, purpose, and community. Currently, more than 325 clubhouses are in operation globally, and individuals who participate in them are called “members.” The clubhouse offers a wide range of onsite community-based volunteer work as well as supportive services for housing, financial planning, and continuing education, among other resources. For a complete list of programs, clinicians can visit the International Center for Clubhouse Development.

CONTROVERSIES IN THE TREATMENT OF ACUTE AND CHRONIC PSYCHIATRIC ILLNESS

1. **Is the family in treatment, a part of treatment, or a member of the treatment team?** Our position is that good treatment involves all three. First, most families have problems coping with the identified patient’s illness. Many families have problems separate from the identified patient. Second, the family’s presence in the treatment process, as compared with individual or drug treatment, makes the family a de facto part of the treatment. (As a result, the therapist should obtain the family’s consent for treatment.) Finally, Wynne et al.[37] argue that the long-term nature and seriousness of recurrent or chronic mental illness and the family’s experience with dealing with a particular member requires that the family’s expertise be harnessed.

   At first, most families feel most comfortable as partners with the treatment team. Later the family may feel ready to become part of treatment or enter into treatment itself. Often this occurs after the patient has stabilized. Over time, clinicians will need to blend all three positions to foster the best outcome for patients and families.
2. **Should the initial goals of family therapy be oriented around family change or family consultation?** This long-standing controversy emanates from the traditional model in which the family is blamed for the patient’s illness. The best way to engage family members

is to contact them "where they are" (i.e., at their level of understanding of the illness), provide psychoeducation, and respond to requests for information and support. The initial consultation serves as a means to ally with the family. Change cannot occur without this first step.

3. **A few family therapists still believe that schizophrenia and other major functional psychoses are purely family systems (i.e., psychological and social but not biologic problems). Are they?** This belief is based in part on the inference that improvement (or recovery) is possible without medication. We agree with Stein[38] (p. 134) that mental illnesses, "like virtually every disease, are influenced by biologic, psychological, and social factors." Treating schizophrenia or any other major mental disorder requires biologic, psychological, and social approaches and anything else that will help.
4. **Many families believe that major mental illnesses are solely brain illnesses.** This belief creates confusion in the minds of some families when they are offered a psychosocial treatment such as family therapy. Why would a biochemical problem be treated with a psychosocial treatment? The answer is that any family, living with a member who has sustained cognitive and other brain function defects, will have major problems in the management of the disorder and with the feelings associated with chronic illness.
5. **How much does family intervention add to medication in the treatment of acutely ill patients?** Most studies indicate that each modality is additive.[26] Medication is effective for positive (and probably negative) symptoms, and family intervention helps with the complicating interpersonal problems of illness.[39] An interesting question is whether family intervention can result in lowered doses of medication and thereby reduction in the risk of tardive dyskinesia (e.g., a side effect of some antipsychotic medications). The Treatment Strategies in Schizophrenia Collaborative Study[6] has addressed this question. The study involved the use of a standard-dose neuroleptic, a low-dose neuroleptic, or an early intervention strategy (i.e., use of medication once the patient starts to relapse) coupled with one of two kinds of family strategies (a weekly, applied, behaviorally oriented family treatment or a monthly supportive group). The greater the family involvement in either applied or supportive treatment, the fewer the patient's symptoms and the lesser the need for medication; however, the addition of family intervention did not interact with the drug conditions. Neither family condition lowered the amount of medication needed, and the targeted strategy was not efficacious for patients with chronic schizophrenia. Conversely, long-term drug maintenance often helps the patient participate more meaningfully in family therapy.
6. **Family treatment in the acute setting lacks evidence of effectiveness; therefore, the enormous resources in time, staff, and money should not be allocated to this modality.** Clinical experience and our study,[22] (referred to earlier in the chapter) suggest that the controversy about the effectiveness of family treatment should be reformulated. The central questions are, Who requires intervention? and What is an effective intervention? Our work indicates that intervention works best for female patients with mood disorder (especially bipolar disorder) and female patients with chronic schizophrenia. The families of all patients with schizophrenia and bipolar disorder seem to derive some benefit from family intervention (as opposed to family therapy). Consequently, our position is that until further studies are done, family intervention should be considered for all patients and prescribed on the basis of available knowledge and a case-by-case evaluation of the patient and the family. Other studies show consistent patterns of effectiveness.[40,41]

CLINICAL PRACTICE IMPLICATIONS

Although the focus of treatment has shifted from inpatient to outpatient settings, the principles of family-oriented care described in this chapter are essential to improving long-term outcomes for patients with psychiatric illness and their families.

Given the chronicity of most psychiatric illnesses, we are not overstating the following treatment guidelines. For the family, it may be "life or death" to work with the psychiatric treatment team before, during, and especially after hospitalization to stabilize and/or improve the posthospital trajectory of the identified patient. Too often, even in 2024, another psychiatric team will not work with a family therapist and family, citing HIPAA reasons. For reference, see our case above.

REFERENCES

1. Glick ID, Hargreaves WA. *Psychiatric Hospital Treatment for the 1980s: A Controlled Study of Short Versus Long Hospitalization*. Lexington; 1979.
2. Glick ID, Klar HM, Braff D. Guidelines for hospitalization of chronic psychiatric patients. *Hosp Community Psychiatry*. 1984;35:934–936.
3. Leggatt M. Families and mental health workers: the need for partnership. *World Psychiatry*. 2002;1(1):52–54.
4. Bhatti RS, Janikramaiah N, Channabassavanna SM. Family psychiatric ward treatment in India. *Fam Process*. 1980;19:193–200.
5. Anderson C. Family intervention with severely disturbed inpatients. *Arch Gen Psychiatry*. 1977;34:697–702.
6. Schooler N, Keith SJ, Severe JB, et al. Relapse and rehospitalization during maintenance treatment of schizophrenia. The effects of dose reduction and family treatment. *Arch Gen Psychiatry*. 1997;54:453–463.
7. Heru AM. Cultural research deconstructs the psychosocial construct "expressed emotion". *Br J Psychiatry*. 2000; 219(4):1–4.
8. Glick ID, Clarkin JF, Goldsmith SJ. Combining medication with family psychotherapy. In: Beitman B, ed. *Combined Treatments, the American Psychiatric Press Review of Psychiatry*. American Psychiatric Press; 1993a: 585–610.
9. Goldstein MJ, Rodnick EH, Evans JR, May PR, Steinberg MR. Drug and family therapy in the aftercare of acute schizophrenics. *Arch Gen Psychiatry*. 1978;35:1169–1177.
10. Doody O, Butler MP, Lyons R, Newman D. Families' experiences of involvement in care planning in mental health services: an integrative literature review. *J Psychiatr Ment Health Nurs*. 2017;24(6):412–430.
11. Kahn EM, White EM. Adapting milieu approaches to acute inpatient care for schizophrenic patients. *Hosp Community Psychiatry*. 1989;40:609–614.
12. Vaughn CE, Leff JP. The influence of family and social factors in the course of psychiatric illness. A comparison of schizophrenic and depressed neurotic patients. *Br J Psychiatry*. 1976;129:125–137.
13. Munuera C, Compagnone P, Husky MM, Lebourleux P, Petit F, M'bailara K. Improving the assessment process of family functioning in adult bipolar disorders: a PRISMA systematic review. *J Clin Med*. 2022;11(3):841.
14. Falloon IRH, Boyd J, McGill C, et al. Family management in the prevention of morbidity of schizophrenia: clinical outcome of a two-year longitudinal study. *Arch Gen Psychiatry*. 1985;42:887–896.
15. Bursten B. Family dynamics, the sick role, and medical hospital admissions. *Fam Process*. 1965;4:206–216.
16. Grunebaum H, Friedman H. Letter. *Hosp Community Psychiatry*. 1989;4:20.
17. Glick ID, Clarkin JF, Spencer JH, et al. A controlled evaluation of inpatient family intervention; a controlled evaluation of practice: preliminary results of the six-months follow-up. *Arch Gen Psychiatry*. 1985;42:882–886.
18. Akhtar S, Helfrich J, Mestayer RF. AMA discharge from a psychiatric inpatient unit. *Int J Soc Psychiatry*. 1981;27:143–150.
19. Goldstein E. The influence of parental attitudes on psychiatric treatment outcome. *Soc Casework*. 1979;60: 350–359.
20. Greenman DA, Gunderson JG, Canning D. Parents' attitudes and patients' behavior; a prospective study. *Am J Psychiatry*. 1989;146:226–230.
21. Heru AM, Drury LM. Working with Families of Psychiatric Inpatients. *A Guide for Clinicians*. Johns Hopkins University Press; 2007.
22. Glick ID, Clarkin JF, Haas GL, Spencer JH Jr. Clinical significance of inpatient family intervention, VII: conclusions from the clinical trial. *Hosp Community Psychiatry*. 1993b;44:869–873.
23. Clarkin JF, Glick ID, Haas GL, et al. A randomized clinical trial of inpatient family intervention, V. Results for affective disorders. *J Affect Disord*. 1990;18:17–28.
24 Glick ID, Spencer JH, Clarkin JF, et al. A randomized clinical trial of inpatient family intervention, IV. Follow-up results for subjects with schizophrenia. *Schizophr Res*. 1990;3:187–200.
25. Spencer JH, Glick ID, Haas GL. A randomized clinical trial of inpatient family intervention, III: Effects at 6-month and 18-month follow-ups. *Am J Psychiatry*. 1988;145:1115–1121.
26. Glick ID, Burti L, Minakawa K, et al. Effectiveness of psychiatric care; II. Outcome for the family after hospital treatment for major affective disorder. *Ann Clin Psychiatry*. 1991a;3:187–198.
27. Greenberg L, Fine SB, Cohen C, et al. An interdisciplinary psychoeducation program for schizophrenic patients and their families in an acute care setting. *Hosp Community Psychiatry*. 1988;39:277–282.

28. World Schizophrenia Fellowship. Families as partners in care. 1998.
29. Hatfield AB. Coping effectiveness in families of the mentally ill: an exploratory study. *J Psychiatr Treat Eval.* 1981;3:11–19.
30. Terkelsen KG. *No Proof that Families Cause Mental Illness.* FAMI Newsletter; 1982.
31. Hibler M. The problem as seen by the patient's family. *Hosp Community Psych.* 1978;29:32–33.
32. Boggs EM. Contrasts in deinstitutionalization. *Hosp Community Psych.* 1981;32:591.
33. Segal SP. Community care and deinstitutionalization: a review. *Soc Work.* 1979;37:521–527.
34. Kanter J, Lin A. Facilitating a therapeutic milieu in the families of schizophrenia. *Psychiatry.* 1980;43:106–119.
35. Dixon LB, Lucksted A, Medoff DR, et al. Outcomes of a randomized study of a peer-taught family-to-family education program for mental illness. *Psychiatr Serv.* 2011;62(6):591–597.
36. Koenig G, Larson H. Religion and mental health: evidence for an association. *Int Rev Psychiatry.* 2001;13(2): 67–78.
37. Wynne L, McDaniel SH, Weber TT. Professional politics and the concepts of family therapy, family consultation, and systems consultation. *Fam Process.* 1987;26:153–166.
38. Stein L. The effect of long-outcome studies on the therapy of schizophrenia: a critique. *J Marital Fam Ther.* 1989;15:133–138.
39. Glick ID, Dulit RA, Wachter E, Clarkin JF. The family, family therapy, and borderline personality disorder. *J Psychother Pract Res.* 1995;4:237–246.
40. Postrado L, Lehman AF. Quality of life and clinical predictors of rehospitalization of persons with severe mental illness. *Psychiatr Serv.* 1995;46:1161–1165.
41. Walling DP, Dott SG. Quality of life: a pilot study—comparison of crisis stabilization and hospitalization (abstract). *Psychopharmacol Bull.* 1994;30:725.

21 Working with Families in the Medical Setting

OBJECTIVES FOR THE READER

- Understand the mutual influence of family functioning and medical illness
- Recognize family coping styles and different ways of family adaptation to illness
- Understand the needs of caregivers
- Know what additional family assessment questions to ask when medical illness is present
- Recognize the range of evidence-based family interventions; family inclusion, family psychoeducation and systemic family therapy

For easier reading, we emphasize that the descriptors "couples" or "marital" are used nearly interchangeably in this chapter.

> *Family therapy is at the top of any list of things psychiatrists know are important and yet avoid. There are many reasons for this. Psychiatry residency requirements mention the need to expose residents to family therapy, but they are vague as to what or how much this exposure should be. Thus, with limited training in family interventions, the average practicing psychiatrist is often reluctant to venture beyond the doctor–patient dyad, citing theoretic stances or confidentiality concerns. This tendency to ignore family members belies common sense, given the degree that most of us depend on our loved ones for both practical and emotional support when we are ill.*
>
> *—Boland (2014)*[1]

INTRODUCTION

Working with families with medical illness means that the family therapist must have a good understanding of the impact of the illness on the family and the impact of the family on the illness. A family therapist also needs to be cognizant of three stages: the life stage of the person with the illness, the current family life stage, and the stage of the illness. The interactions between these three stages must be understood for a family therapist to be effective (Rolland, 1994).

Treatment implications follow the background of how family functioning impacts illness and vice versa, family coping, and adaptation to the illness and caregiving.[2]

HOW FAMILY FUNCTIONING IMPACTS ILLNESS
Gender Matters
Family Health Beliefs
Family Adherence

HOW ILLNESS IMPACTS FAMILY FUNCTIONING
FAMILY COPING AND ADAPTATION TO ILLNESS
Learning to Cope and Adapt
Providing a Therapeutic Space
CAREGIVING
A FAMILY SYSTEMS INTERVIEW FOR FAMILIES WITH MEDICAL ILLNESS
Problem Solving
Communication
Roles
Affective Responsiveness
Affective Involvement
Behavior Control
FAMILY INTERVENTIONS
Family Support
Family Psychoeducation
Family Systemic Interventions
Multifamily Groups
CLINICAL PRACTICE IMPLICATIONS

HOW FAMILY FUNCTIONING IMPACTS ILLNESS

Understanding the patient's family dynamics is a key factor in psychiatric treatment. It is crucial that mental health care providers understand how family systems affect the psychiatric outcomes of patients. Having an understanding of family relationships gives a context for the patient's value systems, which are important aspects to consider when assessing the present mental health status.[3]

A literature review of family factors that influence medical illness outcomes identifies factors that contribute to good family functioning.[4] These factors are (1) good communication, (2) the ability to encourage individual family members, (3) expressing appreciation, (4) having clear family roles, and (5) spending time together as a family. Several possible protective factors, where the evidence is only suggestive, include the ability to talk about emotional issues, the integration of ritual and routine in family life, secure attachments for children, good problem-solving ability, and family recreation time. Family research also identifies families that function poorly as having (1) intrafamilial conflict, (2) blame, (3) rigidity, and (4) high levels of criticism. Criticalness and hostility are the most influential risk factors on disease outcome.

A family needs to be able to manage the medical illness effectively. Their capabilities can be revealed through the story they tell about the illness. If their story is coherent and reveals an understanding of the illness, including a plan for managing illness relapse, they can be considered to have good illness management. Families whose illness story is disorganized are likely to have poor illness management. Paying attention to these factors in the family's story is an evidence-based way of identifying families who will benefit from family intervention.[5]

Family functioning is particularly challenging at the time of family life-stage transition. Even for a family without medical illness, transition is often difficult in adolescence. For example, maintaining good blood sugar control may be less important to an adolescent than participating in an important peer group activity. During adolescence, family conflict and poor diabetic control can be prevented with family intervention.[6]

Gender Matters

In the Healthy Women Study, women with better marital quality had superior cardiovascular risk profiles and illness trajectories.[7] Similarly, in patients with heart failure, good marital quality was associated with substantially better outcome, even at 8 years follow-up, especially for women.[8] The marital components most predictive of good outcome were the frequency of the couple's "useful discussions" about the patient's illness and the ratio of positive to negative exchanges.[9]

Family Health Beliefs

Health care decisions are influenced by family's health beliefs. Patient's perception of pain and adjustment to pain are impacted by their spouse's beliefs about disability, emotion, control, and medication.[10] When a couple has congruent beliefs about the women's ability to control her pain in rheumatoid arthritis, the patient has improved psychological adjustment.[11] A family's decision to use pain medication is influenced by their beliefs about pain control. Parents give less pain medication to their children if they believe that learning to cope with pain is beneficial for their children.[12]

Family Adherence

Family adherence to treatment improves patient outcome. However, family adherence is made up of a variety of family factors. How a family performs on one adherence measure can differ markedly from how they perform on other adherence measures.[13] The assessment of a family's adherence includes asking questions about practical issues. Practical issues include a family's ability to pay for treatment and to transport the patient to appointments. Adherence is also influenced by psychological factors. Psychological factors include the health beliefs of each family member, and the family's ability to solve problems together. One significant factor that is often overlooked is the family's experience of traumatic medical events. When a life-threatening event occurs, such as an asthma attack, families may avoid situations that remind them of the traumatic medical event. This avoidance can result in missed doctors' appointments or "forgetting" to use needed inhalers. Avoidance worsens asthma and increases the likelihood of a life-threatening event and the experience of trauma is then reinforced. Traumatic stress symptoms might be more prevalent in poor and minority families where there is less access to health care, and therefore more likelihood of experiencing traumatic medical events.[5] It is worth asking families if they have this experience.

HOW ILLNESS IMPACTS FAMILY FUNCTIONING

It has been found in medicine that in order to optimize outcomes, family support is necessary. Each illness has specific psychosocial demands.[14] These demands include coping with life-threatening events, role change, or impending death. Adjustment is most difficult if the course of illness is unpredictable. Rolland's Family Systems–Illness Model integrates three processes: the psychosocial illness demands, the developmental phases of the illness type, and key family variables.[14] The psychosocial demands of illnesses vary with the acuteness or chronicity of the illness. Illnesses that have an acute onset require the family to be in constant crisis mode. Illnesses that have a relapsing course, such as asthma, require the family to switch between being in crisis mode and normal functioning. Illnesses that are progressive, requires the family to make steady incremental changes. A well-functioning family strives to attend to normal developmental tasks, in spite of the impact of the illness.

FAMILY COPING AND ADAPTATION TO ILLNESS

Family coping and adaptation to illness is a constantly changing process. Family research is mostly cross-sectional and therefore does not address a family's adaptive progress. Family research often lacks Rolland's insight about the interaction between the developmental stages of the person, family, and illness. The family therapist must, nevertheless, enquire about adaptation across time, and focus on how families make adaptive changes.

Families that cope well are known as resilient families. Resilient families have good problem-solving skills, good communication, and a shared belief system.[15] Resilient families are able to change health behaviors such as improving their diet, increasing exercise, and stopping smoking. Resilient families are flexible about family roles, for example, a family member may give up a job to stay home or older children may give up some childhood activities to take on caregiving responsibilities. Resilient families are well-organized emotional systems and provide as-needed emotional support. When illness robs a family of their customary ways of being together, resilient families find new ways of being together as a family.

Families pass ways of managing symptoms and illness down through the generations. Families who have managed chronic illness by allowing the ill member to retreat to bed and be nursed by the youngest family member may perpetuate this health care behavior in the next generation. Illustrating how family health behaviors can be passed along can be achieved by using a genogram.[16]

Illness management is often punctuated by crises; when change happens without the family having time to deliberate on what coping styles might work best. Coping strategies can become automatic: "Things I have always done to cope." Family changes can become fixed, not by choice, but by happenstance. Families do not usually think about what strategies or coping skills they use to manage illness; they just get along the best they can. Each family member has their own individual coping style that may or may not mesh with the coping styles of others in the family. The "best coper" in the family usually drives the family coping style.[5] However, women are more likely than men to change their coping strategies to a communal style.[17]

When couples view the illness as "our problem," this is described as dyadic coping. Such couples usually have prior experience working together as a team on issues such as parenting and division of roles within the house. They are also able to relax together, provide emotional support such as mutual calming and expressions of solidarity. Couples who use dyadic coping usually share an understanding of the illness. Patients with heart disease have better health outcomes when they and their spouses have dyadic coping. This is identified as high levels of "we-talk."[18] Table 21.1 illustrates the type of questions a family therapist can ask to identify dyadic coping.

Coping styles can be culturally determined. In Korean mothers of children with cancer, "hope" and "less frequent information-seeking" are associated with lower maternal psychological distress and better family relationships.[19] These mothers state that they cope by "believing that my child is receiving the best medical care possible," "believing that my child will get better," and "believing that things will work out." There is clearly no single correct way of coping and a family therapist must ask, "How does this style of coping work for your family?"

Table 21.1 Dyadic coping questions

- It is important that you both agree about the cause of this illness. Can I answer any questions that might help you reach this understanding?
- Are there times in the past where you have successfully solved difficult problems? How did you do that?
- What can your spouse do that will help you get better?
- Can you ask your spouse for help and support?
- Can you work on your spouse's health problem together?
- When you think about problems related to your heart condition, to what extent do you view those as "our problem" (shared by you and your spouse equally) or mainly your own problem?
- When a problem related to your medical condition arises, do you and your partner work together to solve it?
- How do you respond when your spouse gets ill?
- When you both talk about the illness, how much do you use "we-talk"?

Of course, a couple may not want to work together to manage illness. It is important to clarify the family's view on individual versus dyadic or family coping. The therapist can ask: "Do either of you feel that they should do this alone?" If the answer is yes, it will be difficult to move the couple to a dyadic coping style. A second question: "Do your efforts to work together result in greater conflict?" followed by "How much do you want this to change?" can clarify a family's motivation to work together.

Learning to Cope and Adapt

Based on the above discussion, it is evident that each family will have specific adaptive needs. When there is an acute crisis, families move into "crisis mode." Routine family tasks can be neglected. Just as all families are dysfunctional for a few months after the birth of a baby,[20] all families may be dysfunctional for a short period of time after the diagnosis of a serious illness. The "trauma of diagnosis" occurs for a family after a diagnosis of cancer.[21] Clinical experience suggests that families are more likely to engage in treatment at the time of crises. Support to the family can be augmented with questions about the family's future plans for coping and adaptation. Families should be encouraged to think beyond the crisis.

Family members often ask how they should respond to their loved one's symptoms. When complaints of pain become chronic, family members ask; "What is the best way to help my spouse manage pain? Should I give in and do things for them, or encourage them to do more themselves?" Couples research sheds light on this common dilemma. Research shows that patients who try to elicit support from others by a heightened display of pain end up with more severe pain and more disability. Spouses correctly perceive that "helping" does not reduce pain, but rather increases helplessness, dependence, and poorer functioning. Pain catastrophizing elicits short-term support but, over time, family members withdraw. On the other hand, patients may interpret a family member's solicitousness as a sign of their inability to do things, and come to see themselves as a burden. Spouses can also respond to their family member with anger, irritation, and frustration which can result in increased pain, disability, and psychological distress.[22] Family therapists should elicit transactional patterns that occur around the complaints of pain, and move the couple toward effective coping.

Providing a Therapeutic Space

Families frequently present in distress with no clear understanding of the cause of their difficulties. Family members may be unable to differentiate between emotional difficulties such as "I am the primary caregiver and I feel overburdened," and more general practical problems such as "I am happy to be the primary caregiver but I need some extra help getting him to his appointments." It is important to note that family stress can also increase the severity of illness. For example, in children, many times high levels of distress in the family may lead to somatic symptoms expressed by the child. Additionally, in psychiatric studies of adopted children, some of which had mother with a schizophreniform disorder versus without, it was found that these children were more prone to stressful family rearing as compared to those whose mothers did not have a schizophreniform disorder.[23] Family therapists can provide a therapeutic space for families to reflect on how they choose to cope as individuals and how they choose to cope as a family. The family therapist can provide a therapeutic space to reflect on the past, the present, and future changes.

CAREGIVING

One-third of the U.S. population provides care for a chronically ill, disabled, or aged family member. Two-thirds of caregivers are women and 13% of family caregivers are providing at least 40 hours of care a week (http://www.apa.org/pi/about/publications/caregivers/faq/statistics.aspx). There are also 1.3 to 1.4 million child caregivers nationwide (National Alliance of Caregiving, http://www.caregiving.org/). The most common activities reported by children are keeping the care recipient company (96%), helping with chores (85%), grocery shopping (65%), and meal preparation (63%). The demands experienced by family caregivers increase their own vulnerability to stress-related conditions. The Caregiver Health Effects Study demonstrated a strong link between caregiving and mortality risk. Compared to noncaregivers, elderly spouses were 63% more likely to die within 4 years.[24] Due to a perceived lack of time and energy, family caregivers frequently neglect their own care, including adequate meal preparation and exercise. The American Psychological Association (APA) has posted an online "Caregiver Briefcase" (http://www.apa.org/pi/about/publications/caregivers/index.aspx). The briefcase contains caregiving facts, a practice section with common caregiver problems and interventions, and sections on research, education, and advocacy. Research has been conducted on family interventions for caregivers. For dementia caregivers, supportive family intervention programs are able to prevent caregiver illness.[25]

A FAMILY SYSTEMS INTERVIEW FOR FAMILIES WITH MEDICAL ILLNESS

Before beginning an interview with a family where a member has a serious medical illness, the family therapist should consider the following topics:

1. What is the family life-cycle stage? Has chronic illness derailed the family's progression through its normal developmental stages?
2. What is the stage of illness? Is the family in the acute phase of illness, and struggling to find a cure or treatment that "will take the illness away"? With chronic illness, has the family considered how best to adapt? If it is a child or young adult who is ill, is the family grieving?
3. What is the family's experience of health care? Has the family had negative experiences with health care providers leading to suspiciousness or mistrust?
4. What is it like to be in their shoes? Reflecting on the family life stage, the type of illness, and the current situation increases the therapist's empathy and understanding.
5. What are the family's beliefs about illness and treatment? How does their cultural background influence their experience of illness and the health care system?
6. What are the family's strengths?

The family therapist should begin the family meeting with an orientation. For families with limited resources, their ability to attend the family meeting together is a strength to be acknowledged. "Thank you all for coming. Illness takes its toll on everyone, the patient AND the family. This is an opportunity to look at how you all are doing together, as a family. It is important to acknowledge what you are doing well, so you can keep doing it, and to identify areas that can be improved. Is that OK with everyone?" "I know it is difficult because your symptoms are hard to manage. How DO you manage these symptoms, as a family?"

Clarify that you will be assessing family functioning across several dimensions in order to ensure a comprehensive evaluation. As aspects of family functioning are discussed, the family may see the possibility of change. The seeds of intervention are often identified in the process of a thorough assessment. Remember that "family" may include neighbors or church members. The model used in this chapter is the Problem-Centered Systems Therapy of the Family[26] which covers six main areas of family functioning, problem solving, communication, roles, affective responsiveness, affective involvement, and behavior control. Each dimension is discussed in detail.

Problem Solving

A family can usually manage to solve practical problems such as getting to appointments. It is more difficult to identify and talk about the emotional aspects of caregiving. Women are frequently the family health managers, and the emotional barometers in the family. The family therapist helps the family clarify the emotional impact of the illness on the family. Once identified, the family works together to communicate and come up with strategies to solve their problems.

Communication

If family members have busy work schedules, they may not have time to interact with each other. Important decisions may get deferred. When the family does interact, assess the quality of their communication: Do you communicate clearly with each other? Do you sometimes have to guess what other people in the family mean? Has this changed since you became ill? How much time do you spend talking about illness? Is this enough time or too much time? Do family members want to spend more time away from their sick relatives? Do family members communicate about feelings? Is it clear how everyone is feeling? Does the person with the illness try to hide when they are not feeling well? Do they do this to protect others? If so, how does the family respond?

Communication is affected by cultural differences. For example, compared to White families, Latino families tend to communicate indirectly with less emphasis on discussing death and dying. Latino caregivers may want to protect the patient from the knowledge of illness, to deny that death is imminent, and to act as if the patient is getting well. In many Latino families, discussion about the family member's death is minimal because they do not want to "hurt" each other.

Roles

Traditional families divide up roles by gender, but families can negotiate any preferred allocation of roles. Women traditionally cook and prepare the family meals. For many women, their role as household manager and meal preparer can trump their ability to attend to their own dietary needs.[17] General questions about roles include: Who works outside the home and for how many hours? Who handles the money? Who buys the groceries and prepares the meals? Who looks after the home and car? Who oversees the children's education? Do any of you feel overburdened by your roles? How would you like roles divided up differently?

Illness-related questions identify who has the role of the caregiver and the impact of caregiver burden. Ask: Who helps with medications and transportation? Who provides emotional support? How have things changed since you became ill? Are you intimate with each other? Has that changed since your illness? Who is the primary caregiver? Some people like being caregivers and others do not, how do you feel? Are there other people in the family who are caregivers? Do you feel guilty that someone has to care for you? In what ways has the illness changed your roles in the family? What are your expectations of your family?

Roles are affected by cultural difference, with non-White cultures placing a higher value on the role of family in caregiving. African–American (AA) elders have stronger expectations for intergenerational coresidence and filial responsibility. Compared with men, AA female elders have larger, more intricate social networks and frequently exchange caregiving services. However, AA women do not necessarily utilize their supports because of the strong cultural value placed on independence. Churches play a central role in the AA community, providing spiritual comfort, and both practical and emotional support. In Latino cultures, the role of the elders is to educate younger generations and pass along cultural values and elders are generally held in high esteem.

Latinos, like AAs, are more likely to live in multigenerational households compared to Whites, although most elders would prefer to live independently. Compared with Whites, Mexican–American women, like AAs, provide more childcare and assistance to extended family members. Similarly, Native Americans (NA) view the needs of their family and community as more important than their own needs and place great responsibility on caring for family and extended tribal members. In Chinese cultures, caring for the sick is considered a family responsibility and caregiving is an important role.

Affective Responsiveness

Affective responsiveness focuses on how each person experiences and communicates their feelings to other family members. Ask: Are you a family that overresponds or underresponds to situations with a lot of feeling? Are there feelings that you experience more intensely than reasonable, given the situation? Is your spouse mostly happy/sad/angry/critical? Does your spouse agree with that assessment? Have things changed since you became ill? If so, how have they changed? Do you have specific fears? Do you feel angry about how things have changed? Are you able to express your feelings and talk openly about how you feel? Are there feelings that you cannot express or talk about?

Affective Involvement

Affective involvement assesses the intensity of each family's emotional commitment and involvement with each other. Ask: Who cares about what is important to you? Do you think other family members are interested in you? Do they ever show too much interest? Do you feel that they are truly interested in you because it is important to you, or only because they think they should be? Do you feel that other members of the family go their own way and do not care or notice what happens to you? Does the family spend time together? Does the illness prevent the family from doing things together? When the illness gets in the way, are there alternative activities that the family can do together? Is the primary caregiver able to take time for themselves?

Anger at the limitations imposed by illness can be a barrier to family closeness. Questions derived from narrative therapy can identify barriers: "This illness is not only robbing you of what you like, but also stopping your whole family from being close. Are there ways that you, as a family, have been able to prevent this illness from controlling your lives?"

It is worthwhile to help the family identify new interests. Who knew that the family would enjoy building birdhouses together? Sending the family to the library to look at books on hobbies can be an effective homework task.

There may be cultural differences in how families perceive closeness and emotional commitment. A patient noted that his family members did not say much, but diligently cooked various kinds of nourishing food and soup, and that these actions were more powerful than any words.[27] The questions to ask are: "Do you feel that your family cares? How do you know this? How does your family show they care?" Each family has its own way of caring and showing caring feelings; there is no right or wrong way.

Behavior Control

Behavior control seeks to understand the rules in a family. Compared to healthy children in the family, different rules may be applied to an ill child. Ask: Do you have rules in your family about how to handle different situations? Are the rules clear? Are the rules the same for everybody? Can you discuss the rules? Are there rules about smoking, drinking, or curfews? Do the rules get enforced or do you let things slide? What about exercise and diet? How have things changed since you became ill? Does anyone try to stop you from enjoying the things you used to enjoy, because of your health? Are there rules about what you can do and what you can eat? Who nags you the most?

For an adolescent with a medical illness, the parental concern for "what is best for your health" can conflict with the adolescent's drive for independence. Questions about meal times, how blood sugars are monitored, and rituals around administering insulin can highlight the family dynamics about diabetic care. A positive framework works best: How do you keep such good control most of the time? What accounts for the episodes of lack of control? What prevents you from managing your diabetes well, on those days? What happens in the family when you have a bad day? How many times a day does your parent ask if you have checked your blood sugar? How many times do they ask about what you ate or did not eat each day? Does their worrying and caring about you feel like too much nagging? Does anyone express concern for you at school? Do your parents' concerns about your illness affect other aspects of your life?

FAMILY INTERVENTIONS

When evidence-based family interventions are examined, they naturally fall into three categories: family support, family psychoeducation, and family systemic interventions.

Family Support

All family support, both practical and emotional, improves outcome. Practical support includes helping patients keep appointments, adhere to medications, a healthy lifestyle, and the recommendations of the physician. Emotional support, specifically, improves patient outcome.[28] It is important to note that patients do not always recognize having received support even when they have benefitted from support.[29] A lack of understanding of the illness and managing symptoms can result in unsupportive family attitudes and behaviors. Routinely including the family in patient appointments can increase family understanding, in a natural way. If the family needs specific intervention, an appropriate next step is family psychoeducation.

Family Psychoeducation

Psychoeducation provides in-depth illness education, explores the meaning of the illness for each family member, and promotes a broad repertoire of coping skills. It is imperative that families also need to have support when they are caretaking for family members with mental illness. Psychoeducation also addresses difficult family emotional reactions, such as anger, sadness, or frustration. Psychoeducation can be provided as single-family psychoeducation or as multifamily psychoeducation. In multifamily group (MFG) psychoeducation, families have access to other families' successes and failures, which benefits all families. It is also important to include psychoeducation not only during crisis but also preventatively as well.

Family psychoeducation improves both patient and family outcomes. A successful component of psychoeducation is teaching families how to solve problems. The stages of problem solving are (1) problem identification, (2) communication about the problem, (3) generation and evaluation of alternative solutions, (4) choosing a solution, and (5) follow-ups to assess the effectiveness of the intervention. Psychoeducation helps couples reach a common understanding of the patient's actual abilities. For example, three weekly diabetes psychoeducational sessions improved family beliefs about diabetes, psychological well-being, diet, exercise, and family support.[30]

Family Systemic Interventions

In addition to what has caused a problem, a family systems therapist seeks to understand what keeps a problem going, that is, problem maintenance. In order to focus family members on what keeps a problem going, a family therapist asks circular questions. A family systems assessment illustrates to the family how symptoms are maintained and reinforced by particular family transactions. Describing transactional patterns to a family means explaining a problem systemically[31]: "Johnny's illness affects everyone in the family and everyone in the family affects Johnny's illness." After a family systemic conceptualization, the family understands how they influence Johnny's feelings, thoughts, and behavior and Johnny can understand how he influences other family members. Relational patterns have cognitive, behavioral, and affective components, all of which can be good targets of intervention.

Several family systems assessment models are effective with medically ill patients and their families. Medical Family Therapy (MedFT) is a biopsychosocial approach to medical illness which emphasizes the mind–body interaction.[32] The family therapist engages patients and their families in a discussion about the mutual influence of psychological and physical symptoms. Their mutual influence is captured in the phrase “Both-And.” MedFT is practiced by family therapists alongside the physicians providing medical care. An important goal for medical family therapists is to improve the family’s ability to manage the patient’s illness symptoms and behaviors. To start this process, the illness story is solicited, with special emphasis on the beliefs of family members. The medical family therapist works to improve the family’s understanding of their emotional responses to chronic illness in the family, to encourage them to attend to normal family developmental issues, to increase their sense of agency, and to challenge unhealthy coping skills. Ongoing communication is maintained with the family, with an open-door policy for family consultation.

Strategic models, such as the Family Consultation (FAMCON) model, are useful when the goal of the family therapist is to interrupt problem-maintaining behavior.[33] This model identifies important truths about change-resistant health behaviors: (1) How a problem persists is more important than how it begins, (2) investigate what people DO rather than what they HAVE, that is, the type of illness, (3) the path to clinical change is not necessarily continuous and smooth, and (4) the more entrenched a problem, the more helpful are indirect, strategic interventions.

Another useful strategic therapy model is Narrative Therapy.[34] In this approach, the illness is “externalized.” A narrative therapist asks: In what way has diabetes controlled this family? Has diabetes stopped you from enjoying your time together? How has it been able to do that? How has diabetes made you forget about the good times? The family is then asked to give examples of when they have not allowed the illness to control the family: “Are there times when you didn’t let diabetes make you forget about the good times?” This stimulates the family to use their strengths and resources to work together “against the illness.”

Multifamily Groups

MFGs can be psychoeducational or systemic (MFSGs). Psychoeducational MFGs provide education and support by allowing families to share feelings and attitudes about managing illness, reduce feelings of blame and self-criticalness, and promote problem solving. By contrast, MFSGs use specific family systems techniques to clarify family processes and to help families make changes in relational patterns.[35] MFGs are found to be useful for diverse illnesses such as childhood cancer, breast cancer, adolescents with poorly controlled Type 1 diabetes, multiple sclerosis, heart failure, and head and neck cancer. Mothers of children with cancer, who attended an MFG, reported improvements in problem-solving skills and mood.[36] Most benefit was reported by single and younger mothers, who perhaps face the greatest challenges. A family psychoeducational intervention for patients with nonepileptic seizures provides education and support in the face of medical stigma. Witha very positive attendance rate, the patients and families commented on satisfaction with the intervention, noting enhanced understanding of the illness, improved communication about the illness, and reduction in family conflict.[37]

CLINICAL PRACTICE IMPLICATIONS

A successful family therapist must understand the intersection of the stage of illness, the stage of the family, and the developmental stage of the individual with the illness.[14] A detailed family assessment helps differentiate a well-functioning family that is having adjustment difficulties but has the skills to problem solving, from a family which lacks problem-solving skills. A focus on improving coping and adaptation over time encourages a family to move forward. Family interventions must be tailored to the family's needs. Couples and families that are functioning well may only need information and to be included in decision-making. Couples and families, who are struggling, can benefit from a psychoeducational intervention that focuses on teaching problem-solving skills. Couples and families who have deeper conflicts or dysfunction may benefit from a family systems intervention. It is important to remember that families may have one area of difficulty and many areas of strength. We can learn a great deal from families about their resilience in managing illness.

SUGGESTED READINGS

These three books focus on working with family in the medical setting.

Heru AM. *Working with Families in the Medical Setting: A Multidisciplinary Guide for Psychiatrists and Other Professionals*. Routledge; 2013.

McDaniel SH, Hepworth J, Doherty WJ. *Medical Family Therapy: A Biopsychosocial Approach to Families with Medical Problems*. Basic Books; 1992.

Rolland JS. *Helping Couples and Families Navigate illness and Disability*. Guildford Press; 2018.

REFERENCES

1. Boland RJ. Working with families in medical settings: a multidisciplinary guide for psychiatrists and other health professionals. *Am J Psychiatry.* 2014;171(3):372.
2. Ee C, Lake J, Firth J, et al. An integrative collaborative care model for people with mental illness and physical comorbidities. *Int J Ment Health Syst.* 2020;14:83.
3. Saroca K, Sargent J. Understanding families as essential in psychiatric practice. *Focus (Am Psychiatr Publ).* 2022;20(2):204–209.
4. Weihs K, Fisher L, Baird MA. Families, health, and behavior: a section of the commissioned report by the committee on Health and Behavior: Research, Practice and Policy, Division of Neurosciences and Behavioral Health and Division of Health Promotion and Disease Prevention, Institute of Medicine, *National Academy of Sciences. Fam Syst Health.* 2002;20(1):7–47.
5. Wambolt FS, Wamboldt MZ. Family factors in promoting health: the case of childhood asthma. In: Heru AM, ed. *Working with Families in the Medical Setting*. Routledge; 2013.
6. Anderson BJ, Vangsness L, Connell A, Butler D, Goebel-Fabbri A, Laffel LM. Family conflict, adherence, and glycaemic control in youth with short duration type 1 diabetes. *Diabet Med.* 2002;19:635–642.
7. Gallo LC, Troxel WM, Matthews KA, Kuller LH. Marital status and quality in middle-aged women: associations with levels and trajectories of cardiovascular risk factors. *Health Psychol.* 2003;22:453–463.
8. Rohrbaugh MJ, Shoham V, Coyne JC. Effect of marital quality on eight-year survival of patients with heart failure. *Am J Cardiol.* 2006;98:1069–1072.
9. Coyne JC, Rohrbaugh MJ, Shoham V, Sonnega JS, Nicklas JM, Cranford JA. Prognostic importance of marital quality for survival of congestive heart failure. *Am J Cardiology.* 2001;88:526–529.
10. Cano A, Miller LR, Loree A. Spouse beliefs about partner chronic pain. *J Pain.* 2009;10(5):486–492.
11. Sterba KR, DeVellis RF, Lewis MA, DeVellis BM, Jordan JM, Baucom DH. Effect of couple illness perception congruence on psychological adjustment in women with rheumatoid arthritis. *Health Psychol.* 2008;27(2):221–229.
12. Forgeron PA, Finley GA, Arnaout M. Pediatric pain prevalence and parents' attitudes at a cancer hospital in Jordan. *J Pain Symptom Manage.* 2005;31:440–448.
13. Wamboldt FS, Bender BG, Rankin AE. Adolescent decision-making about use of inhaled asthma controller medication: results from focus groups with participants from a prior longitudinal study. *J Asthma.* 2011;48(7):741–750.
14. Rolland JS. *Helping Couples and Families Navigate illness and Disability*. Guildford Press; 2018.
15. Walsh F. Family resilience: a framework for clinical practice. *Fam Process.* 2003;42(1):1–18.
16. McGoldrick M, Gerson R, Petry SS. *Genograms: Assessment and Intervention*. 3rd ed. WW Norton & Co.; 2008.
17. Knudson-Martin C, Mahoney AR. *Couples, Gender, And Power: Creating Change in Intimate Relationships*. Springer; 2009.
18. Rohrbaugh MJ, Mehl MR, Shoham V, Reilly ES, Ewy GA. Prognostic significance of spouse we talk in couples coping with heart failure. *J Consult Clin Psychol.* 2008;76(5):781–789.
19. Han H-R, Cho EJ, Kim D, Kim J. The report of coping strategies and psychosocial adjustment in Korean mothers of children with cancer. *Psychooncology.* 2009;18:956–964.

20. Gustafsson PA, Björkstén B, Kjellman NI. Family dysfunction in asthma: a prospective study of illness development. *J Pediatr.* 1994;125(3):493–498.
21. Kissane D. *Presentation at the American Association of Psychiatrists Annual Meeting*. American Psychiatric Association; 2012.
22. Romano JM, Jensen MP, Turner JA, Good AB, Hops H. Chronic pain patient partner interactions: further support for a behavioral model of chronic pain. *Behav Ther*. 2000;31:415–440.
23. Tienari P, Wynne C, Sorri A, et al. Genotype-environment interaction in schizophrenia-spectrum disorder: long-term follow-up study of Finnish adoptees. *Br J Psychiatry*. 2004;184:216–222.
24. Schulz R, Beach SR. Caregiving as a risk factor for mortality: the caregiver health effects study. *JAMA*. 1999;282:2215–2219.
25. Mittelman M. Taking care of the caregivers. *Curr Opin Psychiatry*. 2005;18:633–639.
26. Epstein NB, Bishop DS, Levin S. McMaster model of family functioning. *J Marital Fam Ther.* 1978;4(4):19–31.
27. Liu JE, Mok E, Wong T. Perceptions of supportive communication in Chinese patients with cancer: experiences and expectations. *J Adv Nurs*. 2005;52(3):262–270.
28. Reblin M, Uchino BN. Social and emotional support and its implication for health. *Curr Opin Psychiatry*. 2008; 21:201–205.
29. Bolger N, Zuckerman A, Kessler RC. Invisible support and adjustment to stress. *J Pers Soc Psychol*. 2000; 79:953–961.
30. Keogh KM, Smith SM, White P, et al. Psychological family intervention for poorly controlled type 2 diabetes. *Am J Manag Care*. 2010;17(2):105–113.
31. Varghese M, Kirpekar V, Loganathan S. Family interventions: basic principles and techniques. *Indian J Psychiatry*. 2020;62(suppl 2):s192–s200.
32. McDaniel SH, Hepworth J, Doherty WJ. *Medical Family Therapy: A Biopsychosocial Approach to Families*. Basic Books; 1992.
33. Rohrbaugh MJ, Shoham V. Family consultation for couples coping with health problems: a social cybernetic approach, In: Friedman HS, ed. *Oxford Handbook of Health Psychology*. Oxford University Press; 2011;480–501.
34. White M, Epston D. *Narrative Means to Therapeutic Ends*. WW Norton; 1990.
35. Steinglass P. Multiple family discussion groups for patients with chronic medical illness. *Fam Syst Health*. 1998;16:55–70.
36. Sahler OJ, Dolgin MJ, Phipps S, et al. Specificity of problem-solving skills training in mothers of children newly diagnosed with cancer: results of a multisite randomized clinical trial. *J Clin Oncol*. 2013;31(10):1329–1335.
37. Libbon R, Rothberg B, Baker S, Heru A. Multifamily group psychotherapy for patients with nonepileptic seizures and their families. *Am J Psychother*. 2023;76(2):62–68.

The question we are asked most frequently is, "What are the guidelines—that is, indications and contraindications—for family therapy?" Now that we have discussed what family therapy is, how to do it, and with whom, we can discuss these issues. In Chapter 22, we describe our version of a decision tree for differential diagnosis and therapeutics. We describe when to do evaluation and the different therapies, including the choices of type, length, and modality. In Chapter 23, we examine complicated situations and guidelines for addressing them. These guidelines are modified by factors such as the family's ethnicity, gender issues involving both family and therapist, and the family's economic status (usually meaning the money and time the family can spend on treatment).

Finally, we present in Chapter 24, a summary of the results of family therapy outcome studies. These studies and accumulated clinical experience in the field provide both the underpinnings for the family therapy guidelines and for the treatment intervention described in Chapter 18.

Section

VII Results of and Guidelines for Recommending Family Therapy

22 Indications for and the Sequence of Family Therapy Evaluation and Treatment 319

23 Controversies and Relative Contraindications 329

24 Results: The Outcomes of Couples and Family Therapy 337

22 Indications for and the Sequence of Family Therapy Evaluation and Treatment

OBJECTIVES FOR THE READER

- To learn decision-making processes in choosing family therapy
- To be able to use the general indications, contraindications, and enabling factors in order to practice family therapy

For easier reading, we emphasize that the descriptors "couples" or "marital" are used nearly interchangeably in this chapter.

INTRODUCTION

A recommendation for family therapy, and a particular form of family therapy, is the result of a sequence of clinical decisions. In this chapter, we present a decision tree to guide the clinician's thinking. Decisions about the choice and timing of treatment are complex. Some well-controlled outcome studies have examined the effectiveness of family therapy for certain problems, but in many circumstances a number of approaches are available and clinicians must use their best judgment.[1]

Family therapy is strongly indicated in the following situations:

- Couple or family problems, discord, or disorders
- Schizophrenia
- Bipolar and related disorders
- Depressive disorders
- Substance use disorder to enhance treatment adherence and implement treatment
- Medical conditions (i.e., psychosocial difficulties arising in conjunction with physical illness)
- Medical or psychiatric illness in children

A variety of situations make choice of treatment more complex today (in 2024) than it used to be, including pressure from managed care for efficient and low-cost treatment, the lessened availability of hospitalization for other than very short–term crisis management, newly available medications, and the variety of new psychotherapeutic approaches. Nevertheless, these guidelines provide a rationale for the treatment choices a therapist will make.

SEQUENCE OF EVALUATION AND TREATMENT PLANNING

STEP 1: IS FAMILY EVALUATION INDICATED?

STEP 2: IS FAMILY TREATMENT INDICATED?
Family Therapy Versus Individual Therapy
Managed Care
Individual, Couples, or Sex Therapy for Sexual Problems
Family Crisis Therapy Versus Hospitalization
STEP 3: WHAT SHALL BE THE DURATION AND INTENSITY OF FAMILY THERAPY?
Family Crisis Therapy
Brief Family Therapy
Long-Term Family Therapy
STEP 4: WHAT MODEL OF FAMILY INTERVENTION IS INDICATED?
CLINICAL PRACTICE IMPLICATIONS

SEQUENCE OF EVALUATION AND TREATMENT PLANNING

Evaluation and treatment planning involves four major steps or decisions:

1. Is a family evaluation indicated? If the family requests treatment, an evaluation is always indicated. If an individual requests treatment, a decision must be made as to whether family evaluation is necessary.
2. Based on the evaluation, is family treatment indicated? If so, should other forms of treatment also be given (e.g., individual psychotherapy, pharmacotherapy), and should they be concurrent or sequenced?
3. Presuming that family therapy is indicated, on the basis of evaluation and differential therapeutics (i.e., deciding on which treatment with which situation rather than giving the *same* treatment regardless of the situation), what shall be its duration and intensity?
4. What model of family intervention is indicated?

We examine each of these decisions in more depth in the sections that follow.

STEP 1: IS FAMILY EVALUATION INDICATED?

Family evaluation as described in Section III is conducted to determine how the family functions, how the system influences and is influenced by the behavior and symptoms of its individual members, and whether family work is possible and appropriate.

Family evaluation is indicated in the following situations:

- When the family or couple request treatment or define the problem as a family issue
- When the problem obviously involves two or more people in the family (e.g., when child abuse, marital conflict, or severe parent–child conflict is present)
- When the presenting patient is a child or adolescent
- When the presenting problem is sexual difficulty or dissatisfaction
- When recent stress or disruption in the family is caused by family crisis or a milestone (e.g., when the couple are approaching the empty-nest stage of their relationship)

Some therapists believe that marital evaluation is indicated for all married patients seeking individual therapy, in that the patient may not accurately report psychiatric symptoms in the spouse or problematic marital interactions that are affecting the partners' lives or mental health. As long as the evaluation is conducted in a respectful manner as a search for information and family strength rather than pathology, most couples appreciate the chance to review issues.

Other therapists believe that this is intrusive and counterproductive to the individual therapy process. In most cases we recommend the former position.

Whenever psychiatric hospitalization or acute treatment for emergencies is being considered, a family evaluation is usually indicated for one or more of the following reasons:

- For history gathering
- To clarify how the family interaction is influenced by and has influenced the course of illness
- To negotiate the treatment plan with the whole family (i.e., Is hospitalization necessary, or can the family manage with outpatient help? If hospitalization is necessary, what role will the family play?)
- When more than one family member is simultaneously in psychiatric treatment
- When improvement in the individual patient is correlated with symptom formation in another family member or deterioration in their relationship
- When individual or group treatment has been tried and is failing or has failed and (1) the patient is much more involved with family problems, (2) the patient has difficulty dealing with family issues unless they are demonstrated directly in the room, (3) the transference to the therapist is too intense or actualized (i.e., the transference and countertransference becomes acted out, or played out, in the session and can be brought back to realistic proportions by including family members), or (4) family cooperation seems necessary to allow the individual to change
- When the therapist decides during the individual evaluation that, although the patient presents with symptoms that are not immediately related to family issues, the primary or secondary gain of the symptoms is an important expression of family systems pathology (e.g., a wife's agoraphobia worsens when her husband works overtime)

Family evaluation is contraindicated in the following situations:

- When any family member strongly prefers or insists on the privacy of an individual evaluation (e.g., because of a family secret)
- When it appears that the individuation of a family member would be compromised by family evaluation (e.g., the therapist might want to wait until time has passed before including the family of a young adult who has recently left home for the first time)
- When a childless marriage is breaking up with little or no desire for reconciliation
- When the presenting problem is clearly the result of repetitive intrapsychic conflicts that recur in many of the individual's relationships and seems more amenable to individual intervention
- When the patient won't trust a therapist who has also seen their family
- When extreme schizoid or paranoid pathology is present—unless hospitalization is indicated in the context of the patient being (still) involved and (usually) dependent on their family (in such a case, we advise therapists to continue working on getting the family to come in, especially if the patient's condition worsens or the patient is decompensating). Many treatment facilities are structured in such a way as to unwittingly preclude the serious consideration of conducting a family evaluation when a prospective patient seeks assistance. Although family clinics, by their name and reputation, attract those who see themselves as having family problems, most clinics are organized to deal with individuals (not family or marital units) who seek help. In such contexts, the secretaries, for example, ask on the first phone call for the name of the patient and a description of the individual's problems. They routinely give an appointment time to the individual, not the family. There may be no format for a family chart. Likewise, private practitioners often have reputations as being primarily marital and family therapists or individual therapists. If care is not given to the initial steps in the help-seeking sequence, the decision to complete a family evaluation can be made by accident rather than in a deliberate manner.

STEP 2: IS FAMILY TREATMENT INDICATED?

The process of choosing a type of therapy is complex. Research is just beginning to develop guidelines for such decisions. The therapist most often must base their judgment on clinical intuition, general clinical opinion, and the wishes and judgments of the people involved.

Family Therapy Versus Individual Therapy

One of the most common questions for clinicians who are fluent in both therapies is the decision about type and timing of therapy. The basic theoretical premise of family therapy is that many problems are purely relational and that individual symptoms in one person can be viewed as interpersonal in terms of etiology or problem maintenance and that these symptoms can be changed by altering the system. The basic principle of individual therapy is that problems or symptoms develop because of the brain psychopathology and subsequent psychodynamics of the individual and that change occurs in the individual (either behaviorally or because of cognitive understanding of the problems) in the presence of an intense and exclusive relationship with the therapist. Table 22.1 summarizes the relative selection criteria for both types of therapy. For many patients, both forms of therapy may be useful or necessary. **Self-knowledge does not always help the person understand the complex family system and how one's behavior affects and is affected by family members, and family therapy does not allow for intense exploration of psychodynamic issues.** Individual therapy also does not allow the clinician to see how the problems of other family members may be affecting the system.

Table 22.1 Relative selection criteria for treatment format: family versus individual

	Family	Individual
Relative indications	Family problems are presented as such, without either spouse or any family member designated as the identified patient; symptoms are predominantly within the marital relationship.	The patient's symptoms or character is based on firmly structured intrapsychic conflict that causes repetitive life patterns more or less transcending the particulars of the current interpersonal situation (e.g., family, job relationships).
	Family presents with current structured difficulties in intrafamilial relationships with each person contributing collusively or openly to the reciprocal interaction problems.	The patient is an adolescent or young adult who is striving for autonomy. Psychiatric problem is of such a private or embarrassing nature that it needs the privacy of individual treatment, at least for the beginning phase.
	Family has fixed and severe deficits in perception and communication: (1) projective identification so that each member blames another for all problems; (2) family using paranoid or schizoid functioning (i.e., boundaries are vague and fluctuating, parts of self are projected readily onto other family members, trading of ego functions occurs); (3) a relentless fixity of distance is maintained by pseudomutual and pseudohostile mechanisms; (4) collective cognitive chaos and erratic distancing; (5) amorphous, vague, undirected forms of communication are pervasive.	

Table 22.1 Relative selection criteria for treatment format: family versus individual (*Continued*)

	Family	Individual
	Adolescent acting-out behavior (e.g., promiscuity, drug abuse, delinquency, perversion, vandalism, violent behavior).	
	Another form of treatment is stalemated or has failed (e.g., the patient has been unable to utilize intrapsychic mode of individual therapy or uses most of sessions to discuss family problems).	
	Improvement of one family member has led to symptoms or signs of deterioration in another.	
	Reduction of secondary gain in one or more family members is a major goal.	
	More than one person needs treatment, and resources are available for only one treatment.	
Enabling factors	Motivation is strongest to be seen as a couple or family, or an individual patient will accept no other format.	The patient is uncomfortable in dyadic situations and is able to handle the potential intimacy of the individual treatment setting.
	No family member has psychopathology of such proportions that family therapy would be prevented (e.g., extreme agitation, mania, paranoia, severe distrust, dangerous hostility, or acute schizophrenia).	Financial and temporal resources are available for individual treatment.
	Crucial members of a defined functional social system are available for family treatment.	
Relative contraindications	The presenting problem of the individual does not have a significant etiology in or effect on the family system.	The only issue of real importance is a family problem. The patient regresses in individual therapy relationships.
	Marital problems, if present, are chronic and ego-syntonic. Family therapy is used to deny individual responsibility for major personality or character illness. Massive but minimally relevant or unworkable parental pathology is present that indicates symptomatic child or adolescent should be treated alone. Individuation of a family member requires that the member has their own and separate treatment. Family treatment has stalemated or failed and has resolved what crises it can, and one or more individual members require additional individual treatment. There is a need for another modality of treatment prior to family therapy (e.g., detoxification, medication, individual sessions to establish trust). Motivation exists to be seen alone (e.g., an adolescent states emphatically that they have personal problems for which they want individual help).	

Consider the following case example:

Mrs. A requested individual treatment for "depression." On family evaluation, the therapist learned that Mrs. A's husband had an untreated bipolar disorder (i.e., he had manic symptoms). Much of Mrs. A's depressive symptoms resulted from Mr. A's behavior when he was in a manic or hypomanic state, and a key factor in treating Mrs. A's "depression" was treating Mr. A's symptoms and having him acknowledge the truth of his wife's concerns about him.

For many people, however, symptoms occur regardless of the different systems around them over time.

Because people tend to pick partners at similar stages of differentiation, it is not unusual for people with psychological difficulties to have spouses with similar or complementary but equally severe problems. In addition to evaluating the partner, the therapist must also address directly other problems such as the couple's problems and how they relate to symptoms such as depression or substance misuse. Children in such families often have genetically based similar illnesses (such as depression), or they experience symptoms as a result of dealing with parental problems. These illnesses and symptoms are often best treated with family therapy, but this does not rule out scheduling special meetings just for the children. For many people, both types of therapy are helpful, allowing for increased pleasure with the partner and providing a context for personal and private growth.

For more severely ill patients, family therapy may be one component of a comprehensive treatment plan that includes several other modalities such as medication, individual treatment, and family group treatment. The treatment of schizophrenia is a prominent example. Because schizophrenia in a family member produces long-term effects on the family, many therapists focus the therapeutic management of this disorder around the family as a unit. It is clear from many decades of research that although medication is essential in the treatment of such illnesses, it alone will not completely alter preexisting family relationships or ways of coping with stress.[2] In recent research if sessions were greater than two including all type of family therapy interventions, extra sentences significantly reduced the relapse rates.

The timing of therapy is another important consideration. If the identified patient is highly symptomatic and has a problem that is usually amenable to medications, it is often helpful to begin medication and family therapy first, in order to reduce the symptoms, educate the family, and eliminate family sources of stress.

In general, the therapist tries to deal with the most acute problems first. If possible in terms of timing and finances, individual and family therapy can be conducted at the same time. Some senior clinicians recommended that different therapists do the individual and family therapies; however, it is imperative that the therapists remain in contact to avoid splitting or conflicting treatment. Some therapists, including us on occasion, have treated both the family and an individual (or individuals) in the family. There are few controlled data to settle this question.

Our guidelines depend more on the characteristics of the family and how the members function than on the particular diagnosis or problem area.

Managed Care

Depending on the type of program, there may be a strong bias toward one type of therapy over another. For example, on inpatient units, medication is preferred over psychotherapy (because it usually has a more rapid effect). In general, managed care companies have been encouraging more medication and less of any kind of exploratory therapy. When only a few sessions are possible, brief family therapy often can stabilize the system and support the development of other family resources most quickly. However, the therapist must put their own sense of the patient's and

Table 22.2 Criteria for sex and couple therapy

Sex therapy	Couple therapy
The couples' problem is clearly focused on sexual dysfunction.	Sexuality is not an issue, or it is one of many issues in couples' dysfunction.
Enabling factors:	*Enabling factors:*
The couple are willing and able to carry out the sexual functioning tasks that the therapist would assign.	Anger and resistance are too intense to carry out extra-session tasks around sexual functioning.
The partners are strongly attached to each other; both partners are interested in reversing the sexual dysfunction.	The couple are not committed to each other; covert or overt behaviors are occurring to dissolve the marriage.

family's needs first over biases about treatment—especially when definitive data are lacking. Unfortunately, many patients do not become "cured" in 10 sessions, and our goal must be to prevent, as much as possible, undertreatment or a "revolving door" (i.e., frequent readmission of the patient).

Individual, Couples, or Sex Therapy for Sexual Problems

This distinction was more clear in the late 1980s, when sex therapy was focused primarily on a specific and highly detailed behavioral protocol. Sex therapy more recently has moved in the direction of further understanding of the physiologic causes of sexual dysfunction on the one hand and the cognitive behavioral issues involved on the other. In general, sexual problems do not disappear with couples therapy unless specific attention is paid to the nature and quality of the sexual problems. We provide a more complete discussion of treatment in Chapter 20, on sex and marital therapy (see also Table 22.2). It is most effective to deal with severe conflict in a couple before beginning to deal with sexual issues directly. Sex therapy includes education, a focus on the intimacy and power aspects of sex, and usually homework assignments that in some way deal with sexual anxiety and expansion of sexual options.[3] Sex therapy has been found to be helpful for women with loss of sexual desire and orgasmic dysfunction, as well as for couples with sexual problems. Additionally, patients with severe mental illness can benefit from sexual therapy to promote sexual health. Individual therapy is indicated if the problems are clearly related to the partner's history (e.g., sexual abuse, hatred of women) or if the problems have occurred in multiple relationships and are not amenable to being worked on in the couple. Individual therapy is the most inefficient way of dealing with most couples-centered sexual problems. It is also important to consider the possible role of organic problems in any dysfunction. It is most effective to deal with severe conflict in a couple before beginning to deal with sexual issues directly.[4]

Family Crisis Therapy Versus Hospitalization

In most settings, hospitalization is now the only setting for triage for people who are dangerous to self or others. Keeping a very ill patient at home requires considerable support and, when possible, a crisis team. As such, family crisis intervention in outpatient settings, such as emergency rooms or clinics, may still be a crucial intervention (see below). Table 22.3 summarizes the criteria and enabling factors for family crisis therapy and hospitalization.

STEP 3: WHAT SHALL BE THE DURATION AND INTENSITY OF FAMILY THERAPY?

To address this question, we have outlined criteria for family crisis intervention and for short- and long-term family therapy.

Table 22.3 Criteria for family crisis therapy and hospitalization

Family crisis therapy	Hospitalization
The risk of destructiveness to self or others is within assumable limits.	The patient is dangerous to self or others or is gravely disabled.
The level of family disruption is relatively low.	Presence of the psychotic patient has harmful effects on the family or society.
A need exists to preserve job and family relationships.	Thorough evaluation requires 24-hour observation and medical facilities. The patient gets worse when with the family.
Enabling factors: The family is intact, available, and motivated.	Enabling factors: The family is highly resistant, not available, or intact enough to carry on treatment and manage the patient.

Family Crisis Therapy

Family crisis therapy is an intense (as often as daily) family intervention performed during a time of crisis and for a brief duration (usually less than 1 month) to help prevent the imminent disintegration of family relationships or decompensation of one or more family members and, it is hoped, to reestablish the family equilibrium at a level equal to, or higher than, before the crisis.

This modality is indicated when an immediate crisis in the family is causing severe and urgent family or individual symptoms or grief that could result in hospitalization or risk to life, limb, sanity, or the family's ability to continue as a unit. The crisis may be triggered by a stress that is:

- Developmental—for example, birth of a child, departure of a child for college, marriage of a family member, responsibility of caring for extended family, aging and retirement, return of the wife to work, acting-out behavior on the part of a teenager
- Accidental—for example, injury, sickness, death, job loss
- Interpersonal—for example, an affair, a bitter argument

Brief Family Therapy

Brief family therapy can be any type of therapy that has a specific endpoint, usually in less than 10 sessions, or it can refer to a specific type of problem-oriented strategic therapy with a duration of 6 to 10 sessions. Most research investigations of family and marital therapy involve treatment that is short term. In general, brief family therapy is present focused, problem focused, and very directive.

Long-Term Family Therapy

Therapists vary in terms of whether they focus exclusively on the problem brought by the family or on a more general review of family functioning. For example, if a child is brought to treatment, should the therapy end when the couple is parenting more effectively, or should it press to address the couple's long-term issues and sexual dysfunction even though the child problem has been solved? Brief therapy in particular is problem focused rather than growth focused and, when possible, leaves the definition of the problem to the family. We believe that when time and families allow, it is best to offer the couple and family the possibility of working on whatever seems necessary.

For example, a couple may present with a complaint of the wife's depression.

A family evaluation that includes the children may reveal that even though the couple did not complain about it, one of the children is also depressed or has attention-deficit/hyperactivity disorder (which sometimes produces a sense of ineffectiveness and depression in the parents). The therapist should feel free to shift the focus to allow for treatment of the child.

We believe that when time and families allow, it is best to offer the couple and family the possibility of working on whatever seems necessary.

Long-term family therapy is a treatment without time limit, when short-term intervention is inadequate or goals for the family are more ambitious. Indications for long-term family therapy may be classified as those arising directly from evaluation or as those arising through referral from brief or crisis therapy.

- Directly from evaluation:
  When a family with multiple problems is inherently unstable and will require long-term external support and integration
  When the family is highly motivated for treatment but problems are complex and not reducible to a manageable, short-term focus
  When the family is not highly motivated for treatment and will require an induction period to establish an adequate therapeutic alliance
  When problems are likely to be chronic and not amenable to brief intervention (e.g., intense marital difficulties with mutual projection, fusion, or long-standing disagreement)
  When short-term therapy was not sufficient in the past
- Through referral from brief or crisis therapy:
  When brief therapy was not complete enough nor sufficiently successful; if the family is motivated to continue work, there is some hope for success
  When the family is especially receptive and responsive to family work and has enough problems to warrant continued treatment and has sufficient resources
- Long-term family therapy is contraindicated when it appears that extended therapy encourages the family to avoid focusing on problems or to delay therapeutic change, or when the cost–benefit ratio is too high.

STEP 4: WHAT MODEL OF FAMILY INTERVENTION IS INDICATED?

Research has demonstrated that no one school of therapy is definitively superior to another. The trend in recent years has been toward a more integrative approach, drawing from a variety of models and allowing for a more fluid type of work. Integrative models such as the one we present in this book are likely to combine some form of here-and-now work (i.e., cognitive or behavioral) with some type of historical understanding of the patterns that led to the current problem.

Child-focused problems must include some structural work; most couple's problems need some attention to the family of origin; and most work with seriously psychiatrically ill patients requires some psychoeducation.

CLINICAL PRACTICE IMPLICATIONS

As we have emphasized in this chapter, family therapy is usually prescribed as part of a multimodal package. The guidelines above should help in making a choice of "what to do next." We discuss the data for these indications in Chapter 24.

REFERENCES

1. Pinsof WM, Wynne LC. The efficacy of marital and family therapy: an empirical overview, conclusions and recommendations. *J Marital Fam Ther.* 1995;21:585–613.
2. Rodolico A, Bighelli I, Avanzato C, et al. Family interventions for relapse prevention in schizophrenia: a systematic review and network meta-analysis. *Lancet Psychiatry* 2022;9:211–221.
3. Weeks GR. *Integrating Sex and Marital Therapy: A Clinical Guide*. Routledge; 2013.
4. Landmark BF, Almås E, Brurberg KG, et al. *The Effects of Sexual Therapy Interventions for Sexual Problems [Internet]*. Knowledge Centre for the Health Services at The Norwegian Institute of Public Health (NIPH); 2012.

23 Controversies and Relative Contraindications

OBJECTIVES FOR THE READER

- To be able to describe general situations in which there is controversy in the field around the indications for marital and family therapy
- To recognize specific problems that make the choice of modality more complex

For easier reading, we emphasize that the descriptors "couples" or "marital" are used nearly interchangeably in this chapter.

INTRODUCTION

Although we feel strongly that marital (or more broadly, couples) or family therapy is indicated for most marital or family problems, and that it should be included at some point in the treatment of many psychiatric conditions (including severe disorders), many questions remain unresolved in the field of family therapy. For persons with significant personal and family issues, what is the relationship among individual therapy, family therapy, group therapy, and medication? If other treatment modalities are indicated, how does the therapist decide whether to use them concurrently or consecutively? We discussed these issues in the context of "couples therapy" in Chapter 15; here we discuss them in the context of "indications and contraindications." In Chapter 22, we reviewed the situations in which family treatment is indicated; in this chapter, we consider specific clinical dilemmas.

COUPLES THERAPY
- Couples Conflict and Dissatisfaction
- Sexual Issues
- Families in the Process of Divorce
- Unmarried Couples

THE CHILD AS THE IDENTIFIED PATIENT
THE ADOLESCENT AS THE IDENTIFIED PATIENT
FAMILY OF ORIGIN ISSUES
SITUATIONS IN WHICH FAMILY THERAPY IS DIFFICULT AND PERHAPS CONTRAINDICATED
- When Psychopathology in One Family Member Makes Family Therapy Ineffective
- When the Family or Therapist Thinks the Risks of Therapy Outweigh the Advantages

When the Family as a Whole Denies Having Family Problems
When Cultural or Religious Prejudices Are Present
SKILLS AND ATTRIBUTES OF THE THERAPIST AS THEY AFFECT FAMILY WORK
CLINICAL PRACTICE IMPLICATIONS

COUPLES THERAPY

Couples Conflict and Dissatisfaction

A growing body of research has produced consistent results in the area of marital treatment. For many years, it has been a prevalent clinical opinion that marital therapy is the treatment of choice for marital difficulties.[1,2] Hurvitz[3] wrote of the dangers of doing individual therapy with only one spouse in such a situation.

- Gurman and Kniskern[4] reviewed research results that indicated conjoint marital therapy was superior to conjoint plus individual therapy, concurrent therapy, and individual therapy. We now know that another criterion for differential therapeutics is the comparative deterioration effects (i.e., worsening of symptoms or function or behavior, in contrast to lessening of positive effects over time or of not improving) of various modalities of treatment. This approaches the question of treatment choice from the negative side, that is, which treatment does the most harm? **Gurman and Kniskern[5] found that the rate of deterioration for conjoint, group, and concurrent–collaborative marital therapies is half that of individual therapy of marital problems.[6]**

Although marital conflict and dissatisfaction seem to lend themselves especially well to conjoint marital treatment, such problems historically have been dealt with individually, especially when one partner requests individual therapy and the therapist is uncomfortable or unfamiliar with conjoint models.

However, it is also true that one or both partners may have independent issues more effectively worked on in private. Consider the following case example:

Mr. and Mrs. A sought treatment because of a sense of distance and sadness in their relationship. History revealed that Mr. A had depression precipitated by his father's death 2 years earlier. Mr. A's relationship with his father had been poor and was unresolved at the time of the father's death.

Possible treatment plans include the following:

- Couples work, including an in-depth discussion of both partners' early history and of Mr. A's grief and loss; medication might be included in this plan, if indicated
- Concurrent individual and couples work
- Individual work with Mr. A first, perhaps including medication, dealing with issues around his father, followed by couples therapy, if still indicated
- Family of origin therapy with Mr. A and his mother and his brother in order to do grief work and help resolve remaining family issues

Guidelines in this case include making the decision with the couple's participation and doing the most urgent thing first. Mr. and Mrs. A felt that unless the marriage was attended to, they were headed rapidly for divorce. The therapist chose to begin with couples therapy that focused on ways in which Mr. A could share his feelings with Mrs. A and; how he could be there for her despite his sadness; and on Mrs. A's grief and anger at having a depressed husband, given her own history of growing up with a depressed father. The couple then began to discuss both families of origin. Mrs. A, who knew Mr. A's family conflict well, was able to offer a number of suggestions about the origin of the problem and how grieving might begin. The therapist later saw Mr. A alone for several sessions and had two family of origin sessions with him, his mother, and his brother.

Had Mr. A presented as an individual patient requesting treatment for depression, he would in all probability have been seen individually with attention given to his depression and early life. This approach likely would not have addressed his issues with his wife, whom he was already ignoring because of his own pain. Lack of attention to couples issues in this case could have slowed Mr. A's recovery because Mrs. A's anger and withdrawal were contributing to his depression and would not have been dealt with. If the individual therapy moved slowly, and Mrs. A were not involved, she might well have reached the point of asking for a separation before too long. Even if Mr. A had presented for individual therapy, a couple's evaluation was certainly indicated.

More complex situations occur when the couple is in serious conflict over goals. Such a situation is most difficult when one partner wants to preserve the marriage, and the other is very ambivalent but probably wants to divorce. In this case, is it best to see the ambivalent person alone to sort out their feelings, or is it best to work on the marital relationship directly and deal with ambivalence within the couples work? No research is available to help the therapist sort out this kind of dilemma, and it is left to them to determine the best direction, on the basis of information at hand. Many therapists believe that dealing with the ambivalent partner alone supports the ambivalence and a tendency to move out of the marriage, so that a direct trial of couples therapy is often recommended, asking the ambivalent partner to behave as if the marriage is definitely going to continue so that the couple try as hard as possible to make it work. If the ambivalence seems to be part of a lifelong pattern of ambivalent behavior, if the ambivalent partner is in the midst of a transitional crisis, or if the ambivalent partner is having an affair that they will not give up, the indications for individual work become stronger.

Sexual Issues

Sexual issues are almost always dealt with conjointly if possible, and research suggests the therapy must be directed at both couples dynamics and the sexual symptoms (see Chapter 20). Therapy does not have to include sensate focus exercises unless indicated for specific problems. Again, however, some people need time alone to consider their previous sexual experiences, fantasies, and feelings.

Families in the Process of Divorce

Families in the process of divorce require a complicated mix of individual and family work. Although the grief work involved in a separation is best done alone, attention to the details of establishing childcare, new routines, and a way to communicate requires joint work. In some middle-class families that have experienced years of conflict, the family members have acquired a sizable number of therapists by the time the divorce proceedings are impending—we have seen families involved with four or five therapists, one for each parent and one for each of the children. The goal is to reduce the number of therapists to a manageable level or at least to promote clear communication among all of them. All persons involved in the care of the children must have a chance to get together and plan so that they do not lose the sense of the entire family's needs and positions.

In couples who are considering but are not yet at the point of divorce, the issue of couples versus individual therapy is complex. Individual therapy, which promotes personal growth in one partner without including or even informing the other, is more likely to lead to a split. Equally important, if individual therapy is indicated, the other partner (and the partner's therapist, if there is one), should be kept informed.

Unmarried Couples

Unmarried couples presenting for therapy related to commitment and communication problems are treated the same as any couples. More complex situations emerge when one member of the couple is still married to someone else, or when the relationship is inappropriate or in its very early stages. Consider the following case example:

A couple requested therapy after a dating relationship of 6 weeks. The young man of the couple had been in therapy for most of his life since early adolescence and used therapy in part to cope and in part as a solution for most life problems. The therapist stated that she felt a relationship of so short a duration should stand or fall on its own merits, and if the couple were still together in a few months and wanted help she would see them then. The couple broke up shortly afterward.

THE CHILD AS THE IDENTIFIED PATIENT

When the identified patient is a child, it has long been the practice of child guidance clinics to involve at least one of the parents (most often the mother), usually in collateral treatment in which both the patient and the parent are in individual treatment but with different therapists. This at least represents token recognition of the importance of the family in the problem and its resolution.

A more thorough approach seems indicated in these cases, however, with evaluation of the possible role of the child as the symptom bearer of more general family problems (e.g., unresolved marital issues). Usually the marital partners are seen as a couple for a major part of the treatment. The child may benefit from some individual attention addressed to their particular symptoms and psychosocial difficulties. A common sequence of events is for the entire family to start out in treatment together, and then for various individual dyads and triads to be separated out for special attention after an interval of time. Of these, the marital dyad is unquestionably the most important. Some family therapists suggest that whenever a symptomatic prepubescent child is involved, family treatment is indicated unless specific contraindications are present.

Since the early 1990s, there have been marked changes in the field of child psychiatry. Most institutions have shifted from an individual psychoanalytic focus to a family systems approach. An increasing number of childhood disorders are now being treated with family therapy. For example, school phobias are often treated with family therapy plus antidepressants. The causes of child psychopathology are complex. Biologic and genetic differences in temperament, intelligence, and ability (including attention-deficit/hyperactivity disorder and inherited tendencies to develop psychiatric disorder) interact with family dynamics and the child's cognitive and emotional development to produce child psychopathology. Controversies in this area persist as to the relative contribution of each factor in specific problems.

Within the area of parent–child interactions, conflict between child psychiatrists and family therapists has been over whether the child is best treated alone, using the relationship between therapist and child as the major change agent, or whether most attention should focus on supporting the family system to deal with the child better. In terms of family dynamics, there is also controversy over whether one must pay the most attention to the child's developmental task completion and the family's history, or whether direct attention to the here-and-now family patterns is the best focus.

The trend has been toward including the parents in treatment at some point. Part of the problem in the transition in model has been that many family therapists have not had enough training to identify psychopathology or developmental delay in children, and many child psychiatrists are not trained sufficiently in family dynamics to recognize problems and to produce change.

Another issue in choosing a treatment modality is whether the parents, even with therapy, can support the child emotionally or whether another adult is needed. In some situations, the parents are troubled enough, or their relationship conflicts are bitter enough, that family therapy cannot significantly alter the child's living situation, so that the child needs the outside support of caring adults. Although adult connections already established in the child's life (e.g., other family members, teachers) are always preferable, a troubled child may need the privacy and support offered by an individual therapist. Particularly as children get older they may need a place to consider their issues in private in addition to the public space of the family.

The therapist's recommendation should be based on an awareness that couples distress leads to deleterious effects on children including their mental health and academic performance.[7] Many such patients remain at an impaired level of function (as in childhood), and some get worse as they age as adults. For others, there is a marked discontinuity between child and adult psychopathology; that is, childhood illness does not go into adult life. With or without treatment many childhood psychiatric disorders are self-limiting. Children who are very impaired may show dramatic improvement as adults, and only 13% of children who were treated as children were rated more disturbed than controls in adult life.[8,9] Of course, the reverse is also true—many people who show normal development as children develop psychiatric illness in later life. Many patients remain ill or get worse as adults.

THE ADOLESCENT AS THE IDENTIFIED PATIENT

When the identified patient is an adolescent, a focus on the family is still indicated, especially while the adolescent is living at home, before they have established psychosocial autonomy. A good deal of attention must often be focused on the marital partnership. The adolescent often benefits from individual attention and from the encouragement of peer-group relationships. In treating a family that has an adolescent with an "authority problem," inclusion of the entire family group can dilute the adolescent's feelings about the therapist as an authority figure, making it easier for the therapist to make intervention(s).

With the family therapy field, a difference of opinion exists regarding the treatment of adolescents involved in symbiotic, mutually destructive parent–child relationships. Some therapists view this type of relationship as an indication for family treatment in order to facilitate the weaning of the teenager.[10] Other therapists believe it is difficult to promote further separation and individuation in family treatment, which brings all members together and may involve them even more in one another's lives. These latter therapists recommend that such adolescents receive individual or group treatment to demonstrate concretely their individuation and promote their growth outside the family, and that perhaps the parents be seen together to solidify their attachment to each other and their ability to tolerate the loss of their child. There seems to be some growing consensus that family therapy is most indicated when the symptomatic adolescent is exhibiting acting-out behavior (e.g., substance use or delinquent behavior). Some adolescents are seen in treatment who are not able to benefit from insight-oriented individual modes of treatment. A more focused, action-oriented family model is often more helpful.

FAMILY OF ORIGIN ISSUES

The idea of seeing adult children with their parents is little known outside the family therapy field. Adults are presumed to be able to report correctly about their childhood, and parents who have unfinished business with their children are expected to work on their own issues. Whatever the dynamics of childhood, the real relationship of adult children and their parents is very meaningful and is best worked on by the people involved. This is particularly true because the parent and the child may have changed greatly in the 20 or 30 years since the child grew up. This approach is in direct conflict with classic psychoanalytic models, which proposes that the agent of change is the transference relationship with the therapist and that little or no communication should be had with other family members. Years of clinical experience suggest strongly that family sessions, if respectful and supportive, can powerfully turn around many highly dysfunctional family dynamics and allow parents and children to make some kind of peace with one another. In addition, the process of learning about one's past from one's parents, and seeing them as the flawed but real people they are and were, rather than as the monsters of one's childhood, often speeds the process of one's own therapy.

SITUATIONS IN WHICH FAMILY THERAPY IS DIFFICULT AND PERHAPS CONTRAINDICATED

When Psychopathology in One Family Member Makes Family Therapy Ineffective

Dishonesty or manipulation of the therapy for secondary gain would constitute a serious barrier to effective treatment. For example, a partner might use therapy as a way to keep a spouse involved while continuing to have an affair and conceal it. There does exist specifically developed forms of family therapy focused on couples whose partner had infidelity.[11] Additionally, some persons, such as those with antisocial personality disorders, may be savvy at convincing others of the honesty of their position while engaging in very destructive behavior (e.g., using the family's money to gamble, engaging in crime). Additionally, children who are lying or stealing are most likely responding to family issues, which must be addressed in therapy.

If one family member is extremely paranoid, manic, or agitated, medication might be initiated for behavior that is too disruptive to control, before family therapy begins. As we pointed out in Chapter 18, even quite psychotic people can be active members of the family and can profit from family work. Lastly, controversy remains over the role of family therapy for individuals who are abusing substances.[12] There does exist couple-based treatments for couples in which at least one partner has a substance use disorder.[13] In some cases, particularly when the user is an adolescent or young adult who is not physically dependent on the drug, family therapy may be a primary treatment modality. For more deeply addicted people, family therapy must be part of a larger treatment plan including detoxification, group treatment, and specific alcohol and drug treatment. In doing family therapy with this population, it is critical not to blame the drug use on other family members or to allow the user to blame them. For example, statements such as "I wouldn't drink if you didn't nag" are not acceptable explanations for drinking. Family therapy in which a family member is abusing substances must involve the goal of the family member stopping the substance abuse. It is ineffective to continue couples therapy with an actively using partner without dealing with the alcohol abuse and its destructive effects on the marriage. Many therapists originally believed that if they could improve communication, or the couple's sex life, the alcoholism would stop. Because the addicted person would usually prefer to keep the addiction, this model simply perpetuated the problem.

When the Family or Therapist Thinks the Risks of Therapy Outweigh the Advantages

Family members may be concerned that treatment will leave them in a worse state than when they began. This possibility should be explored at the outset, and therapy should be sensitive to this concern whenever possible. This concern commonly arises when families apply to a child guidance clinic. Many children develop problems in relation to parental conflicts. For example, a child may develop a school phobia, may become abusive to other children, or maybe encopretic whenever the parents have severe fights. The parents may want the child "fixed" but are determined not to address their own conflicts because they are afraid that divorce will result. This is particularly true if the parents believe that one of them would become suicidal or psychotic if they admitted to their problems. In these cases, the therapy should be addressed only to parenting issues, and couples issues should be tabled at least until the child is better. In most cases, it is possible to find some way of uniting the parents around the child even when they are still in conflict. Consider the following case example:

A 10-year-old girl whose problems included severe tantrums at home described her evenings. She would be doing her homework in the kitchen, and her parents would have screaming fights in the next room, threatening each other with divorce. Needless to say, she did not get much homework done. She would often try to stop the fights, and sometimes the parents would appeal to her to settle their arguments. The parents admitted they fought but downplayed the significance or level of verbal violence. The therapist framed the child as sensitive and told her to go to her room upstairs and close the door if her parents began to disagree. Her parents were asked to reward her when she did this, so that she would not feel she was deserting them. Because they wanted her to do her homework more than they wanted a referee, they complied. Although the child's home life remained difficult, this approach removed her from the middle of things and allowed her some safe time, and she calmed down considerably. The parents' concerns could then be addressed, to the extent they were willing to do so. They chose to end therapy shortly thereafter.

A family that truly believes that therapy will result in divorce will not enter treatment. For couples and families in pain, the real issue is how hard and when to push issues they are afraid to discuss. For example, encouraging a woman who has been subservient to stand up for herself may provoke serious reprisals from a husband who needs a very acquiescent wife. As we describe in Chapter 25, on ethics, this is both an ethical decision and a therapeutic one. It is best to discuss with the couple the pros and cons of relationship change. Often the couple will elect to stop therapy at the time and return to treatment later when the situation has deteriorated to the point that change is inevitable.

When the Family as a Whole Denies Having Family Problems

In some families, their whole way of life is oriented around denial of difficulties. Such families make therapy extremely problematic and may best be treated by brief therapy using systemic and strategic models that emphasize restraint of change and positive reframing of symptoms, what Karpel[14] (p. 181) calls defiance-based therapy.

When Cultural or Religious Prejudices Are Present

Unyielding, inflexible cultural or religious prejudices against any sort of outside intervention in the family system would make family therapy difficult. In these cases, other alternatives can be offered, including working with a clergyperson, community worker, or educator, with the family therapist acting as a consultant.

SKILLS AND ATTRIBUTES OF THE THERAPIST AS THEY AFFECT FAMILY WORK

Many therapists are uncomfortable with family groups, or with particular types of families, and should not force themselves to treat them. Therapists can refer patients for family therapy if needed.

Mr. B, age 35 years, was in individual treatment for 6 years for his depression. His therapist believed he was passive and encouraged him to learn to speak up for what he wanted. Mr. B and his wife went to couples therapy with an unrelated therapist at the point at which his wife was ready to leave the marriage. Mrs. B said her husband had always been self-centered, but in the years since therapy started he had been impossibly critical and demanding. In the couples session, far from being passive, he was angry, condescending, and completely unempathetic to his wife. The individual therapist's disinterest in Mr. B's wife's perception of the problem had led to an increasingly dysfunctional marriage and near divorce.

A decision to treat an individual should not mean ignoring couples issues. If a therapist has strong emotional ties to a family (e.g., a spouse's or friend's relative) or significant countertransference to a particular family, they should refer the family.

The age, sex, and race of the therapist can have significant effects on treatment, and these issues need to be considered. For example, a 50-year-old educated and status-conscious couple is not likely to respond to a 25-year-old therapist who has an MSW rather than a PhD. Many families of color, having experienced serious oppression, are reluctant to allow a middle-class White therapist to treat them without a long period of trust building.

CLINICAL PRACTICE IMPLICATIONS

Family therapy is an approach and a worldview in addition to being a specific technique. Research has defined situations in which family therapy is the treatment of choice (see Chapter 22). In other situations, where there is no scientific data, the therapist must use their clinical judgment to consider all aspects of the problems and to formulate the best intervention. We also recommend second opinions from other colleagues as necessary.

REFERENCES

1. Avallone S, Aron R, Starr P, Breetz S. How therapists assign families to treatment modalities: the development of the treatment method choice set. *Am J Orthopsychiatry*. 1973;43:767–773.
2. Greene BL, Lee RR, Lustig N. Treatment of marital disharmony where one spouse has a primary affective disorder (manic-depressive illness), I: general overview—100 couples. *J Fam Couns*. 1975;1:39–50.
3. Hurvitz N. Marital problems following psychotherapy with one spouse. *J Consult Psychol*. 1967;31:38–47.
4. Gurman AS, Kniskern DP. Research on marital and family therapy. In: Garfield SL, Bergin AE, eds. *Handbook of Psychotherapy and Behavior Change: An Empirical Analysis*. 2nd ed. Wiley; 1978:817–901.
5. Gurman AS, Kniskern DP. Deterioration in marital and family therapy: empirical, clinical, and conceptual issues. *Fam Process*. 1978;17:3–20.
6. Lebow J, Snyder DK. Couple therapy in the 2020s: current status and emerging developments. *Fam Process*. 2022;61:1359–1385.
7. Berent JE, Jacobson CH. Ethical and legal issues in family and couple therapy. In: Fiese BH, Celano M, Deater-Deckard K, Jouriles EN, Whisman MA, eds. *APA Handbook of Contemporary Family Psychology*. American Psychological Association; 2019:53–68.
8. Cass LK, Thomas CB. *Childhood Pathology and Later Adjustment: The Question of Prediction*. Wiley-Interscience; 1979.
9. Vaillant GE. Book review. *Am J Psychiatry*. 1980;137:387.
10. Haley J. *Leaving Home: The Therapy of Disturbed Young People*. McGraw-Hill; 1980.
11. Scheinkman M. Intimacies: an integrative multicultural framework for couple therapy. *Fam Process*. 2019; 58(3):550–568.
12. Stanton MD. Family therapy for drug abuse. *Paper presented at the National Conference on Marital and Family Therapy Outcome and Process Research*. State of the Science; 1995.
13. McCrady BS et al. Alcohol-focused behavioral couple therapy. *Family Process*. 2016;55(3):443–459.
14. Karpel M. *Evaluating Couples: A Handbook for Practitioners*. WW Norton; 1994.

24 Results: The Outcomes of Couples and Family Therapy

OBJECTIVES FOR THE READER

- To become familiar with the scientific criteria for family psychotherapy research
- To be able to critically review modern studies on the outcomes of family therapy
- To be able to compare the outcomes of family therapy with other therapies and no-treatment conditions
- To be able to formulate clinical generalizations from both process and outcome family therapy data

For easier reading, we emphasize that the descriptors "couples" or "marital" are used nearly interchangeably in this chapter.

INTRODUCTION

Does couples and family therapy work? In this chapter, we provide an overview of the results of family therapy outcome studies. We also present several studies in some detail to give the reader a fuller sense of the designs, problems, and results found in family therapy research and of the criteria used to judge the quality of a research project. Finally, we draw clinical generalizations from this existing research database. These summaries are crucial to be aware of for every family therapist in clinical practice.

OVERVIEW OF PSYCHOTHERAPY OUTCOME RESEARCH
1. Specificity
2. The Difference between Efficacy and Effectiveness
3. The Difference between Qualitative and Quantitative, or Exploratory and Confirmatory, Research
4. The Difference between Process and Outcome Research
WHAT THE STUDIES SHOW?
COUPLES TREATMENTS FOR ADULT DISORDERS
Insight-Oriented Marital Therapy for Marital Distress
Integrative Behavioral Couple Therapy for Marital Distress
Emotionally Focused Couples Therapy for Marital Distress
Behavioral Marital Therapy for Depression
Behavioral Couples Therapy for Alcoholism
Couples Therapy for Posttraumatic Stress Disorder

FAMILY TREATMENTS FOR ADULT DISORDERS
Schizophrenia and Major Mental Illness
Focused Family Therapy for Bipolar Disorder
FAMILY TREATMENTS FOR CHILD AND ADOLESCENT DISORDERS
Brief Strategic Family Therapy for Children and Adolescents with Externalizing Disorders
Functional Family Therapy for Delinquent Adolescents
Multidimensional Family Therapy for Adolescent Substance Abuse
Multisystemic Therapy for Youth at Risk
Functional Family Therapy for Adolescents with Bipolar Disorder
Family-Based Treatment for Anorexia Nervosa
FAMILY INTERVENTIONS FOR MEDICAL ILLNESSES
THE EFFECTIVENESS OF COMBINING MEDICATION AND FAMILY THERAPY
LIMITATIONS OF FAMILY THERAPY
NEGATIVE EFFECTS OF FAMILY THERAPY
INABILITY TO ENGAGE AND PREMATURE TERMINATION OF FAMILY THERAPY
CLINICAL IMPLICATIONS OF DATA FROM COUPLES AND FAMILY THERAPY OUTCOME STUDIES
CLINICAL PRACTICE IMPLICATIONS

OVERVIEW OF PSYCHOTHERAPY OUTCOME RESEARCH

Couples therapy has emerged as the standard of care evidenced-based treatment for marital strain. In 2005 in a large international study, it was found that 70% of therapists treat couples.[1] Couples therapy has now become a mainstay line of treatment and much more common given the increased number of marriages ending in divorce and the higher level of expectations people have for satisfaction in their relationships in the modern day and age.[2] **Studies have shown that family therapy is equal to or better than individual therapy over a wide variety of treatment areas.** In understanding family therapy research, and in thinking about what research can tell us and what it cannot, there are several helpful areas to consider.

1. Specificity

The concept that therapy works is a comforting one, but ultimately the therapist and the therapy consumer (i.e., the patient) need to know what kind of therapy works for what patient under what conditions. This area is difficult to research, and only now are outcome studies addressing it. This research is conducted primarily with between-group studies (e.g., a treatment group and a waiting-list group), but it is difficult to do well, because it requires specificity in treatment with a homogeneous group of people. Although no specific school of therapy has proven more effective in general than others in reasonably large-scale testing, we know from clinical practice that some therapies, or therapists, work better with specific patients. Many patients have gone to multiple therapists before finding one with whom they clicked. It is not clear whether the finding of no differences between modalities is because nonspecific factors in therapy (e.g., personality match) are key, or because we have not been specific enough in matching type of problem with type of therapy.

Because most therapies function at several different levels, it may be that almost all therapies provide a new way of looking at the problem and a set of possible new solutions. We must also consider cost effectiveness, that is, what is the briefest and least expensive way to get the same results? Cost effectiveness will be a key issue in the future as cost containment efforts dominate practice.

2. The Difference between Efficacy and Effectiveness

The classic distinction between efficacy and effectiveness in the public health literature is that "efficacy denotes the degree to which diagnostic and therapeutic procedures used in practice can be supported by scientific evidence of their usefulness under optimum conditions. Whether or not these procedures are applied adequately in practice and whether they produce the intended results when so applied are matters of effectiveness."[3] This has been the ongoing struggle in trying to bring research into everyday clinical practice. In therapy done as part of a research project, subjects are recruited by the researcher and are most often homogeneous in their personal characteristics compared with the heterogeneous kinds of patients treated in clinical therapy.

In clinical research, treatment is usually provided for one focal problem, and people who have multiple issues (e.g., marital conflict with coexisting medical illness or alcoholism) are screened out. Usually, the therapist does one specific type of therapy, often from a manual that restricts the therapist's ability to mix methods. In the clinic or the private office, things are much messier. Patients or clients enter with multiple problems, widely differing in age and culture, and they are often less committed to the process. Treatment tends to be much more variable in length in general clinical practice. Clinicians vary greatly in their experience and are not supervised. They are specifically less likely to use behavioral marital therapy (BMT), the most studied marital and family therapy (MFT) method.

Clinicians in practice often are frustrated by research findings, which seem less applicable to their specific day-to-day needs. They often use the methods with which they personally feel compatible (i.e., those they believe intuitively will work). Clinicians over time seem to become more eclectic as they struggle with complex and multilevel problems. Researchers often feel that clinicians are sloppy thinkers and uninterested in really finding out what works. It is likely that as outcome studies become more comprehensive and widely known, we will begin to see rapprochement.

3. The Difference between Qualitative and Quantitative, or Exploratory and Confirmatory, Research

Qualitative research is used to generate hypotheses—it is exploratory, open ended, and directed more at discovery than confirmation. It involves studying a few cases intensively with in-depth interviewing, audiotapes and videotapes, and observations of therapy through a one-way mirror. It emphasizes context, multiple perspectives, and client perspectives. The researcher is often a participant observer. This research is designed to answer questions about the process of how therapy works. Because of its small sample size, this research cannot be considered confirmatory. Quantitative research is concerned with proving things—which requires data collection and analysis, objectivity, large samples, controlled conditions, and statistical analysis. Quantitative research is the method most of us think of as research. Because conditions must be controlled, this approach differs from office-based clinical work.

Both types of research must be part of the therapeutic endeavor, and the reader of a particular research article must be clear on what each type of research can and cannot do. Meta-analysis is a special type of qualitative research in which the results of studies (usually with small numbers of patients) are pooled and then conclusions are drawn. Of course, the better the quality of each of the studies, the more confident one is of the conclusions drawn.

4. The Difference between Process and Outcome Research

Process research describes the interactions among individuals (i.e., the process), whereas outcome research describes the end result (i.e., the outcome) for the family system and the individuals in the system. In family therapy research, the issues are particularly complex because there are so many variables. We are trying to understand how an entire system changes and to describe that change in order to improve the efficacy of our treatments. Part of the problem in outcome studies of family therapy is determining how one decides the criteria for a good outcome.

For example, in some marital cases, divorce is a good outcome, but few studies have considered that or even defined a good divorce. Another question is whether the outcome is determined only by changes in the presenting problem (which is usually labeled as an individual problem) or by changes in family interaction patterns. Also, if multiple changes are possible, and changes occur but not in the presenting problem, is that a good outcome? For example, if a couple come in because of marital strife, and after therapy they are still unhappy but their parenting skills have improved so that their children are doing better, how do you describe this? If we assume that we are using family therapy because the problem is in some way embedded in the family, then changes in the couple and family interaction are necessary for a good outcome.

WHAT THE STUDIES SHOW?

Every clinician should be prepared to answer the question, "Do couple and family interventions work?" Lebow et al.,[4] in a "clinician's response" to their excellent review of the literature, contends that couples therapy works:

> Distressed couples enter treatment demoralized about their relationships. This state of demoralization with which couples enter treatment often leads to questions of "Can this relationship be helped?" The data from research allow for a strong and unambiguous answer: "Yes, you may not feel hopeful now but three of four couples who complete therapy do emerge much happier in their relationship." In a world in which increasingly people want evidence to make realistic appraisals of their present circumstance, the evidence is available that most treatment helps and that distressed relationships can and do improve.

To make sense of the current research on treatment efficacy, it is helpful to examine the first wave of couples and family outcome studies, summarized by Shadish et al.,[5] who looked at 163 randomized studies (62 couples therapy and 101 family therapy). They found that:

1. Family treatment was more effective than no treatment. This conclusion is manifest in studies that contrast family and marital treatment to no-treatment control groups. Roughly 67% of marital cases and 70% of family cases improved. The outcome was slightly better if the identified patient is a child or an adolescent than if they were an adult, and no one therapeutic method was demonstrated clearly to be better than another.
2. The deterioration rate (i.e., the percentage of patients who become worse or experience negative effects of therapy) was estimated at about 10%—lower than for individual. Pinsof and Wynne[6] believed the rate was lower than 5% to 10% and described family therapy as not harmful.
3. In some areas (e.g., schizophrenia, depressed women in distressed marriages, marital distress, alcoholism, anorexia nervosa), evidence indicated that family treatment was the preferred intervention strategy. In other areas, marital/family therapy and individual therapy were equally efficacious—often in situations in which the identified patient had a serious Axis I problem.

More recently, Shadish and Baldwin[7] reviewed six previous meta-analyses of couples therapy and found that a couple receiving treatment is better off than 80% of couples who did not receive treatment. It is important to note that marital distress does not seem to improve without treatment.[8] In a German study, Klann et al.[9] found improved ratings of marital satisfaction after couples therapy. Carr[10] also highlighted the effectiveness of family therapy and systemic interventions for a range of adult-centered problems. Snyder and Halford[11] show that couple therapy produces large and clinically significant effects for both relationship distress as well as couples dealing with physical health problems. Current research has displayed that couples therapy is very effective in improving relationship satisfaction in the short term.[12] Finally, summarizing most up to date couples treatment research, Lebow et al.[4] report that couples therapy has an impact, with roughly 70% of cases showing improvement.

COUPLES TREATMENTS FOR ADULT DISORDERS

While Lebow et al.[4] comment that couples and family therapies work is borne out by these large-scale studies, clinicians often wonder about the efficacy of specific approaches that have been tailored to treat specific populations. While it is impossible to provide a thorough review that summarizes every study, the following section offers an overview of the most current findings in the field.

Insight-Oriented Marital Therapy for Marital Distress

Snyder et al.[13,14] compared their insight-oriented approach to couples therapy, focusing on examining the developmental sources of relationship distress and affective reconstruction, with a traditional behavioral approach emphasizing communication skills training and behavior exchange techniques. After approximately 20 sessions, couples in both treatment modalities showed statistically and clinically significant gains in relationship satisfaction compared to a wait-list control group. However, at 4 years following treatment, 38% of the behavioral couples had experienced divorce compared to only 3% of couples treated in the insight-oriented condition. These findings suggest that once individuals examine and resolve emotional conflicts from their own family and relationship histories, the risk of subsequent relationship dissolution decreases. These studies have not yet been replicated.

Integrative Behavioral Couple Therapy for Marital Distress

Developed by Christenson and Jacobson,[15] integrative behavioral couple therapy (IBCT) integrates goals of both acceptance and change as positive outcomes for couples in therapy. In other words, couples who succeed in therapy usually make some concrete changes to accommodate the needs of the other but they also show greater emotional acceptance of the other. IBCT integrates a variety of treatment strategies under a consistent behavioral theoretical framework. In a study of 134 distressed couples, both IBCT and traditional behavioral couple therapy (TBCT) produced clinically significant change at posttreatment, 71% of IBCT, 59% of TBCT couples reliably improved or recovered.[16] Throughout treatment, TBCT improved more quickly but plateaued while IBCT produced slower yet stable change. At 2-year follow-up, both IBCT and TBCT produced lasting clinical changes, although IBCT was statistically superior.[17] However, at 5 years, clinically significant changes were maintained but differences between IBCT and TBCT disappeared.[18]

Emotionally Focused Couples Therapy for Marital Distress

Emotionally focused couples therapy (EFT) was originally developed by Johnson and Greenberg,[19] and this approach emphasizes emotional regulation and attachment theory to understand what is happening in couple relationships and to guide therapists in helping couples improve their functioning. In a study examining the effectiveness of emotionally focused therapy using a within-subject design in which couples were placed in both the experimental condition and the control condition, couples experienced significant changes in adjustment, intimacy, complaint reduction, and goal attainment after receiving the eight-session treatment. Johnson et al.[20]

conducted a meta-analytic study of EFT looking at EFT's efficacy on treating marital discord, and Johnson and Wittenborn[21] summarized past and most recent research that supports EFT. They found that 70% to 75% of couples move from distress to recovery and approximately 90% show significant improvements.

Behavioral Marital Therapy for Depression

O'Leary and Beach[22] showed in a randomized controlled trial (RCT) that cognitive behavioral therapy (CBT) and BMT were equally effective for women at reducing depressive symptoms, BMT was more effective in improving relationship quality. Beach et al.[23] examined the utility of marital therapy in the treatment of depression and concluded that BMT is a viable and useful form of intervention for a substantial subpopulation of depressed persons. Barbato and D'Avanzo[24] conducted a meta-analysis of clinical trials of couple therapy for depression in which the authors reviewed eight controlled trials. Here again, couple therapy and individual therapy appeared to be equally effective for addressing depressive symptoms, while couple therapy significantly reduced relationship distress. Finally, Whisman and Beach[25] take the reader through their cognitive behavioral-based, three-stage therapy, which focuses on psychoeducation about depression, decreasing negative and increasing positive interactions, teaching communication skills, exploring the role of criticism, and emphasizing relapse prevention. This study outlines an approach to therapy for couples who are experiencing marital discord and at least one of the partners is depressed.

Behavioral Couples Therapy for Alcoholism

O'Farrell et al.[26] showed that for alcoholism, behavioral couples therapy is effective in reducing alcohol use as well as having positive effects on the spousal relationship, specifically reducing family violence. For alcoholics in remission, the prevalence of violence dropped to about 12%, nearly identical to the comparison group. Behavioral couples therapy establishes a daily "sobriety contract" with the patient and spouse in which the patient states their intent not to drink or use drugs, and the spouse expresses support for the patient's efforts to stay abstinent. Behavioral couples therapy also teaches communication skills and increases positive activities.

O'Farrell et al.[26] also found that partner violence before and after behavioral couples therapy. They found that before BCT, 60% of alcoholic patients were violent to their female partners. After 1 to 2 years of BCT, violence decreased significantly. Violence still decreased even if patients remitted into alcoholism after BCT. Powers et al.[27] found in their meta-analysis on 12 RCTs that BCT has better outcomes than controls across domains including relationship satisfaction, frequency of substance use, and consequences of use.

Couples Therapy for Posttraumatic Stress Disorder

Monson's cognitive behavioral conjoint therapy (CBCT) for posttraumatic stress disorder (PTSD) has shown promise in reducing the symptoms of PTSD while also improving relationship satisfaction.[28,29] Forty couples were randomly assigned to undergo immediate CBCT treatment or to a wait-list control condition. In the study, 40 couples were selected in Boston and Toronto, with one partner in each study diagnosed with PTSD. Half of the couples received treatment (CBCT) while the other half remained on a waiting list. After the 15 sessions, the couples who received the therapy showed significant improvement across multiple measures: clinician-rated PTSD symptom severity, intimate relationship satisfaction, and partner and patient ratings of PTSD.[29] The effects of the treatment, when tested 3 months later, still existed. The findings of this study seem to be reliable, especially because of the diversity of the participant pool. The patients reflected different genders, trauma experiences, and sexual orientations.

Strategic approach therapy (SAT)[30] is a 10-session manualized BCT which targets avoidance/numbing symptoms of PTSD. Sautter et al.[30] initially demonstrated that significant improvements in avoidance/numbing symptoms of PTSD were reported by the clinician, partner, and veteran, as well as veteran self-reported total PTSD symptoms, but not for reexperiencing or hyperarousal symptoms. IBCT for combat veterans with PTSD was able to decrease relationship conflict and experiential avoidance.[31] Finally, Johnson and Williams-Keeler[32] conducted a study of emotionally focused couple therapy with a small sample of couples in which one partner had a history of child sexual abuse, and EFT resulted in increased marital satisfaction and decreased PTSD symptoms.

FAMILY TREATMENTS FOR ADULT DISORDERS

Schizophrenia and Major Mental Illness

McFarlane et al.[33] reviewed how family psychoeducation has emerged as a treatment of choice for schizophrenia, bipolar disorder, major depression, and other disorders. More than 30 randomized clinical trials have demonstrated reduced relapse rates, improved recovery of patients, and improved family well-being among participants. Interventions common to effective family psychoeducation programs have been developed, including empathic engagement, education, ongoing support, clinical resources during periods of crisis, social network enhancement, and problem-solving and communication skills. Jewell et al.[34] looked at whether multiple-family groups (MFG) therapy were effective for treating patients with schizophrenia in comparison to single-family treatment. Results showed that overall, the MFG therapies were much more effective, especially in patients with higher risk for relapse. In an RCT, Breitborde et al.[35] showed that MFG psychoeducation reduced relapse rates among individuals with first-episode psychosis. However, given the cognitive demands associated with participating in this intervention, the cognitive deficits that accompany psychotic disorders may limit the ability of certain individuals to benefit from this treatment.

Focused Family Therapy for Bipolar Disorder

With regard to bipolar disorder, the results of including family interventions are more varied. An RCT of focused family therapy versus pharmacotherapy alone was conducted among 101 patients with bipolar disorder. Focused family therapy[36] was effective in preventing depressive but not manic relapse. The patients were assigned to 21 sessions of focused family therapy over 9 months or to a comparison treatment of two family education sessions and crisis management. Both groups received pharmacotherapy. The patients receiving focused family therapy had a significantly better outcome at 1 year (71%) than those receiving crisis management help alone (47%). Results show that family-focused treatment (FFT) subjects had fewer relapses and longer periods between relapses. Moreover, FFT helped increase drug adherence in patients and helps increase the frequency of positive communication between family members. At the same time, the study showed that the frequency of negative communication between family members did not vary between the two types of therapies. This study is important because it helps further show that family-focused therapy can have positive effects on bipolar I patients. Moreover, the study suggests that these positive results are related to better drug adherence and more positive family communications.

Miklowitz[37] showed in an RCT that FFT helps decrease relapse rates in patients with bipolar disorder. The results are notable because patients in all three psychotherapy groups showed improvements and did much better compared to the collaborative care group. However, it is important to note that results between the three psychotherapy groups were not statistically different, thus suggesting that other forms of therapy, not just FFT, are beneficial to bipolar disorder patients.

FAMILY TREATMENTS FOR CHILD AND ADOLESCENT DISORDERS

Emotional and behavioral symptoms and disorders are prevalent in children and adolescents. There has been a burgeoning literature supporting evidence-based treatments for these disorders. Increasingly, family-based interventions have been gaining prominence and demonstrating effectiveness for myriad childhood and adolescent disorders. Carr[38] reviewed the noteworthy effectiveness of family therapy and systemic interventions for a range of child-focused problems. In a review of studies looking at the treatment of internalizing disorders (including mood disorders, eating disorders, and psychological factors in somatic illness), Retzlaff et al.[39] summarized 38 trials, in which 33 showed that family or systemic therapy to be efficacious. There is some evidence for ST being also efficacious in mixed disorders, anxiety disorders, Asperger disorder, and in cases of child neglect. Results were stable across follow-up periods of up to 5 years.

Von Sydow et al.[40] also reviewed current studies looking at the efficacy of systemic therapy for externalizing disorders. A total of 42 trials showed systemic therapy to be efficacious for the treatment of attention-deficit/hyperactivity disorders (ADHDs), conduct disorders, and substance use disorders. Results were stable across follow-up periods of up to 14 years. There is a sound evidence base for the efficacy of systemic therapy for children and adolescents (and their families) diagnosed with externalizing disorders.

Brief Strategic Family Therapy for Children and Adolescents with Externalizing Disorders

Szapocznik et al.[41] compared three treatment conditions (brief strategic family therapy [BSFT], psychodynamic child therapy, and control) in their effectiveness of retention as well as the reduction of behavioral and emotional problems in children with emotional and behavioral problems. The results suggest that BSFT and psychodynamic child therapy are equally effective in retaining cases, reducing behavioral and emotional problems, and improving child functioning. At 1-year follow-up, BSFT was more effective than psychodynamic child therapy in protecting the integrity of the family. Santisteban et al.[42] investigated the efficacy of BSFT with Hispanic behavior problem and drug using youth. One hundred and twenty six Hispanic families participated in the study, and randomized into BSFT or group treatment control. Results showed that BSFT cases showed significantly greater improvement in the following areas: parent reports of adolescent conduct problems and delinquency, adolescent reports of marijuana use, and observer ratings and self-reports of family functioning.

Functional Family Therapy for Delinquent Adolescents

Sexton and Turner[43] showed that functional family therapy administered by highly adherent therapists was much more effective in reducing crime rates and recidivism, as compared to other comparable therapies. In addition, highly adherent therapists had a significantly lower rate of recidivism than low adherent therapists, and there was a significant interaction between youth risk level and adherence level, showing that functional family therapy was more successful for at-risk youth if therapists adhered to the treatment protocol.

Multidimensional Family Therapy for Adolescent Substance Abuse

Liddle et al.[44] conducted an RCT of multidimensional family therapy (MDFT) with marijuana- and alcohol-abusing adolescents and showed that participants in the MDFT group has superior improvement over participants in the other two approaches—adolescent group therapy (AGT) and multifamily educational intervention (MEI). In an RCT, Liddle et al.[45] compared MDFT to a peer group intervention. MDFT demonstrated superior effectiveness over the 12-month follow-up in reducing substance use, substance use problems, and in reducing risk in family, peer, and school domains among young adolescents. Liddle et al.[46] also compared CBT to MDFT and demonstrated that substance use-related problem severity decreased from intake through the 12-month follow-up period regardless of treatment. Fewer substance use-related problems were reported by MDFT participants than by CBT participants at the 6-month follow-ups.

Multisystemic Therapy for Youth at Risk

Henggeler and Sheidow[47] looked at multisystemic therapy (MST) and other empirically supported, family-based treatments (FBTs) for conduct disorder. These treatments include functional family therapy, multidimensional treatment foster care, and BSFT. In addition to summarizing the clinical and theoretical basis for these treatments, the authors highlight the empirical research for each, including mechanisms of change and long-term outcomes. This article is highly recommended, as it provides a clear overview of the main, contemporary treatments for conduct disorder, exploring their foundations, theories, and efficacy.

Functional Family Therapy for Adolescents with Bipolar Disorder

Miklowitz et al.[48] described the family-focused treatment for bipolar adolescents (FFT-A). The authors provided research background of FFT and then presented how FFT is applied to teens with bipolar. Authors identified early onset bipolar as a major public health hazard as it is highly associated with suicide, hospitalization, substance use, and conduct disorder. While pharmacotherapy is the cornerstone of treatment for bipolar youth, adherence to medication is low. FFT is developed as an adjunctive psychosocial treatment to address family environmental factors that are correlated with the course of mood disorders. Authors provided a comprehensive overview of the selection criteria, goals, structures, and modules for FFT-A. Additionally, the article includes the result of a 1-year open trial of FFT-A and pharmacotherapy for adolescent bipolar patients and their families which shows an outcome of 38% of improvement on the K-SAD depression subscale from baseline to 12-month follow-up and 46% improvement on the mania subscales. Authors proposed future research on identifying mediating and moderating mechanisms to refine existing treatment and increase the duration of the effect.

Family-Based Treatment for Anorexia Nervosa

Lock et al.[49] found FBT as effective for children as for adolescents. Lock et al.[50] compared FBT with adolescent-focused individual therapy for adolescents with anorexia nervosa and showed improvement over alternative treatment. Loeb and le Grange[51] summarized FBT for both anorexia and bulimia nervosa, reviewing the history, core elements, and key findings for each treatment. Also notable are the clinical questions and controversies addressed, including whether FBT is clinically appropriate for all adolescents (e.g., older adolescents, patients with comorbid conditions) and whether it can be indicated for all types of families (e.g., critical, enmeshed, and nonintact families).

FAMILY INTERVENTIONS FOR MEDICAL ILLNESSES

Family interventions in medical illnesses are of benefit to patients and their family members although the effect size is small.[52] Three meta-analyses that assessed RCT and required a treatment as usual comparison have been completed. In the first, family interventions improved patient mortality in five studies.[53] In the second meta-analysis, family interventions resulted in improved patient health.[54] The effect size was small (odds ratio [OR] of 1.72 to 1.84), but stable, across 52 RCTs. This means that patients had a 72% to 84% higher chance of improved health, with the intervention. Overall, there were higher effect sizes for relationship-focused interventions than for psychoeducational interventions. Family members showed improved outcome in 18 studies (OR 1.84), with improved physical health, less caregiver burden, anxiety, etc. A third meta-analysis reviewed 25 couples interventions.[55] The interventions resulted in reduced patient depression, enhanced marital functioning and reduced perception of pain. Couples interventions were more successful than psychoeducational interventions. More refined research is needed in developing family interventions for medical illnesses. Many studies did not take into account the life stage of the family or the individual, nor the stage of illness.

In that context, Shields et al.[56] reviewed how intervention research for couples and families managing chronic health problems remains at an early developmental stage. Randomized clinical trials of family interventions conducted for common neurologic diseases, cardiovascular diseases, cancer, and diabetes have tended to be time-limited therapeutic interventions that trained families to improve their communication and problem-solving skills, individual and family coping skills, and medical management. Family interventions show promise to help patients and family members manage chronic illnesses.

THE EFFECTIVENESS OF COMBINING MEDICATION AND FAMILY THERAPY

Research continues to show the efficacy of combining medication with family interventions in a number of disorders. In their review of three meta-analysis of psychoeducational family therapy for schizophrenia, Pfammatter et al.[57] found that compared with medication alone, multimodal programs which included psychoeducational family therapy and antipsychotic medication led to lower relapse and rehospitalization rates, and improved medication adherence. In a comparative study of depressed inpatients, Miller et al.[58] found that family therapy combined with antidepressant medication led to more rapid recovery and a higher improvement rate than antidepressants combined with cognitive therapy. In a comparative trial of depressed inpatients, Lemmens et al.[59] found that when offered to single families, or in multifamily groups, systemic couples therapy (with some additional family sessions involving children) combined with antidepressant medication led to a significantly higher rate of treatment responders and to fewer patients being on antidepressants at 15-month follow-up, compared with standard treatment.

LIMITATIONS OF FAMILY THERAPY

Not all problems are the result of problematic patterns in the family. In many families, the overall family structure and function are relatively healthy; nevertheless, one member has a problem that affects other family members. Patterns emerge, in turn, that can maintain the original problem. Consider the following case example:

> *Mrs. A is a 48-year-old patient who came in with her husband and four children seeking therapy. She said that her parents died in a plane crash when she was 1 year old. Throughout her life she was raised by a series of adoptive parents and relatives. Each time one of her adoptive parents left the family, for example, when an adoptive father was drafted into the army, she would become very depressed, tearful, and angry, blaming other family members for their various deficiencies.*
>
> *Family therapy was sought at this time because the family was having trouble living with Mrs. A in her depressed state—a problem that had been present for 30 years. The family therapist's task was to see what could be changed. It turned out that the precipitant was the oldest daughter going away to college. The family therapist helped the mother and the rest of the family cope with the derivatives of the mother's classical separation experience (i.e., loss of the parents at an early age as it now affected the family structure). The family therapist could not change*

> *the fact that the mother would have a strong and dysfunctional reaction to loss, but she could help the children understand it was not their fault and keep Mrs. A's husband from becoming angry and absent.*

The family therapist commonly assumes that when a family comes for help with a specific problem, the cause is generally found in system problems of a more serious nature. It follows that the treatment strategy is to treat the system. The assumption is that treating the system will cause the symptom to change. Treating the system and even changing the system to function better does not necessarily mean that all symptoms in the family will improve. In practice, some symptoms will be left untreated. The degree of improvement varies from family to family. Framo[60] has written from long experience in the field.

> *Now that I have a more sober appreciation of clients' fears, of the complexities and difficulties involved, of the potential pitfalls, of the hard realities of intergenerational work—I have toned down my enthusiasm. For instance, I now caution that the sessions are not likely to change people's lives drastically, and I moderate some clients' unrealistic expectations about what the sessions can accomplish. For example, clients need to be prepared for not being able to fulfill fantasies of what they can get from parents or siblings.*

What are the variables that limit change in families? To the extent that families or couples have not been able to cope with and master previous stages of development, they may have limitations in coping with a current phase. Other limiting factors include the degree of rigidity of chronic character traits; the couple's style (e.g., are they "screamers" or "compromisers"); and biologic, physical, and social variables. As Snyder and Halford[11] report, 25% to 30% of couples show no benefit from couples therapy.

NEGATIVE EFFECTS OF FAMILY THERAPY

Any treatment that induces beneficial results must also be capable of producing harmful effects.[61] Although not a great deal has been written about this subject in family therapy literature, most experienced clinicians would agree that family therapy can sometimes induce negative effects. Table 24.1 expands on the following five categories of negative effects.

1. **Exacerbation of presenting symptoms during or after treatment.** In most cases, there is a phase of family therapy in which problems may worsen.
2. **Appearance of new symptoms in another family member.** All members do not benefit equally. For example, if the mother challenges the father, he may become depressed. New symptoms may occur in a family member other than the identified patient.
3. **Patient abuse or misuse of therapy.** Most commonly one family member tries to use the family therapy for one-upmanship. For example, the father might say, "the doctor said that I seemed to have the best judgment in the family," and then proceed to blast his spouse and children.
4. **The family's overreaching itself.** Some therapists believe that anything is possible and encourage families to attempt tasks and try for goals that clearly are beyond their reach. Such attempts are destructive and should be avoided.
5. **Disillusionment with the therapy, the therapist, or both.** The family may try family therapy as a last resort. When the therapy does not produce beneficial change (at least in the family's terms), the family may be worse than at the start, because the members have lost their last hope.
6. As we mentioned earlier in this chapter, the precise incidence of negative effects resulting from family therapy is not known, but it probably occurs in 5% to 10% of all cases.

Table 24.1 What constitutes a negative effect?

Exacerbation of presenting symptoms	Appearance of new symptoms	Patient's abuse or misuse of therapy	Patient "overreaching" self	Disillusionment with therapy or therapist
1. "Worsening," increase in severity, pathology, etc.	1. *Generally* may be observed when a. psychic disturbance is manifested in a less socially acceptable form than previously b. symptom substitution occurs when a symptom that had fulfilled an imperative need is blocked	1. Substitution of intellectualized insights for other obsessional thoughts	1. Two forms: a. undertaking life tasks (marriage, graduate school, etc.) that require resources beyond those of patient b. undertaking life tasks prematurely	May appear variously as a. wasting of patient's resources (time, skill, money) that might have been better expended elsewhere b. hardening of attitudes toward other sources of help c. loss of confidence in therapist, possibly extending to any human relationship general loss of hope, all the more severe for initial raising of hopes that may have occurred at onset of therapy
2. *Generally* may take form of or be accompanied by a. exacerbation of suffering b. decompensation c. harsher superego or more rigid personality structure	2. *Specific* examples a. erosion of solid interpersonal relationships b. decreased ability to experience pleasure c. severe or fatal psychosomatic reactions d. withdrawal e. rage f. dissociation g. drug/alcohol abuse h. criminal behavior i. suicide j. psychotic breaks	2. Utilization of therapy to rationalize feelings of superiority or expressions of hostility toward other people	2. May be related to a. intense wishes to please therapist b. inculcation of unachievable middle-class "ideals" c. increased "irrational" ideas	

3. *Specific* examples of symptom exacerbation a. depressive breakdown b. severe regression c. destructive acting-out d. increased anxiety e. increased hostility f. increased self-doubting g. increased behavioral shirking h. increased inhibition i. paranoia j. fixing of obsessional symptoms k. exaggeration of somatic difficulties l. extension of phobias m. increased guilt n. increased confusion o. lowered self-confidence p. lowered self-esteem q. diminished capacity for delay and impulse control		3. Therapy becomes an end in itself; a substitute for action	3. May result in any or all of the following: a. excessive strain on patient's psychological resources b. failure at task c. guilt self-contempt	
		4. Fear of "intellectualization" prevents patients from examining their ethical and philosophical commitments 5. Participation in more radical therapies encourages belief in irrationality in order to avoid painful confrontation with realities of life 6. Sustained dependency on therapy or therapist		

Source: Hadley and Strupp.[61] Reproduced with permission of American Medical Association.

What happens if the outcome of marital treatment is separation or divorce? One might automatically assume that such an outcome is deleterious and that MFT should be designed to hold the families together. On reflection, experience seems to indicate otherwise. **Marital therapy allows the partners to examine whether it is to their advantage to stay together, and it gives them permission to separate if that is what they need to do.**

Dr. and Mrs. B were in their 30s. He was a dentist, she was a homemaker who had previously been a teacher. Mrs. B described her father as a philanderer, and she married her husband because he appeared to be reliable and stable. Dr. B described his mother as dull and masochistic, and he married his wife because she seemed exciting and interesting.

The couple came to therapy after 5 years of marriage, when Mrs. B discovered that Dr. B was having extramarital affairs. (He had left several notes from girlfriends lying around the house.) Exploration of the situation revealed that soon after marriage Mrs. B had become slowly and imperceptibly disillusioned with her husband when she found that he was very insecure about himself, was very unreliable, and characteristically lied and cheated. Dr. B perceived after a few years that his wife was not as exciting as he had thought and would not fulfill the role he had envisioned for her—that is, being enslaved to her professional husband.

The therapy allowed the couple to examine some of the original premises on which they had gotten together, and they found them faulty. The process of therapy, and not the therapist's values, gave them the necessary permission to separate.

INABILITY TO ENGAGE AND PREMATURE TERMINATION OF FAMILY THERAPY

The dropout rate in the early phases of family therapy is relatively high.[62] In one study, about 30% of all the families referred for family therapy failed to appear for the first session (so-called defectors) and another 30% terminated in the first three sessions, leaving about 40% who continued.[63] The main reason families gave for termination was a lack of activity on the part of the therapist, whereas defectors in general had a change of heart and denied that a problem existed. The motivation of the husband appeared to play a crucial role—the more motivated he was, the more likely the family was to continue treatment. The few studies that report dropout in couples therapy have reported 35% to 40% dropout by the third session[64] and up to 57% dropout at some point.[65]

Most prior research on the factors that impact dropout has focused on the demographic characteristics of individuals in treatment. Although the pretherapy patient characteristics related to dropout have not been consistent, some serve as indicators of vulnerability to dropout: living a significant distance from the clinic, current illicit drug use, young age, low income, or being an ethnic minority.[66–74] Prior psychiatric hospitalization appeared to decrease the likelihood of dropout.[67] Level of education and number of children appear to have an inconsistent relationship to dropout.[71,74,75]

Nonetheless, there is little question that the therapeutic alliance between a couple or family and therapist is generally understood as a requirement for therapeutic work to proceed[76] and building this alliance is considered a fundamental task of early therapy.[77] Therapist behavior is thought to influence alliance, and dropout is a problem for the clients who continue to suffer, miss appointments, and squander scarce mental health resources.[62,68,78–80] Weak alliance and increased dropout have been linked by both theory and prior research.[81–83] Weak alliance has been associated with higher dropout rates for individuals in therapy,[69,72,84] and for couples in conjoint alcoholism treatment.[85] Knobloch-Fedders et al.[65] analyzed husbands as a group and wives as a group and found lower alliances at session 1 for couples who left treatment by session 8.

Catherall,[86] Pinsof, and Wynne,[6] and Pinsof et al.[87] first proposed that a "split," a significant difference between each partner's assessment of alliance, could be detrimental to success in couples therapy. As groups, men and women have rated alliance similarly, however when specific husband–wife pairs are compared, spouses often differ.[65,88] In family therapy, Robbins et al.[89] found that imbalances between adolescent–therapist and parent–therapist alliances were more prevalent in those families that dropped out of treatment. Preliminary evidence suggests that differences, including differences defined here as split relate to outcome.[86] Furthermore, Symonds and Horvath[90] concluded that agreement about the alliance was more important than strength of the alliance for positive outcome.

CLINICAL IMPLICATIONS OF DATA FROM COUPLES AND FAMILY THERAPY OUTCOME STUDIES

We return to the clinical implications of the data that emerge from couples and family research studies and consider the thoughtful review by Lebow et al.[4] as well as Pinsof and Wynne's[6] overview. Both focused on the research data for the family therapist. We present the following important implications for family therapists.

The following conclusions are based on an overview of the field of MFT research primarily as presented in the articles in this Special Issue. These conclusions are provisional—the field of MFT research is not ready for definitive conclusions at this stage of its development. Even though a considerable body of empirical evidence has been accumulated, most of the findings have not been replicated systematically. Additionally, even though the field has made great progress, many methodologic problems still plague the research and hinder the accumulation of a coherent and clear body of knowledge about the efficacy and effectiveness of MFT. A strong conclusion requires confirmation from at least two controlled studies.[6]

1. MFT works. A clear and consistent body of evidence has been accumulated and reviewed that indicates that MFT (MT/FT) is significantly and clinically more efficacious than no psychotherapy for the following patients, disorders, and problems: adults schizophrenia (FT); outpatient depressed women in distressed marriages (MT); marital distress and conflict (MT): adult alcoholism and drug abuse (FT/MT); adult hypertension (MT); elderly dementia (FT); anorexia in young adolescent girls (FT); adolescent drug abuse (FT); child conduct disorders (FT); aggression and noncompliance in ADHD children (FT); childhood autism (FT); chronic physical illnesses in children (asthma, diabetes, etc.) (FT); child obesity (FT); and cardiovascular risk factors in children (FT).
2. MFT is not harmful. MFT does not appear to have negative or destructive effects. In all of the research reviewed, there has not been one replicated and controlled study in which patients and families receiving family or marital therapy had poorer outcomes than patients receiving no therapy.
3. MFT is more efficacious than standard and/or individual treatments for the following patients, disorders, and problems: adult schizophrenia; depressed outpatient women in distressed marriages; marital distress; adult alcoholism and drug abuse; adolescent conduct disorders; adolescent drug abuse; anorexia in young adolescent females; childhood autism; and various chronic physical illnesses in adults and children. Additionally, involving the family in engaging alcoholic adults in treatment is more efficacious than just working with the individual adults. Similarly, family involvement in aftercare for alcoholic adults is more efficacious than standard individual or group aftercare.
4. There are no scientific data at this time to support the superiority of any particular form of marital or family therapy over any other. The meta-analyses of MFT, when controlled from methodologic confounds, failed to reveal any consistent effects of one type of MFT over another. Similarly, reviews do not reveal any consistent effects of one MFT approach over any other. The one trend and very preliminary hypothesis that emerged fairly consistently is that treatments that combined conventional family or marital therapy sessions with

other interventions were more efficacious than standard family therapy approaches alone for severe disorders. It is premature to draw firm conclusions from this trend since it has not been formally tested in replicated controlled trials.

5. Data from a small number of studies indicate that MFT is more cost effective than standard inpatient and/or residential treatment/placement for schizophrenia and severe adolescent conduct disorders and delinquency. There are some preliminary data that suggest it is more cost effective than alternative treatments for adult alcoholism and adult and adolescent drug abuse. From the perspective of the health care providers and managed care, marital and family therapies may be more cost effective than individual treatments in that more clients or patients are treated by a therapist in a single session. Additionally, the broader systemic focus of many marital and family therapies means that the therapist is focused not only on the mental and physical health of the individual client but also on the health of the other family members. This broader scope of concern theoretically expands the impact of MFT.
6. MFT is not sufficient in itself to treat effectively a variety of severe disorders and problems. More than half of the treatments that have demonstrated efficacy involve components that go beyond the standard and conventional "family therapy session" format of MFT.

Similarly, the most effective treatments for childhood autism, severe adolescent conduct disorders, adult and adolescent drug abuse, and adult alcoholism involve additional treatment (group and/or individual and/or medication) and education components.

The research on these problems and treatments suggests that family involvement is a critical and necessary component in the treatment of these problems but is not sufficient in itself. An emerging hypothesis from these data is that multicomponent, integrative, and problem-focused treatments may be necessary to treat severe behavioral disorders effectively in adults, adolescents, and children. In fact, the more severe, pervasive, and disruptive the disorder, the greater the need to include multiple components in effective treatments.

CLINICAL PRACTICE IMPLICATIONS

Outcome research has continued to elucidate indications and contraindications for family treatment, the clinician has a much better idea of when to do what now than they did in the past. A reason for continuing the push for treatment assessment is that the public is demanding proof of the efficacy of all psychotherapies. Because we practice in a more cost- and evidence-oriented health care environment, every mental health clinician should be able to respond to queries about whether couple and family interventions have demonstrated efficacy. We believe the implication for the family therapist is that the day is approaching when third-party payers will attempt to reimburse for only those treatments demonstrating efficacy.

REFERENCES

1. Orlinsky DE, Rønnestad MH, Ambühl H. *How Psychotherapists Develop: A Study of Therapeutic Work and Profession Growth*. American Psychological Association; 2005.
2. Cherlin AJ. *The Marriage-go-around: The State of Marriage and the Family in America Today*. Vintage Books; 2009.
3. Starfield B. Is strong primary care good for health outcomes? In: Griffin J, ed. *The Future of Primary Care: Papers for a Symposium Held on 13th September 1995*. Office of Health Economics; 1996:18–29.
4. Lebow J, Snyder DK. Couple therapy in the 2020s: current status and emerging developments. *Fam Process*. 2022;61:1359–1385.
5. Shadish W, Ragsdale K, Glaser R, Montgomery L. The efficacy and effectiveness of marital and family therapy: a perspective from meta-analysis. *J Marital Fam Ther*. 1995;21:345–360.
6. Pinsof W, Wynne L. The efficacy of marital and family therapy: an empirical overview, conclusions, and recommendations. *J Marital Fam Ther*. 1995;21:585–613.
7. Shadish W, Baldwin S. Meta-analysis of MFT interventions. *J Marital Fam Ther*. 2003;29:547–570.

8. Baucom D, Hahlweg K, Kuschel A. Are waiting-list control groups needed in future marital therapy outcome research? *Behav Ther.* 2003;34:179–188.
9. Klann N, Hahlweg K, Baucom D, Kroeger C. The effectiveness of couple therapy in Germany. *J Marital Fam Ther.* 2009;35:1–9.
10. Carr A. The effectiveness of family therapy and systemic interventions for adult-focused problems. *J Fam Ther.* 2009;31:46–74.
11. Snyder DK, Halford WK. Evidence-based couple therapy: current status and future directions. *J Fam Ther.* 2012;34:229–249.
12. Bradbury TN, Bodenmann G. Interventions for couples. *Annu Rev Clin Psychol.* 2020;16:99–123.
13. Snyder D, Wills R. Behavioral versus insight-oriented marital therapy: effects on individual and interspousal functioning. *J Consult Clin Psychol.* 1989;57:39–46.
14. Snyder D, Wills R, Grady-Fletcher A. Long-term effectiveness of behavioral versus insight-oriented marital therapy: a 4-year follow-up study. *J Consult Clin Psychol.* 1991;59:138–141.
15. Christensen A, Doss BD, Jacobson N. *Integrative Behavioral Couple Therapy: A Therapist's Guide to Creating Acceptance and Change.* 2nd ed. W. W. Norton; 2020.
16. Christensen A, Atkins D, Berns S, Wheeler J, Baucom DH, Simpson LE. Traditional versus integrative behavioral couple therapy for significantly and chronically distressed married couples. *J Consult Clin Psychol.* 2004;72:176–191.
17. Christensen A, Atkins D, Yi J, Baucom DH, George WH. Couple and individual adjustment for 2 years following a randomized clinical trial comparing traditional versus integrative behavioral couples therapy. *J Consult Clin Psychol.* 2006;74:1180–1191.
18. Christensen A, Atkins DC, Baucom B, Yi J. Marital status and satisfaction five years following a randomized clinical trial comparing traditional versus integrative behavioral couple therapy. *J Consult Clin Psychol.* 2010;78:225–235.
19. Johnson S, Greenberg L. Emotionally focused couples therapy: an outcome study. *J Marital Fam Ther.* 1985; 11:313–317.
20. Johnson S, Hunsley J, Greenberg L, Schindler D. Emotionally focused couples therapy: status and challenges. *Clin Psychol Sci Pract.* 1999;6:67–79.
21. Johnson SM, Wittenborn AK. New research findings on emotionally focused therapy: introduction to special section. *J Marital Fam Ther.* 2012;38:18–22.
22. O'Leary K, Beach SR. Marital therapy: a viable treatment. *Am J Psychiatry.* 1990;147:183–186.
23. Beach SRH, Whisman MA, O'Leary D. Marital therapy for depression: theoretical foundation, current status, and future directions. *Behav Ther.* 1994;25:345–371.
24. Barbato A, D'Avanzo B. Efficacy of couple therapy as a treatment for depression: a meta-analysis. *Psychiatr Q.* 2008;79(2):121–132.
25. Whisman MA, Beach SRH. Couple therapy for depression. *J Clin Psychol.* 2012;68:526–535.
26. O'Farrell T, Murphy CM, Stephan S, Fals-Stewart W, Murphy M. Partner violence before and after couples-based alcoholism treatment for male alcoholic patients: the role of treatment involvement and abstinence. *J Consult Clin Psychol.* 2004;72:202–217.
27. Powers M, Vedel E, Emmelkamp PMG. Behavioral couples therapy (BCT) for alcohol and drug use disorders: a meta-analysis. *Clin Psychol Rev.* 2008;28:952–962.
28. Monson C, Schnurr P, Stevens S, Guthrie KA. Cognitive–behavioral couple's treatment for posttraumatic stress disorder: initial findings. *J Trauma Stress.* 2004;17:341–344.
29. Monson C, Fredman S, Macdonald A, Pukay-Martin ND, Resick PA, Schnurr PP. Effect of cognitive-behavioral couple therapy for PTSD: a randomized controlled trial. *JAMA.* 2012;308:700–709.
30. Sautter FJ, Glynn SM, Thompson K, Franklin L, Han X. A couple-based approach to the reduction of PTSD avoidance symptoms: preliminary findings. *J Marital Fam Ther.* 2009;35:343–349.
31. Erbes C, Polusny M, MacDermid S, Compton JS. Couple therapy with combat veterans and their partners. *J Clin Psychol.* 2008;64:972–983.
32. Johnson S, Williams-Keeler L. Creating healing relationships for couples dealing with trauma: the use of emotionally focused marital therapy. *J Marital Fam Ther.* 1998;24:25–40.
33. McFarlane W, Dixon L, Lukens E, Lucksted A. Family psychoeducation and schizophrenia: a review of the literature. *J Marital Fam Ther.* 2003;29:223–245.
34. Jewell TC, Downing D, McFarlane WR. Partnering with families: multiple family group psychoeducation for schizophrenia. *J Clin Psychol.* 2009;65:868–878.
35. Breitborde NJ, Moreno F, Mai-Dixon N, et al. Multifamily group psychoeducation and cognitive remediation for first-episode psychosis: a randomized controlled trial. *BMC Psychiatry.* 2011;11:9.
36. Miklowitz D Adjunctive psychotherapy for bipolar disorder: state of the evidence. *Am J Psychiatry.* 2008; 165:1408–1419.
37. Miklowitz D. The role of the family in the course and treatment of bipolar disorder. *Curr Dir Psychol Sci.* 2007;16:192–196.

38. Carr A. The effectiveness of family therapy and systemic interventions for child-focused problems. *J Fam Ther.* 2009b;31:3–45.
39. Retzlaff R, von Sydow K, Beher S, Haun MW, Schweitzer J. The efficacy of systemic therapy for internalizing and other disorders of childhood and adolescence: a systematic review of 38 randomized trials. *Fam Process.* 2013;52:619–652.
40. Von Sydow K, Retzlaff R, Beher S, Haun MW, Schweitzer J. The efficacy of systemic therapy for childhood and adolescent externalizing disorders: a systematic review of 47 RCT. *Fam Process.* 2013;52:576–618.
41. Szapocznik J, Rio A, Murray E, et al. Structural family versus psychodynamic child therapy for problematic Hispanic boys. *J Consult Clin Psychol.* 1989;57:571–578.
42. Santisteban D, Coatsworth JD, Perez-Vidal A, et al. Efficacy of brief strategic family therapy in modifying Hispanic adolescent behavior problems and substance use. *J Fam Psychol.* 2003;17:121–133.
43. Sexton T, Turner C. The effectiveness of functional family therapy for youth with behavioral problems in a community practice setting. *J Fam Psychol.* 2010;24:339–348.
44. Liddle HA, Dakof GA, Parker K, Diamond GS, Barrett K, Tejeda M. Multidimensional family therapy for adolescent drug abuse: results of a randomized clinical trial. *Am J Drug Alcohol Abuse.* 2001;27:651–688.
45. Liddle H, Rowe C, Dakof G, Henderson CE, Greenbaum PE. Multidimensional family therapy for young adolescent substance abuse: twelve-month outcomes of a randomized controlled trial. *J Consult Clin Psychol.* 2009;77:12–25.
46. Liddle HA, Dakof GA, Turner R, Henderson CE, Greenbaum PE. Treating adolescent drug abuse: a randomized trial comparing multidimensional family therapy and cognitive behavior therapy. *Addiction.* 2008; 103:1660–1670.
47. Henggeler S, Sheidow A. Empirically supported family-based treatments for conduct disorder and delinquency in adolescents. *J Marital Fam Ther.* 2012;38:30–58.
48. Miklowitz D, George E, Axelson D, et al. Family-focused treatment for adolescents with bipolar disorder. *J Affect Disord.* 2004;82:S113–S128.
49. Lock J, Couturier J, Agras WS. Comparison of long-term outcomes in adolescents with anorexia nervosa treated with family therapy. *J Am Acad Child Adolesc Psychiatry.* 2006;45:666–672.
50. Lock J, Le Grange D, Agras WS, Moye A, Bryson SW, Jo B. Randomized clinical trial comparing family-based treatment to adolescent-focused individual therapy for adolescents with anorexia nervosa. *Arch Gen Psychiatry.* 2010;67(10):1025–1032.
51. Loeb K, le Grange D. Family-based treatment for adolescent eating disorders: current status, new applications and future directions. *Int J Child Adolesc Health.* 2009;2:243–254.
52. Heru A. *Working with Families in Medical Settings: A Multidisciplinary Guide for Psychiatrists and Other Health Care Professionals.* Routledge; 2013.
53. Martire L, Lustig A, Schultz R, Miller GE, Helgeson VS. Is it beneficial to involve a family member? A meta-analysis of psychosocial interventions for chronic illness. *Health Psychol.* 2004;23:599–611.
54. Hartmann M, Bäzner E, Wild B, Eisler I, Herzog W. Effects of interventions involving the family in the treatment of adult patients with chronic physical diseases: a meta-analysis. *Psychother Psychosom.* 2010;79:136–148.
55. Martire L, Schultz R, Helgeson V, Small BJ, Saghafi EM. Review and meta-analysis of couple-oriented interventions for chronic illness. *Ann Behav Med.* 2010;40:325–342.
56. Shields C, Finley M, Chawla N, Meadors WP. Couple and family interventions in health problems. *J Marital Fam Ther.* 2012;38:265–280.
57. Pfammatter M, Junghan U, Brenner H. Efficacy of psychological therapy in schizophrenia: conclusions from meta-analyses. *Schizophr Bull.* 2006;32(suppl 1):S64–S80.
58. Miller IW, Solomon DA, Ryan CE, Keitner GI. Does adjunctive family therapy enhance recovery from bipolar I mood episodes? *J Affect Disord.* 2004;82:431–436.
59. Lemmens GMD, Eisler I, Buysse A, Heene E, Demyttenaere K. The effects on mood of adjunctive single-family and multi-family group therapy in the treatment of hospitalized patients with major depression. A 15-month follow-up study. *Psychother Psychosom.* 2009;78:98–105.
60. Framo JL. *Family of Origin Therapy: An Intergenerational Approach.* Brunner/Mazel; 1992:44.
61. Hadley S, Strupp H. Contemporary views of negative effects in psychotherapy. An integrated account. *Arch Gen Psychiatry.* 1976;33:1291–1302.
62. Wolfson AN. *Alliance Patterns Related to Dropout in Couples Therapy.* Boston University; 2007.
63. Shapiro R, Budman S. Defection, termination, and continuation in family and individual therapy. *Fam Process.* 1973;12:55–67.
64. Mamodhoussen S, Wright J, Tremblay N, Poitras-Wright H. Impact of marital and psychological distress on therapeutic alliance in couples undergoing couple therapy. *J Marital Fam Ther.* 2005;31:159–169.
65. Knobloch-Fedders LM, Pinsof WM, Mann BJ. The formation of the therapeutic alliance in couple therapy. *Fam Process.* 2004;43:425–442.
66. Berghofer G, Schmidl F, Rudas S, Steiner E, Schmitz M. Predictors of treatment discontinuity in outpatient mental health care. *Soc Psychiatry Psychiatr Epidemiol.* 2002;37:276–282.

67. Bischoff RJ, Sprenkle DH. Dropping out of marriage and family therapy: a critical review of research. *Fam Process.* 1993;32:353–375.
68. Edlund M, Wang P, Berglund P, Katz SJ, Lin E, Kessler RC. Dropping out of mental health treatment: patterns and predictors among epidemiological survey respondents in the United States and Ontario. *Am J Psychiatry.* 2002;159:845–851.
69. Johansson H, Eklund M. Helping alliance and early dropout from psychiatric out-patient care: the influence of patient factors. *Soc Psychiatry Psychiatr Epidemiol.* 2006;41:140–147.
70. Kadzin A, Stolar M, Marciano P. Risk factors for dropping out of treatment among White and Black families. *J Fam Psychol.* 1995;9:402–417.
71. Le Fave M. Correlates of engagement in family therapy. *J Marital Fam Ther.* 1980;6:75–81.
72. Reis BF, Brown LG. Preventing therapy dropout in the real world: the clinical utility of videotape preparation and client estimate of treatment duration. *Prof Psychol Res Pr.* 2006;37(3):311–316.
73. Tucker J, Davison J. Waiting to see the doctor: the role of time constraints in the utilization of health and behavioral health services. In: Bickel WK, Vuchinich RE, eds. *Reframing Health Behavior Change with Behavioral Economics.* Lawrence Erlbaum Associates; 2000:219–264.
74. Wierzbicki M, Pekarik G. A meta-analysis of psychotherapy dropout. *Prof Psychol Res Pr.* 1993;24:190–195.
75. Allgood S, Crane D. Predicting marital therapy dropouts. *J Marital Fam Ther.* 1991;17:73–79.
76. Gurman A, Jacobson N. *Clinical Handbook of Couple Therapy.* Guilford Press; 2002.
77. Rait D. The therapeutic alliance in couples and family therapy. *J Clin Psychol.* 2000;56:211–224.
78. Hampson R, Prince C, Beavers W. Marital therapy: qualities of couples who fare better or worse in treatment. *J Marital Fam Ther.* 1999;25:411–424.
79. Hansen N, Lambert M, Forman E. The psychotherapy dose-response effect and its implications for treatment delivery services. *Clin Psychol Sci Pract.* 2002;9:329–343.
80. Masi M, Miller R, Olson M. Differences in dropout rates among individual, couple, and family therapy clients. *Contemp Fam Ther.* 2003;25:63–75.
81. Bordin E. The generalizability of the psychoanalytic concept of the working alliance. *Psychother Theory Res Pract.* 1979;16:252–260.
82. Frank E, Kupfer D, Siegel L. Alliance not compliance: a philosophy of outpatient care. *J Clin Psychiatry.* 1995;1:11–6.
83. Makinen JA, Johnson SM. Resolving attachment injuries in couples using emotionally focused therapy: steps toward forgiveness and reconciliation. *J Consult Clin Psychol.* 2006;74(6):1055–1064.
84. Mohl P, Martinez D, Ticknor C, Huang M, Cordell L. Early dropouts from psychotherapy. *J Nerv Ment Dis.* 1991;179:478–481.
85. Raytek H, McCrady B, Epstein E, Hirsch LS. Therapeutic alliance and the retention of couples in conjoint alcoholism treatment. *Addict Behav.* 1999;24:317–330.
86. Catherall D. *The Therapeutic Alliance in Individual, Couple, and Family Therapy.* Northwestern University; 1984.
87. Pinsof W. An integrative systems perspective on the therapeutic alliance: theoretical, clinical, and research implications. In: Horvath AO, Greenberg LS, eds. *The Working Alliance: Theory, Research, and Practice.* John Wiley & Sons; 1994:173–195.
88. Heatherington L, Friedlander ML. Couple and family therapy alliance scales: empirical considerations. *J Marital Fam Ther.* 1990;16:299–306.
89. Robbins M, Liddle H, Turner C, Dakof GA, Alexander JF, Kogan SM. Adolescent and parent therapeutic alliances as predictors of dropout in multidimensional family therapy. *J Fam Psychol.* 2006;20:108–116.
90. Symonds D, Horvath A. Optimizing the alliance in couple therapy. *Fam Process.* 2004;43:443–455.

Section

VIII Ethical, Professional, and Training Issues

25 Ethical and Professional Issues in Couples and Family Therapy 359

25 Ethical and Professional Issues in Couples and Family Therapy

OBJECTIVES FOR THE READER

- To be aware of ethical issues in practicing family therapy
- To be able to use informed consent procedures with a family
- To be aware of the family implications of financial issues
- To be aware of the professional issues inherent in family therapy practice
- To be able to specify family therapy training objectives and an optimal family therapy training program
- To be able to describe political and contextual issues in psychiatry residency training programs

For easier reading, we emphasize that the descriptors "couples" or "marital" are used nearly interchangeably in this chapter.

INTRODUCTION

In this chapter, we pull together material discussed in previous chapters to some of the issues that face family therapists currently. They include ethical, financial, professional, and training issues.

ETHICAL ISSUES INHERENT IN FAMILY THERAPY
Conflicting Interests of Family Members
Understanding HIPAA
Secrets and Confidentiality
Issues Involving Gender, Gender Roles, and Sexuality
Ethics in a Managed Care World
INFORMED CONSENT
FINANCIAL ISSUES
PROFESSIONAL ISSUES
The Problem of Boundaries and Dual Relationships
COMPETENCIES
TRAINING ISSUES
CLINICAL EXPERIENCES
TRAINING PROGRAMS IN FAMILY PSYCHIATRY

A MULTIDISCIPLINARY FIELD
Family Therapy Fellowships
TRAINING AND LICENSURE
CLINICAL PRACTICE IMPLICATIONS

ETHICAL ISSUES INHERENT IN FAMILY THERAPY

The fundamental ethical dilemmas inherent in psychotherapy—confidentiality, limits of control, duty to warn/reporting of abuse, and therapist–patient boundaries—become more complex when the treatment involves more than one person. The family therapist has an ethical responsibility to everyone in the family. In some cases, individual needs and family system needs may be in conflict. For example, a husband may wish to conceal a brief episode of unprotected sex with another woman, whereas his wife is better off, for health and psychological reasons, if she knows about it. A wife's wish to be divorced from a psychiatrically ill and demanding husband may conflict with his need for her care. Such clinical situations provide a set of ethical dilemmas for the therapist.

> The family therapist has an ethical responsibility to everyone in the family. In some cases, individual needs and family system needs may be in conflict.

The therapist must be clear that their job in most cases (such as impending divorce) is to help the partners sort out their values, obligations, and options rather than to make a decision for them. In some cases (e.g., with the reporting of child abuse), the ethical decision must be the therapist's. Sometimes the therapist faces difficult gray areas that must be decided on a case-by-case basis. The therapist also has certain unalterable ethical obligations such as not engaging in dual relationships with patients (described later in this chapter) or not exploiting patients for their own benefit.

This section reviews common ethical dilemmas from the point of view of the family therapist. Although the operative concept is first do no harm, the questions of how one defines harm and who will be harmed by a certain action are complex and difficult to answer.

Conflicting Interests of Family Members

It is not unusual for the interests of each family member to conflict at some point. Boszormenyi-Nagy and Spark[1] years ago emphasized the contractual obligations and accountability between persons in the multiple generations of a family. The family therapist in this view is uniquely attuned to the well-being of each family member (who will be affected by the treatment process) via their deep-rooted relatedness over time and through many generations. *Relational ethics* is concerned with the balance of equitable fairness between people. To gauge the balance of fairness in the here and now, and across time and generations, each family member must consider their own interests and the interests of each family member. The basic issue is one of equitability. That is, everyone is entitled to have their welfare and interests considered in a way that is fair to the related interests of other family members.

As we discussed earlier in this book, it may not always be clear who the "patient" is in family therapy (see the case example in Chapter 23). The symptomatic family member is often thought by the family to be the patient, but the family therapist may designate the whole family system as the patient or as involved persons in the treatment. The family therapist must be aware of the ethical issues implied in involving the family in the treatment process and in considering its contribution to the problem and the solution when it did not originally see itself as such or explicitly contract for treatment.

The family therapist must be aware of the ethical issues implied in involving the family in the treatment process. Our advice is to never be above asking a colleague for a consultation. In some situations, clinicians may require legal guidance during the course of treatment.

Because family therapy often involves meetings with all or most of the family members present, the family therapist may be in the position of asking nonsymptomatic individuals to attend sessions against their wishes. This may involve urging both resistant adults and minors to attend. This situation may become particularly troublesome if a previously nonsymptomatic individual comes to family therapy and becomes distressed.

There may be times when it is difficult to decide whether a therapeutic action or suggestion may be helpful for one individual but not helpful or even temporarily harmful to another individual. In their concern for the healthy functioning of the system as a whole, therapists may inadvertently ignore what is best for one individual. An ethical issue is how the decision is made. Should it be the therapist's concern alone, or should it be shared with the family? How much information should the family be given on the pros and cons of modalities? Our bias is to negotiate and give the family all the relevant information so that it can make the most informed decision possible (for review, see Hare-Mustin[2] and Hare-Mustin et al.[3]).

Understanding HIPAA

By definition, family intervention always includes family members and/or significant others. What should clinicians who work with families do when patients don't give permission to contact their families? Many psychiatrists erroneously believe that the sharing of information with others, without the patient's explicit consent, is prohibited by the Health Insurance Portability and Accountability Act (HIPAA). HIPAA violations may have serious consequences, so it is important to have a clear understanding of what the HIPAA 45 CFR 164.510(b) rule entails as well as its intended use.[4] The following information is extracted from the website of the U.S. Department of Health and Human Services and provides guidance for health care providers. Here are some guidelines:

1. Health care information may be shared with relevant individuals present when the patient has given prior approval, or simply does not object.
2. Asking a friend to be in the interview room provides the implicit right to disclose information in their presence.
3. Clinicians also have the authority within the Privacy Act to share information based on their professional judgment, believing that there would be no objection to its discussion. For example, a clinician may share information about medication with those providing transportation from the hospital.
4. If the patient is not present but has requested an individual to gather information for them, or is incapacitated by an emergency, a physician may once again use best judgment in sharing or gathering information. This may include a proxy picking up of medications from the pharmacy or receiving other protected information. **We strongly recommend that clinicians err on the side of families in emergency situations especially when suicidal or homicidal behavior is likely.**
5. Physicians should be aware of state laws within their region of practice that may affect the use of the Privacy Act within scenarios of emergency or safety concern.

Using these guidelines, family members (or friends) who accompany the patient can be invited into the interview and the benefits of their inclusion explained. Most evidence-based family interventions are psychoeducational, where illness symptoms and treatments are explained and feelings and beliefs about the illness are explored. When patients understand the goal of family intervention is psychoeducational, they are more likely to agree.

Family involvement is often misunderstood as being a hindrance to individuation, when in fact family-oriented interventions can improve patient functioning, agency, and autonomy. This is often the case when young adults are forced, because of illness, to return home to live with their parents.

The use of shared decision-making may help the patients frame their long-term goals in line with the goals of the family.[5] Psychiatrists can help the patient prepare for the family meeting. With a clear agenda, the patient will be less anxious and be more accepting of family members working with them. Psychiatrists can proceed, using one of the most underutilized evidence-based interventions in psychiatry—family psychoeducation.

Secrets and Confidentiality

We discussed "family secrets" in Chapter 14. Let us now return to this issue in the context of ethical concerns.

Unless a therapist sees all members of a family together at all times, they will eventually face a situation in which family secrets are disclosed in individual sessions. Because secrets are a common source of family dysfunction, discovering and dealing with them is a frequent occurrence. As Imber-Black,[6] (p. 15) says, "secrets, decisions about secrecy and openness, and the management of information are woven into the fabric of our society. The paradoxes of what is to be kept secret and what is to be shared and with whom are all around us and are embedded in each encounter between family and therapist."

The family therapist needs to make a distinction between secrecy and privacy. *Privacy* is usually considered to mean information held by one person that they would prefer not to share but that does not directly affect their relationship with others. It usually implies a zone of comfort free from intrusion. *Secrecy* usually relates to feelings or information that would directly affect a relationship. Secrets are most often connected to fear, anxiety, and shame and are often shared—that is, some people in the system know them, whereas others do not. There is also a gray area in which different people have different ideas about whether the information is important. For example, is an affair that ended 10 years ago, that occurred during the marriage, private or secret?

Secrets define hierarchy and relationships, leaving the unaware mystified and out of alliance. Some secrets are helpful in that they promote differentiation and separation in less powerful members of a group. For example, a 6-year-old boy who says to his sister, "Don't tell mom we ate the cookies" is learning that parents can't read their minds and that they (the children) have some autonomy. However, some secrets are dangerous in that proper action will not be taken by the unaware. For example, the adolescent who says to his sister, "Don't tell mom we were drinking and driving without a license" leaves the parents unable to keep the children safe. Some secrets are about the past, such as an affair many years ago, and some are about the present, such as an ongoing affair or an impending bankruptcy. The majority of toxic secrets are in some way related to money, betrayal, or sex (e.g., abortions, illegitimate births).

In general, a secret should be disclosed if it seriously affects connections between people, if it poses a danger to a family member (e.g., sexual abuse), or if it shapes family coalitions and alliances. Keeping secrets is such a serious barrier that it is better to disclose them, even if painful; otherwise, the sense of mystification and isolation in the unaware is very strong. This seems to be true in many areas regarding children, such as adoption, out-of-wedlock birth, and artificial insemination, that were formerly kept secret. The issue of whether to tell depends strongly on the situation. For example, if adult children choose not to disclose their homosexuality to their parents, the matter should be considered private, because an adult's sexuality is considered their own decision. Even so, because such an issue maintains a large barrier between the child and their parents, the child should be encouraged to tell in most cases. In contrast, if a husband is bisexual or homosexual and does not tell his wife but engages in unprotected (or even protected) intercourse with men, the wife is in serious danger and needs to know. Because the husband's sexuality is definitely the wife's concern, not telling her this secret is a serious threat to the relationship.

A secret should be disclosed if it seriously affects connections between people, poses a danger to a family member, or shapes family coalitions and alliances.

The therapist must carefully consider the timing and type of disclosure. Premature disclosure, before the therapist has an alliance with the family, can cause the family to leave therapy with no place to deal with potentially explosive topics. This is particularly true when the family has a history of violence or abuse. It is generally believed that if a family member refuses to disclose a secret so serious that therapy will be derailed, the therapist may terminate therapy but should not disclose the secret. In cases of potential violence to another, especially child abuse or threatened murder, the therapist is required to report the situation to the authorities and the potential victim, so that the secret will have to be disclosed. The confusion many therapists feel when faced with reporting and knowing that this may end their relationship with the family is difficult to manage; these cases must be discussed with a supervisor or mentor. Issues related to disclosure also arise when one partner has not disclosed their HIV-positive status to the other partner. The therapist is not legally obliged to do so; however, ethically it is extraordinarily hard not to. The patient should be urged strongly to disclose HIV status.

Therapists working with families that are involved with multiple caretaking systems (e.g., school, welfare, social services) are faced constantly with decisions about what to share with other caretakers and with the public record. Family members who have individual therapists may or may not want the family therapist to talk with the other therapists involved. It is strongly recommended that a connection be established between all therapists involved with a family to prevent splitting and mixed agendas from complicating treatment.

Confidentiality issues arise with family members outside the "family" as defined in the treatment group. For example, what information can be given to a concerned grandmother about a child who might be abused? What is owed to the noncustodial parent if the custodial parent and children have been the family of treatment? The therapist must help the family consider what is in its best interest. Interested parties are better brought into the therapy room as potential allies than ignored. However, the need to maintain boundaries between the nuclear family and other family members must also be considered carefully. In general, any disclosures should be discussed at length with the family.

Issues Involving Gender, Gender Roles, and Sexuality

Ethical issues connected with unequal treatment of men and women are an underexplored area in family therapy. The most critical areas involve the tendencies to blame mothers for their children's problems and to let fathers off the hook, both conceptually and in treatment strategies. Although paying more attention to the mother than the father is not unethical in the same way that is breaking therapeutic confidentiality or sleeping with a patient, it is important to consider the ethical implications of accepting traditional role assignments when they result in severely unequal treatment of men and women. For example, if a husband and wife have a relationship in which all decisions are made by the husband and the wife behaves in a completely submissive manner, to what extent does the therapist work toward a more egalitarian relationship? Similarly, if the wife is doing all of the childcare and the father is doing none of it, how much should the therapist encourage the husband to take on half the childcare as opposed to dealing only with the symptomatic child?

Treatment of a patient engaged in an affair involves the therapist's value system (e.g., Is it normal to have a one-night stand, or is this a major therapy issue?). Ethical issues in sexuality revolve around areas in which the therapist may have very different values from the patient. Consider the following case example:

A therapist was seeing Mr. and Mrs. A, who requested therapy for the husband's impotence. It developed that the couple were involved heavily in swapping partners and that the husband was potent with his wife but not with their joint sex partners. The therapist in this case refused to treat the problem, on the grounds that the husband's body was giving him a message he needed to listen to. The therapist made it clear that if the couple still wished therapy she would refer them to a therapist who was more comfortable with these types of relationships.

A therapist is not obligated to treat a couple whose values they disagree with, whether this involves abortion, swinging, or any other issues, but the therapist is obligated to make their own value system clear to the couple rather than hiding it and trying to convince them they are wrong. Differences in values between therapist and patient are particularly common in family therapy because so many of the issues have to do with how one lives one's life rather than clear, diagnosable psychopathology.

Ethics in a Managed Care World

The practice of psychiatry is being changed dramatically by managed care policies that encourage brief treatment, discourage long-term psychotherapy, and make it difficult to hospitalize patients for anything other than brief stabilization. These changes have put enormous pressure on therapists to discharge patients early, to use medication as the primary form of treatment, and to treat only the presenting problem while ignoring other, perhaps equally vital, issues such as family issues. They also put great pressure on families of the mentally ill, who are asked to deal with very ill family members.

Confidentiality is difficult to keep when permission must be given by a managed care expert for increased sessions, hospitalization, and so on. Each therapist must consider their own willingness to accept the rules of a given managed care company and to fight for the patient's and family's right to adequate treatment.

Accordingly, we advise family therapists to take a proactive stance based on principles we elucidated earlier in this book. First, the therapist formulates a careful diagnosis of issues relevant to the patient and the family. Second, the therapist lays out a treatment plan based on models of intervention presented in this book. Third, the therapist presents the case to the new "member of the treatment team"—a managed care supervisor. Finally, the therapist fights for (i.e., advocates) the plan.

INFORMED CONSENT

Similar to other psychotherapy formats, family therapy does not require informed consent from the family before initiating treatment. Our bias is to inform the family of possible difficulties of treatment. If the therapist believes problems may occur, for example, in treating a psychiatric disorder, it seems quite appropriate and even necessary for the therapist to clearly state and negotiate the treatment goals with the family so that the family can make an informed judgment about its desire to embark on the therapy. The negotiation should be done both at the outset and throughout the therapy. If during the evaluation the therapist identifies family secrets to be central to the family problem, they may want to inform the family that those issues may need to be a focus. More important, we agree with Gutheil et al.[7] that the sharing of uncertainty through the informed consent procedure can be a focal point in building a therapeutic alliance: "Increasingly, patients and families who experience tragic disappointment in their expectations ... attempt to assuage their grief, helplessness, and despair by blaming ... the physicians." This sharing can be done by understanding the family's wish for certainty and by empathizing with their unrealistic desires.

FINANCIAL ISSUES

Who pays the bill is relatively simple in individual treatment with adult patients, but in marital and family work, the issue is more complicated. The ethical issues of who pays the bill become especially tense in marital treatment of spouses in conflict. For example, if both spouses have insurance coverage from their respective employers, whose insurance should be used? This issue becomes most delicate when the spouses have conflicting views of the matter for any number of reasons (e.g., "I don't want my administrative assistant seeing the insurance forms" or "Using my insurance makes me the patient"). As with many concrete conflicts, the family therapist should approach the matter with a sense of fairness. The symbolic meanings of who pays should be explored thoroughly. When both partners have separate incomes and separate financial arrangements, they should each pay half the bill. Divorced couples may negotiate bitterly over who pays bills for family sessions. If a family session is held between adults and their parents, the question of who pays must be discussed with great care. Most often, the person requesting the session pays for it.

Other financial questions involve sudden changes of fortune. For example, if a woman married to a well-to-do man divorces and her income drops severely and suddenly, is the therapist willing to continue treatment even if the husband refuses to pay? For many therapists and many clients, money is the most taboo subject, even more so than sex. It is the therapist's job to clarify their own understanding and feelings about money so that they can support discussions with patients. Money is often used as power to influence treatment. For example, a spouse who is used to controlling their partner may refuse to pay for treatment when the power dynamic shifts to a more equal role.

PROFESSIONAL ISSUES

The Problem of Boundaries and Dual Relationships

The issue of boundaries and dual relationships is a critical one in all forms of psychotherapy. Because marital and family therapy involves more than one patient in the consulting room, there is less likelihood of inappropriate sexual contact between therapist and patient. However, there have been cases in which a therapist working with a couple began an affair with one of the spouses, either during couples therapy or after the couple separated. Therapists may also have other forms of dual relationships. For example, a therapist may agree to treat the child of a colleague. This makes a very confusing boundary for the child (e.g., the child may wonder what the therapist will tell their parent), and if family sessions are needed, the therapist will have a very difficult time remaining neutral. Therapists who are treating students directly under them in training programs are also engaging in behavior considered to be unethical, because the patient is at a serious disadvantage as a student who must be graded or evaluated.

Other confusing issues may arise because the issues that families face are the same as the issues therapists face in their personal lives, making it very likely that countertransference issues may become ethical ones at some point. For example, it is extremely difficult for a therapist to treat a couple going through a separation at the same time that they are going through the early stages of divorce, and the likelihood of the therapist remaining neutral to both parties is not great. Although it is impossible for a therapist to stop treating patients while going through a divorce, they could certainly choose not to accept a new client whose situation is very similar to their own or who reminds the therapist of their departing spouse. Issues of confidentiality and boundaries are mentioned in the American Association of Marital and Family Therapy Code of Ethics; we include the relevant sections in Table 25.1.

Table 25.1 Excerpt from AAMFT Code of Ethics

Principle I: Responsibility to Clients
Marriage and family therapists advance the welfare of families and individuals. They respect the rights of those persons seeking their assistance, and make reasonable efforts to ensure that their services are used appropriately.
1.1 Non-discrimination. Marriage and family therapists provide professional assistance to persons without discrimination on the basis of race, age, ethnicity, socioeconomic status, disability, gender, health status, religion, national origin, sexual orientation, gender identity, or relationship status.
1.2 Informed consent. Marriage and family therapists obtain appropriate informed consent to therapy or related procedures and use language that is reasonably understandable to clients. The content of informed consent may vary depending upon the client and treatment plan; however, informed consent generally necessitates that the client: (a) has the capacity to consent; (b) has been adequately informed of significant information concerning treatment processes and procedures; (c) has been adequately informed of potential risks and benefits of treatments for which generally recognized standards do not yet exist; (d) has freely and without undue influence expressed consent; and (e) has provided consent that is appropriately documented. When persons, due to age or mental status, are legally incapable of giving informed consent, marriage and family therapists obtain informed permission from a legally authorized person, if such substitute consent is legally permissible.
1.3 Multiple relationships. Marriage and family therapists are aware of their influential positions with respect to clients, and they avoid exploiting the trust and dependency of such persons. Therapists, therefore, make every effort to avoid conditions and multiple relationships with clients that could impair professional judgment or increase the risk of exploitation. Such relationships include, but are not limited to, business or close personal relationships with a client or the client's immediate family. When the risk of impairment or exploitation exists due to conditions or multiple roles, therapists document the appropriate precautions taken.
1.4 Sexual intimacy with current clients and others. Sexual intimacy with current clients, or their spouses or partners is prohibited. Engaging in sexual intimacy with individuals who are known to be close relatives, guardians or significant others of current clients is prohibited.
1.5 Sexual intimacy with former clients and others. Sexual intimacy with former clients, their spouses or partners, or individuals who are known to be close relatives, guardians, or significant others of clients is likely to be harmful and is therefore prohibited for 2 years following the termination of therapy or last professional contact. After the 2 years following the last professional contact or termination, in an effort to avoid exploiting the trust and dependency of clients, marriage and family therapists should not engage in sexual intimacy with former clients, or their spouses or partners. If therapists engage in sexual intimacy with former clients, or their spouses or partners, more than 2 years after termination or last professional contact, the burden shifts to the therapist to demonstrate that there has been no exploitation or injury to the former client, or their spouse or partner.
1.6 Reports of unethical conduct. Marriage and family therapists comply with applicable laws regarding the reporting of alleged unethical conduct.
1.7 No furthering of own interests. Marriage and family therapists do not use their professional relationships with clients to further their own interests.
1.8 Client autonomy in decision-making. Marriage and family therapists respect the rights of clients to make decisions and help them to understand the consequences of these decisions. Therapists clearly advise clients that clients have the responsibility to make decisions regarding relationships such as cohabitation, marriage, divorce, separation, reconciliation, custody, and visitation.
1.9 Relationship beneficial to client. Marriage and family therapists continue therapeutic relationships only so long as it is reasonably clear that clients are benefiting from the relationship.
1.10 Referrals. Marriage and family therapists assist persons in obtaining other therapeutic services if the therapist is unable or unwilling, for appropriate reasons, to provide professional help.
1.11 Non-abandonment. Marriage and family therapists do not abandon or neglect clients in treatment without making reasonable arrangements for the continuation of treatment.
1.12 Written consent to record. Marriage and family therapists obtain written informed consent from clients before videotaping, audio recording, or permitting third-party observation.

Table 25.1 Excerpt from AAMFT Code of Ethics (*Continued*)

1.13 Relationships with third parties. Marriage and family therapists, upon agreeing to provide services to a person or entity at the request of a third party, clarify, to the extent feasible and at the outset of the service, the nature of the relationship with each party and the limits of confidentiality.

1.14 Electronic therapy. Prior to commencing therapy services through electronic means (including but not limited to phone and Internet), marriage and family therapists ensure that they are compliant with all relevant laws for the delivery of such services. Additionally, marriage and family therapists must: (a) determine that electronic therapy is appropriate for clients, taking into account the clients' intellectual, emotional, and physical needs; (b) inform clients of the potential risks and benefits associated with electronic therapy; (c) ensure the security of their communication medium; and (d) only commence electronic therapy after appropriate education, training, or supervised experience using the relevant technology.

Principle II: Confidentiality

Marriage and family therapists have unique confidentiality concerns because the client in a therapeutic relationship may be more than one person. Therapists respect and guard the confidences of each individual client.

2.1 Disclosing limits of confidentiality. Marriage and family therapists disclose to clients and other interested parties, as early as feasible in their professional contacts, the nature of confidentiality and possible limitations of the clients' right to confidentiality. Therapists review with clients the circumstances where confidential information may be requested and where disclosure of confidential information may be legally required. Circumstances may necessitate repeated disclosures.

2.2 Written authorization to release client information. Marriage and family therapists do not disclose client confidences except by written authorization or waiver, or where mandated or permitted by law. Verbal authorization will not be sufficient except in emergency situations, unless prohibited by law. When providing couple, family or group treatment, the therapist does not disclose information outside the treatment context without a written authorization from each individual competent to execute a waiver. In the context of couple, family or group treatment, the therapist may not reveal any individual's confidences to others in the client unit without the prior written permission of that individual.

2.3 Confidentiality in non-clinical activities. Marriage and family therapists use client and/or clinical materials in teaching, writing, consulting, research, and public presentations only if a written waiver has been obtained in accordance with Subprinciple 2.2, or when appropriate steps have been taken to protect client identity and confidentiality.

2.4 Protection of records. Marriage and family therapists store, safeguard, and dispose of client records in ways that maintain confidentiality and in accord with applicable laws and professional standards.

2.5 Preparation for practice changes. In preparation for moving from the area, closing a practice, or death, marriage and family therapists arrange for the storage, transfer, or disposal of client records in conformance with applicable laws and in ways that maintain confidentiality and safeguard the welfare of clients.

2.6 Confidentiality in consultations. Marriage and family therapists, when consulting with colleagues or referral sources, do not share confidential information that could reasonably lead to the identification of a client, research participant, supervisee, or other person with whom they have a confidential relationship unless they have obtained the prior written consent of the client, research participant, supervisee, or other person with whom they have a confidential relationship. Information may be shared only to the extent necessary to achieve the purposes of the consultation.

2.7 Protection of electronic information. When using electronic methods for communication, billing, recordkeeping, or other elements of client care, marriage and family therapists ensure that their electronic data storage and communications are privacy protected consistent with all applicable law.

Source: Reprinted with permission from the AAMFT Code of Ethics. Copyright © 2015 American Association for Marriage and Family Therapy.

COMPETENCIES

In order to protect the public from untrained, incompetent, or unethical family therapists and family intervention, a clear delineation must exist in the competencies needed to do family therapy. In addition, ways of teaching and assessing the presence (or absence) of these competencies must be developed.

Some of the qualities we think are important for the family therapist, and those required to do other therapies, include the following:

- Tolerance of family fighting
- Comfort with family secrets
- Ability to adapt to different technical models or mix different modalities together in a treatment package
- Interest in issues of gender, diversity, class, and culture
- Ability to be active and directive

We have a strong bias that in the training of family therapists, attention should be paid to the humanistic qualities of integrity, respect, and compassion for patients and their families. Our point is that attainment of these qualities is critical to the outcome of therapy. Therapists must come to realize that they are not omnipotent.

For successful long-term outcome, both the family and the therapist must play a part. For example, the therapist may recognize the family's need to be cared for, or the family's inability to make decisions, but it is not their responsibility to take over in these respects. Instead, the therapist must help the family recognize its difficulties and start seeking solutions. Although therapists may decide to accept responsibility for providing a setting, establishing and maintaining a therapeutic alliance, and offering observations and suggestions, those therapists who take considerably greater responsibility for change are diluting what energy and motivation the family might have; these therapists are also likely candidates for burnout.[8] The everyday practice of family therapy is untidy and disorderly. At times, therapists fail, make mistakes, and regret them.[9]

Please see Table 25.2 for the GAP Proposal for Specific Family Systems Competencies. In this Table 25.2, the authors discuss skills needed for a resident to be competent in supporting and working with families, as mandated by the residency review committee (RRC) core competencies.

TRAINING ISSUES

We would be remiss to conclude without discussing issues of training for both psychiatric residents and trainees in family therapy institutes. Although a tad parenthetical to the objectives of a textbook, we believe some key elements need to be mentioned in order for readers to master fully the theory and practice of family therapy described throughout the book.

Just as every faculty member wishes that their area of specialty would assume priority in the competitive environment of residency or graduate training, so too teachers of couples and family therapy imagine every resident developing solid competencies in this approach. In the family therapy training program at Stanford, residents begin their internship/PGY-II training with lectures that introduce the elements of systemic theory and practice, basic interviewing skills, and applications for those training sites that occupy the greatest proportion of their time: emergency room, psychiatric in-patient settings, and consultation/liaison settings. When time permits, it is also helpful to schedule several sessions in the summer crash course for PG-I/IIs focusing on basic family interviewing skills and systemic thinking to help introduce family-systems concepts to new residents.

In some regards, these early training sites require the greatest clinical skill due to the acuity, the time constraints, and the emotionality that often surrounds the presenting situation.

Table 25.2 Group for the advancement of psychiatry (GAP) proposal for specific family systems competencies

GAP proposal for family skills competency

The GAP Family Committee makes the following general observations about the RRC competencies:

1. The RRC states specifically that for the purposes of their document, "family" is defined as those people having a biologic or otherwise meaningful relationship with the patient. Such "significant others" are to be defined from the patient's point of view.
2. The basic tenet of their document is that the family should be included as part of the treatment team, that family members be seen as allies and that it is critical to communicate with, educate, and support family members.
3. All residents should be competent to form an alliance with, assess, educate, and support families.
4. Family skills include being able to see a presenting problem through a systemic as well as an individual lens.

The GAP Family Committee proposes specific family competencies that consist of the knowledge, attitudes, and skills required for a resident to be competent in working with families. These competencies are outlined below.

GAP proposal for specific family systems competencies

Knowledge. The resident is expected to demonstrate knowledge of family factors as they relate to psychiatric and medical illnesses, based on scientific literature and standards of practice. The resident is expected to demonstrate knowledge of:

i. basic concepts of systems applicable to families, multidisciplinary teams in clinical settings, and medical/government organizations impacting the patient and doctor
ii. couple and family development over the life cycle and the importance of multigenerational patterns
iii. principles of adaptive and maladaptive relational functioning in family life and family organization, communication, problem solving, and emotional regulation
iv. family strengths, resilience, and vulnerability
v. how age, gender, class, culture, and spirituality affect family life
vi. the variety of family forms (e.g., single parent, stepfamily, same-sex parents)
vii. how the family affects and is affected by psychiatric and nonpsychiatric disorders (e.g., specific information regarding the impact of parental psychiatric illness on children)
viii. special issues in family life (e.g., loss, divorce and remarriage, immigration, illness, secrets, affairs, violence, alcohol and substance abuse, sexuality, including gay, lesbian, bisexual, transgender [GLBT] issues)
ix. relationship of families to larger systems (e.g., schools, work, health care systems, government agencies).

Residents must be informed about the current research on family functioning and evidence-based treatment and practice. First, the role of family factors that influence the presentation and course of illness must be understood. In schizophrenia spectrum disorders, adoptees at high genetic risk for schizophrenic spectrum disorders are significantly more sensitive to adverse rearing patterns in their adoptive families compared to adoptees without this genetic risk. Maladaptive parental behavior is associated with the increased risk of psychiatric disorders in their children, regardless of the presence or absence of diagnosed psychiatric illness in the parents. Marital violence is correlated with disorganized attachment disorders in infants, and generational transmission of psychopathology has been demonstrated in boys with conduct disorder. Family factors also influence the course of psychiatric illness. Patients with major depression, whose families have significant dysfunction, have a slower rate of recovery. Conversely, good family functioning improves outcomes in major depression. A family construct called expressed emotion (EE) describes the level of criticism, hostility, and emotional overinvolvement in families. Although initially used with schizophrenic patients and their families, EE is studied extensively across the health care spectrum and in many cultures. High (EE) is a "significant and robust" predictor of relapse in many illnesses, such as schizophrenia, depressive disorders, acute mania, and alcoholism. High EE in families can also result from ongoing stressful interaction with a disturbed family member, thus indicating a bidirectional process.

Second, the residents must know about successful family interventions, which range from family psychoeducation to "manualized" family therapy. Family intervention reduces relapse rates and improves quality of life for patients with schizophrenia, bipolar disorder, major depression, alcoholism and borderline personality disorder, obsessive compulsive disorder in children and adolescents and eating disorders. Multifamily groups in the treatment of chronic illness in children, such as bipolar disorder, are also proving effective. These clinical studies are considered to provide strong evidence of efficacy.

Source: Reprinted by permission from Springer: Berman EM, Heru AM, Grunebaum H, et al. Family skills for general psychiatry residents: meeting ACGME core competency requirements. *Acad Psychiatry.* 2006;30(1):69–78. Copyright © 2014 Academic Psychiatry.

Residents must therefore identify the role of families in the maintenance of and recovery from acute and chronic psychiatric conditions, be able to rapidly evaluate an individual problem in the context of the couple or family, and sensitively grasp the patient's and family's difficult experiences while acknowledging assets, strengths, and hope. Observing taped interviews and role-playing common situations are especially helpful adjuncts to training.

In the PGY-III year, typically the year that concentrates on a range of outpatient experiences, residents participate in an intensive seminar introducing them to structural family therapy, family assessment, the leading models and schools (structural, family of origin, experiential, emotionally focused, cognitive-behavioral, psychoeducational), and more advanced techniques and strategies of therapy. Case material comes mostly from couples and families seen primarily in outpatient settings. Here again, the focus is on developing observational and conceptual skills by examining taped interviews, role-playing initial interviews, developing clinical hypotheses, and devising interventions. Residents read primary sources and both examine and adopt the assumptions of the systemic model during the course. The seminar is fast paced, aims to provide an accessible clinical framework based on the structural family therapy model, and focuses on the concepts and skills needed to conduct couples and family treatment.

In the PGY-IV year, typically a half to two-thirds of the residents opt for an elective, year-long supervised training experience in out-patient couples and family therapy, either in the Stanford Couples and Family Therapy Clinic or the Family Therapy Program at the VA Palo Alto Health Care System. In these clinics, residents treat outpatient cases, either marital or family, under supervision. In terms of supervision, residents meet in pairs and present cases, most often by showing clips from videotape sessions. Supervision focuses on hypothesizing, broadening the resident's style, and supporting the development of creative, interventions. The atmosphere of the supervision teams tends to be lively, and residents value the opportunity to observe each other and the opportunity to learn from their peers' experiences. Both generic (e.g., dealing with "resistance") and specific (e.g., special issues in dealing with mood disorders) issues are highlighted in the course of supervision.

CLINICAL EXPERIENCES

In the out-patient clinics, supervision is primarily conducted through videotape review and live supervision. Treatment rooms are equipped with one-way mirror, cameras, observation rooms, VCRS/monitors, and telephone hook-up so that the supervisor and observing team can communicate directly with the therapist in the treatment room. Couples and families sign informed consent, and typically report appreciating the fact that a team is devoted to their care. Although initially anxious, residents find observing themselves on videotape, supervisory feedback, and the experience of live supervision to be direct, genuine, constructive, and fun. As Lieberman and Wolin (2004) observe:

> *Training in family therapy is still the exception rather than the rule in psychiatry residency programs. Such training may seem to impose on already overscheduled programs, but developing specific skills to work with families makes clinical work more interesting and rewarding. Most residents and medical students like this training, which is experiential and includes "live" supervision. Family-inclusive psychiatry adds to the attractiveness of our specialty in an era when technologic approaches threaten to overwhelm its humanistic side (p. 2330).*

Pedagogically, residents recognize that these forms of teaching, while limiting their ability to hide and obfuscate the clinical data, represent invaluable contributions to their overall clinical education. In addition, because residents observe each other, they learn about the struggles of learning through their colleagues' experiences as well. Finally, residents observing sessions with a supervisor behind the mirror or watching videotape can hear the supervisor "think out loud" about therapeutic choice points, interventions, and clinical strategy. The final product of the training is the demonstrated skill of the resident in the conduct of couples and family treatment. The most successful training processes continually focus on the skills that the therapist needs to demonstrate across a range of cases.

The role of the teacher and supervisor is to create an atmosphere in which these skills can be defined, described, demonstrated, and put into effective operation with families in need. For example, systematically isolate and describe critical functions performed by the family therapist, such as engagement, problem identification, facilitation of change, and termination. The generic skills taught can be viewed both within and across the various schools, (e.g., structural, family of origin, experiential, psychodynamic, emotionally focused, cognitive-behavioral, psychoeducational).

Nonetheless, trainees often feel that a single, clearly delineated theoretical model helps them best master the conceptual and technical skills needed for basic couples and family assessment and intervention. In that regard, we teach structural family therapy as the primary clinical model. Structural family therapy's conceptual skills are taught in a seminar format, whereas the executive skills can be modeled either live or on videotape by experienced family therapists, role-played by the trainees, and eventually practiced in supervised work with families. The directness and simplicity of the approach makes it appealing, especially for beginning family therapists. Innovative pedagogical approaches, such as these, help the unfamiliar aspects of couple and family work appear accessible, powerful, and enjoyable.

We agree that residents "be competent to form an alliance with, assess, educate and support families" and "should be able to see a presenting problem through a systemic or an individual basis." While adopting a systemic perspective can be challenging, learning how to intervene systemically requires practice, reflection, and careful attention. Even the strongest residency training programs cannot offer all things equally to all trainees, nor is it clear that this ambition is desirable. Still, the growing role of family members as the context of, as extenders of, and as providers of care cannot be underestimated.

TRAINING PROGRAMS IN FAMILY PSYCHIATRY

Today, with the rise in the popularity of psychopharmacology and the promise of biologic interventions, there are fewer opportunities for family systems training within psychiatric residency programs. In order to receive family systems training, a psychiatrist may decide to enroll in an independent family training institute, such as the Ackerman Institute for the Family in New York. However, there are still some psychiatric residency programs that consider learning to work with families to be an essential psychotherapeutic skill.

A MULTIDISCIPLINARY FIELD

Family systems training occurs in other disciplines: psychology, social work, and marriage and family therapy (MFT) programs. The number of MFT programs across the United States is large, reflecting the demand for family systems therapists.

Psychologists with a special interest in family therapy belong to the American Psychological Association's Division 43. Division 43 supports family-oriented clinical and scientific activities as well as education and public policy, a journal called the Journal of Family Psychology, and a quarterly newsletter called The Family Psychologist. Many psychologists are trained in family therapy work in primary care settings. A past president of American Psychological Association, Nadine J. Kaslow, Ph.D., is a family therapist who helps underserved and underprivileged populations receive culturally competent, evidence-based, biopsychosocially oriented mental health services.

Social workers are required to take two exams: one to be "licensed" as an LCSW (licensed clinical social worker) after graduation with a master's degree. After 3,000 hours of supervised clinical practice, social worker takes second exam for independent licensure LICSW (licensed independent clinical social worker).

Social work schools have a course or two in family therapy. After graduation, students may choose to specialize in couples and family therapy. Like psychiatric and psychological training programs, there is wide variation in the amount of family therapy taught in schools of social work.

MFTs have their own organization, the American Association for Marriage and Family Therapy (AAMFT). This organization's training is specific to families and couples. Members are required to be supervised in clinical practice for 2 years. AAMFT produces the Journal of Marital and Family Therapy. The AAMFT website also lists accredited programs in the United States and Canada.

Two American journals in this area are interdisciplinary: Family Process and Families, Systems & Health. Family Process has broad representation on its board from all disciplines and has a strong focus on family systems research and social justice. Family Process aims to support emerging researchers and clinicians worldwide, and periodically offers grants. Families, Systems & Health is multidisciplinary with a focus on research and clinical practice in medical illness, and health psychology.

The American Family Therapy Academy (AFTA) is the only organization that is interdisciplinary. Founded in 1977, AFTA's objectives include "the advancement of theories, therapies, research, and professional education that regard the family as a unit in a social context, to make information about family therapy available to practitioners in other fields of knowledge and to the public and to foster collaboration among the medical, psychological, social, legal, and other professions that serve families and the science and practice of family therapy."

AFTA is outspoken on issues that affect families. For example, its Immigration Position Statement addresses the negative impact of U.S. immigration policy on families and children. AFTA has strong views about the DSM-5, stating that "the current revision of the DSM continues a long history of ignoring research and excluding vital contributions of nonpsychiatric mental health disciplines resulting in invalid diagnostic categories and treatment protocols. The DSM is dominant in determining mental health diagnosis and treatment and is more harmful than helpful in delineating best practices."

Family therapy has grown from a small group of interested academics, mostly psychiatrists, to a large group of interdisciplinary professionals. Today, psychiatrists have less access to family systems training than in previous decades but can still access training. In addition to attending conferences, psychiatrists interested in this area might see whether training programs would accept them into their courses.

Family Therapy Fellowships

For those trainees in fellowships (i.e., in the family therapy institutes), the emphasis is properly more focused on the family model. Goals include the following:

- Improving clinical skills in interviewing, assessing, and treating families, couples, and family networks
- Developing familiarity with current theory of family process and treatment
- Learning to provide consultation and liaison services to faculty, staff, professionals, and students from other disciplines and community agencies
- Gaining experience in teaching family concepts, and the application of family therapy, to medical students, other professionals, and community groups
- Affording opportunities for research in the general area of family therapy and family process
- Learning the linguistics of the specialty (i.e., learning in depth the basic philosophical constructs, language, and research in the field). Intensive supervision is provided on an ongoing

basis in assessment and therapy with families and couples and includes a weekly clinical caseload of 9 to 12 families, consultation and liaison services with other hospital and community programs, and development of videotapes for training

TRAINING AND LICENSURE

Professional licensure has been a recent development in the field of marital and family therapy. The American Association of Marriage and Family Therapy has developed a consensus about a fundamental knowledge base. As a unique profession, the practice of marital and family therapy involves the application of psychotherapeutic and family system theories and techniques to the delivery of services to individuals, couples, and families in order to diagnose and treat a nervous and mental disorder. Based on this definition, a national examination in marital and family therapy now exists. This examination covers the following domains: (1) joining, assessment, and diagnosis; (2) designing treatment; (3) conducting the course of treatment; (4) establishing and maintaining appropriate networks; (5) assessing the outcome of treatment; and (6) maintaining professional standards. As of 2015, all 50 states required specific licensure for the practice of marital and family therapy.

CLINICAL PRACTICE IMPLICATIONS

A final issue is one we discussed earlier in Chapter 1, that is, the marginalization of the field. The key implication for the trainee is, as Kramer[10] (p. 13) has warned, that family therapy as a modality will not be reimbursed (like other forms of psychotherapy) "because it conforms poorly to contemporary models of research." Of course, the field has been working on issues of reimbursement, and trainees and supervisors need to cover this issue in the course of training so that patients can be treated properly. Historically, as family therapy developed, differences appeared between the basic assumptions and practices of the field and the tenets of the feminist movement. Early papers challenged the family therapy establishment from a feminist perspective.[11] Inevitably, these issues came under scrutiny in the training and supervision of students. The resulting dialogue has enriched the field and has reshaped the focus of many educational programs. Descriptions of the variety of sexuality and gender differences have emerged from marital interaction research, and a rich literature of related training practices has developed. We have discussed these issues throughout the book.

At the end of a family therapy training program, the trainee's education is just beginning.[12] In a rapidly changing field such as family therapy, an individual must begin a program of lifelong self-education based on a continual awareness of the literature and course work, and on the need to evaluate their own work, to entertain new ideas, and to discard old ones. As obvious as this may seem, it is the inculcation of these principles that identifies the inspired and skillful clinician, teacher, or researcher.

SUGGESTED READINGS

These following four articles on training and family therapy can benefit the psychiatric resident.

Berman E, Heru A, Grunebaum H, et al. Family-oriented patient care through the residency training cycle. *Acad Psychiatry*. 2008;32:111–118.

Rait D. Family therapy training in child and adolescent psychiatry fellowship programs. *Acad Psychiatry*. 2012; 36:448–451.

Rait D, Glick I. Reintegrating family therapy training in psychiatric residency programs: making the case. *Acad Psychiatry*. 2008;32:76–80.

Rait D, Glick I. A model for reintegrating couples and family therapy training in psychiatric residency programs. *Acad Psychiatry*. 2008;32:81–86.

REFERENCES

1. Boszormenyi-Nagy I, Spark G. *Invisible Loyalties: Reciprocity in Intergenerational Family Therapy*. Harper & Row, 1973.
2. Hare-Mustin R. Family therapy may be dangerous for your health. *Pro Psy.* 1980;11:935–938.
3. Hare-Mustin R, Marecek J, Caplan K, Liss-Levinson N. Rights of clients, responsibilities of therapists. *Am Psychol*. 1979;34:3–16.
4. U.S. Department of Health and Human Services. Does the HIPAA Privacy Rule permit a doctor to discuss a patient's health status, treatment, or payment arrangements with the patient's family and friends?; 2013.
5. Swindell JS, McGuire AL, Halpern SD. Beneficent persuasion: techniques and ethical guidelines to improve patients' decisions. *Ann Fam Med*. 2010;8:260–264.
6. Imber-Black E. *Secrets in Families and Family Therapy*. WW Norton; 1993.
7. Gutheil TG, Bursztajn H, Brodsky A. Malpractice prevention through the sharing of uncertainty. Informed consent and the therapeutic alliance. *N Engl J Med*. 1984;311:49–51.
8. Lask B. Whose responsibility? *J Fam Ther*. 1986;8:205–206.
9. Spellman D, Harper DJ. Failure, mistakes, regret and other subjugated stories in family therapy. *J Fam Ther*. 1996;18:205–214.
10. Kramer P. Shape of the field. Psychiatric Times; 1995.
11. Hare-Mustin RT. A feminist approach to family therapy. *Fam Process*. 1978;17:181–194.
12. Fadden G. Research update: psychoeducational family intervention. *J Fam Ther*. 1998;20:293–310.

INDEX

Note: Page numbers followed by f indicate figures; those followed by t indicate tables.

A

Abuse, 277
- child, 278–279
- family violence and alcohol/drug, relationship between, 269
- intrafamilial child sexual, 275–278
- sexual, 212–213, 266
- sibling, 276
- verbal, 266

Ackerman, Nathan, 121, 123
Acute family intervention (AFI), 290–292
- common goals of, 290–292
- empirical studies, 295–296
- guidelines for recommending, 294–295
- staffing, 292–293
- timing, 292
- working model of, 294

Acute residential care, 286
Acute team for family, function of, 286–287
Acute treatment, 286–296
- acute family intervention for, 290–292
  - common goals of, 290–292
  - empirical studies, 295–296
  - guidelines for recommending, 294–295
  - staffing, 292–293
  - timing, 292
  - working model of, 294
- acute residential care, 286
- acute team for family, function of, 286–287
- brief acute psychiatric intervention, 286
- controversies in, 298–299
- family burden in psychotic illness, 287–288
- family therapy techniques for, 293–294
- family treatment, process of, 289–290
  - allying with family, 289
  - common goals of, 290–292
  - evaluation of family, 289
  - setting goals, 289–290
- mental illness of family member, family responses to, 287
- rationale for, 288–289
- staffing for, 292–293
- timing, 292

Addiction, 254
ADHD. *See* Attention-deficit/hyperactivity disorder
Adherence to treatment, 304
Adolescent as identified patient, 333
Adolescent group therapy (AGT), 344
Adolescents in family therapy, 178–180
- diagnostic family evaluation, 179–180
- treatment, 180

Adoption, 65
Adult disorders
- couples therapy for
  - behavioral couples therapy for alcoholism, 342
  - behavioral marital therapy for depression, 342
  - emotionally focused couples therapy for marital distress, 341–342
  - insight-oriented marital therapy for marital distress, 341
  - integrative behavioral couple therapy for marital distress, 341
  - posttraumatic stress disorder, 342–343
- family therapy for
  - bipolar disorder, 343
  - major mental illness, 343
  - schizophrenia, 343

Affective involvement, 309
Affective responsiveness, 309
Affordable Care Act (ACA), 8–9
Age-appropriate childrearing techniques, 51
Aging of population, 31–32
Agoraphobia, 249–250
AGT. *See* Adolescent group therapy
AIDS, 213
Alcohol/alcoholism, 213, 269, 276
- behavioral couples therapy for, 342

Alcoholics anonymous (families group)/narcotics anonymous (families group), 255
American Association for Marriage and Family Therapy (AAMFT), 372
American Association of Marital and Family Therapists, 7
American Association of Marital and Family Therapy Code of Ethics, 365, 366t–367t
American family
- function of, 21–22
- structure of, 21–22

American Family Therapy Academy (AFTA), 372
American Family Therapy Association, 7
American marriages, 204
American Orthopsychiatric Association, 7
American Psychiatric Association, 7
American social psychiatry, 7
Amnesia, 251–253
- rationale, 251–252
- treatment considerations, 252–253

AN. *See* Anorexia nervosa
Anorexia nervosa, family therapy for, 345
Anorexia nervosa (AN), 253–254
Antihypertensive medications, 213
Antipsychotic medication, 260
Anxiety, 156

Anxiety disorders, 248–250, 259
  agoraphobia, 249–250
  panic disorder, 249–250
  rationale, 248–249
  treatment, 249–250
ARFD. *See* Avoidant restrictive food intake disorder
ASD. *See* Autism spectrum disorder
Assaultive behavior, 266
Assumptions by therapists, 173
Attention-deficit/hyperactivity disorder (ADHD), 257–258, 344
  children with, 258
  prevalence of, 257
  treatment, 258
Authority, 72
Autism spectrum disorder (ASD), 256–257
Avoidant restrictive food intake disorder (ARFD), 253–254

B

Barbiturates, 213
Basic needs, provision of, 51
Baucom, D., 125
BCT. *See* Behavioral couples therapy
BED. *See* Binge eating disorder
Behavioral couples therapy (BCT), 255
  for alcoholism, 342
  for depression, 342
Behavior control, 104, 309–310
Binge eating disorder (BED), 253–254
Binuclear families, 59–61, 221
  divorce based on age of child, impact of, 59–60
  father-headed single-parent families, 61
  functional single-parent family, 60–61
  mother-headed single-parent families, 61
Biography, family's, 92
Bipolar disorder, 239–242
  focused family therapy for, 343
  functional family therapy for adolescents with, 345
  rationale, 239–241
  treatment considerations, 241–242
    other specific psychosocial interventions, 242
    psychoeducational marital interventions, 242
BN. *See* Bulimia nervosa
Borderline personality disorder (BPD), 246–248
  adolescents and young adults at home, 247
  borderline-partnered and married people, 247
  rationale, 246–247
  treatment considerations, 247–248
Boszormenyi-Nagy, I., 124
Boundary-making techniques, 145
Bowen, M., 121, 123–124
BPD. *See* Borderline personality disorder
Brief family therapy, 326
Brief strategic family therapy (BSFT), 344
BSFT. *See* Brief strategic family therapy
Bulimia nervosa (BN), 253–254

C

Caregivers, 178
Caregiving, 306–307
CBT. *See* Cognitive behavioral therapy
CD. *See* Conduct disorder
Child abuse, 278–279
  accidental *versus* abusive forms, 278
  blunt trauma, 278
  child maltreatment, 278
  child neglect, 278
  consequences of, 278–279
  incestuous trauma, 279
  physical evidence of, 279
  psychosomatic symptoms, 279
  sexual abuse, 279
Child/children, 48–49
  adoption, 65
  of alcoholic parents, 256
  anxiety disorders in, 259
  with CD, 259
  communicating issue of divorce to, 218
  divorce and, 58–59
  in family therapy, 178–180
    diagnostic family evaluation, 179–180
    treatment, 180
  as identified patient, 332–333
  maltreatment, 278
  mood disorders in, 259
  neglect, 278
  obesity in, 260
  with ODD, 259
  parent and, 72
  psychiatry, 178
  psychology, 178
  rearing and socializing of, 79
Child-focused problems, 327
Christensen, A., 125
Chronically ill, families of, 296–299
Circular causality, 69
Clarification technique, 147
Classification of relational disorders (CORD), 115t
Clinical experiences in family therapy, 370–371
Closeness-distance (emotional intensity), 46
CNM. *See* Consensual nonmonogamy
Coaching model, 166
Coercive control, 266
Cognitive–behavioral model, 125–126
Cognitive behavioral therapy (CBT), 254, 342
Cognitive disorders, 251–253
  rationale, 251–252
  treatment considerations, 252–253
Cohabitation, 225–226
Cohabiting couples, 225–226
Collaborative family therapy, 176
Commitment, issue of, 197–198
Communication, 103, 141, 224, 308
Community-based support groups, 298
Community Reinforcement and Family Treatment (CRAFT), 255
Companionship, 47
Competencies in family therapy, 368
Concurrent family therapy, 176
Concurrent individual therapy, 176
Conduct disorder (CD), 259, 344

Confidentiality, 362–363
Confirmatory research, 339
Conflicting interests of family members, 360–361
Conflicts, 42
  of couples, 330–331
  model, 166
Confrontation, 147
Congenital malformation syndrome, 256
Conjoint couples therapy, 176
Conjoint family therapy, 176
Conjoint marital therapy, 330
Consensual nonmonogamy (CNM), 29
Controlling family members, 274
CORD. *See* Classification of relational disorders
Corrective feedback, 14
Co-therapists, 181
Co-therapy, 181
Council on Contemporary Families, 221
Counseling psychology, 8
Countertransference, 123
Couples, 7–10. *See also* Marital coalition
  cohabiting, 225–226
  conflict, 330–331
  depression in, 243–244
  dissatisfaction, 330–331
  evaluation
    case example/formulation, 109–115, 114t
    classification and diagnosis, 105–108, 106f, 107t
    content of, 94–101
    explicit interview data, gathering of, 96–97
    family function, dimensions of, 95
    family genogram, 97f–98f, 101
    family problem, background of, 97–98, 97f–98f
    family's goals and expectations of treatment, 100
    gathering identifying data and establishing current phase of family life cycle, 95–96
    outline, 95–100, 95f
    past treatment attempts, history of, 98–99
    process of, 85–93
  and family life cycle, 42–50
  LGBTQ, 27–28
  life cycle, 44
  personality, 47
  process of
    clinical practice implications, 93
    dimensions of, 87–90
    family life cycle, 89t
    historical material/data, role of, 91–92
    identifying family structure, 90
    individual and family diagnoses, role of, 92–93
    interview, progression of, 87
    joining with couple/family, 88
    members to include in, 86
    overview, 85
    recognizing developmental stage, history, and culture, 88–90, 89f, 89t
    systemic model of change, working with, 90–91, 90f, 91t
    systemic patterns, 88
  remarried, 62
  separation, 215–220. *See also* Divorce; Separation
  setting goals after, 109t
  temperament, 47
  therapeutic approach, 108–109, 108t
  treatment contract, 108–109, 108t
Couples difficulties/problems/dysfunction, 194–197
  from behavioral point of view, 196
  development dysfunction, 197
  from a dynamic point of view, 195–196
  from psychiatric illness point of view, 196–197
  from systems point of view, 196
Couples therapy, 197–203, 338–340
  for adult disorders, 341–343
    behavioral couples therapy for alcoholism, 342
    behavioral marital therapy for depression, 342
    emotionally focused couples therapy for marital distress, 341–342
    insight-oriented marital therapy for marital distress, 341
    integrative behavioral couple therapy for marital distress, 341
    for posttraumatic stress disorder, 342–343
  clinical implications of data from outcome studies, 351–352
  clinical practice implications, 203
  for couples conflict and dissatisfaction, 330–331
  evaluation of partners, 198–199
  for families in process of divorce, 331
  goals of, 199
  guidelines for interviewing couples, 202t
  individual models, 200–201
  intervention
    on patterns of interaction, 199–200
    strategies and techniques of, 199
  issue of commitment, 197–198
  for sexual issues, 331
  strategies and techniques, 201–203
  studies result, 340–341
  for unmarried couples, 332
Course of family treatment, 151–161
  clinical practice implications, 161
  early phase, 152–155
    available time distribution, 153
    distinguishing evaluation from treatment, 154–155
    objectives of, 152
    strategies, 152–153
    styles and techniques of gathering history, 153–154
  middle phase, 155–156
  termination phase, 156
Courtship, 45
Covert power, 274
CRAFT. *See* Community Reinforcement and Family Treatment
Culture, 7
Cybernetics, 13

D

Dance, 124–125
Database, 123

Delinquent adolescents, functional family therapy for, 344
Dementias, 251–253
  rationale, 251–252
  treatment considerations, 252–253
Depression
  in adolescents and young adults, 243
  behavioral marital therapy for, 342
  in parents, 244
  in partnered/married people, 243–244
Detouring, 72
The Diagnostic and Statistical Manual of Mental Disorders, Fifth Edition (*DSM-5*), 92
The Difficult Divorce, 219
Dimensions of couple and family assessment, 87–90
  family life cycle, 89t
  identifying family structure, 90
  joining with couple/family, 88
  recognizing developmental stage, history, and culture, 88–90, 89f, 89t
  systemic patterns, 88
Disclosure, 363
Disconnection in family therapy, 167–173
  clinical practice implications, 174
  family, emanating from, 167–168
  family secrets, 172–173
  in ongoing treatment, 171–172
  stages of treatment, 169–171
  techniques to deal with, 173–174
    assume nothing, 173
    collaboration, 173–174
    emphasizing family responsibility, 174
    focus on present, 174
  at termination phase of therapy, 172
  from therapist–family system, 168–169
    common systems to be considered, 168–169
    disagreement as to treatment goals, 168
    mismatch between therapist and family, 168
  therapists, emanating from, 168
Dissatisfaction of couples, 330–331
Divorce, 25–26, 57–59, 220–221
  children and, 58–59
  issue, communicating to children, 218
  long-term effects of, 220
  marital separation, 57–58
  postdivorce treatment, 220–221
  process, 58
  separation leading to, 217–218
  therapy for families facing, 219–220
Domestic violence, 266
Dysfunctional family system, 68–80
  beliefs and myths, 73–75
  clinical practice implications, 79–80
  implications for treatment, 75–77
  life cycle problems and, 77–78
  social system and, 75
  systems approach to problems and dysfunction, 69–73
    current perspectives, 70–71
    family resilience key processes, 71
    historical perspectives, 69–70
    solution-as-the-problem approach, 72–73
    structural and organizational problems, 71–72
  task performance in, 78–79
    family's basic needs, providing for, 78
    functional marriage, maintaining, 79
    rearing and socializing of children, 79
  toxic secrets, 78
  unresolved grief, 78

E

Early adulthood, 44
Early marriage, 45
Eating disorder NOS (EDNOS), 253–254
Eating disorders, 253–254
  rationale, 253
  treatment of, 253–254
  types of, 253
ED. *See* Erectile disorder
EDNOS. *See* Eating disorder NOS
EE. *See* Expressed emotion
Emotional abuse, 266
Emotional empathy, 141
Emotional experience, 139–140
Emotionally focused couples therapy for marital distress, 341–342
Emotional over involvement (EOI), 287, 291, 296–297
Enactment, 145
EOI. *See* Emotional over involvement
Epstein, N., 125
Erectile disorder (ED), 209
Ethical issues inherent in family therapy, 360–364
  conflicting interests of family members, 360–361
  gender, gender roles, and sexuality, 363–364
  HIPAA violations, 361–362
  managed care policies, 364
  secrets and confidentiality, 362–363
Ethnicity, 22–24
  definition, 22–23
  internalized and structural racism, 23–24
  versus race, examples, 23
Experiential therapy, 126
Exploitation, 276–277
Exploratory research, 339
Expressed emotion (EE), 286, 296–298, 369t
Extended family, 177–178
Extended individual life cycle, 56
Externalizing disorders, 344

F

FAMCON model, 311
Families, 5
  adoption and, 65
  behavior, 14
  binuclear. *See* Binuclear families
  biography, 92
  burden in psychotic illness, 287–288
  changing life cycle, 32
  classification and diagnosis, 105–108, 106f, 107t
  clinical practice implications, 32–33

conflicts, 42
coping and adaptation to illness, 304–306
learning to, 306
therapeutic space, 306
culture, 30–31
definition, 176
in early civilizations, 21
equilibrium for, 14
forms, 55–67. *See also specific family type*
function, dimensions of, 95, 103–105
affective responsiveness and involvement, 104
behavior control, 104
communication, 103
operative family beliefs and stories, 105
problem-solving, 103
recent family events and stresses, 105
roles and coalitions, 103–104
functional, 41–42, 41t
grandparent-headed, 63
health beliefs, 304
homeostasis, 30–31
interracial, 65–66
lesbian, gay, and transgender, 63–64
marriages and, 5, 42
MPF, 65
of origin, 5
race, 30–31
resilience, keys to, 66t
resilient, 305
role in relation to psychic and social distress, 6
single-parent family, 26, 60–61
stepfamilies (blended families), 26–27, 62–63
structure, 49–50, 90
suicidal patient and, 279–282
as system, 40–42
types, 30–31
Families, Systems & Health, 372
Family adherence to treatment, 304
Family belief systems, 53, 73–75
Family coalitions, types of, 143
Family crisis therapy
family intervention performed during, 326
versus hospitalization, 325, 326t
indications for, 326
Family emotional system, 124
Family evaluation
case example/formulation, 109–115, 114t
classification and diagnosis, 105–108, 106f, 107t
content of, 94–101
explicit interview data, gathering of, 96–97
family function, dimensions of, 95
family genogram, 97f–98f, 101
family problem, background of, 97–98, 97f–98f
family's goals and expectations of treatment, 100
gathering identifying data and establishing current phase of family life cycle, 95–96
outline, 95–100, 95f
past treatment attempts, history of, 98–99
indications for, 320–321
process of, 85–93
clinical practice implications, 93
dimensions of, 87–90
family life cycle, 89t
historical material/data, role of, 91–92
identifying family structure, 90
individual and family diagnoses, role of, 92–93
interview, progression of, 87
joining with couple/family, 88
members to include in, 86
overview, 85
recognizing developmental stage, history, and culture, 88–90, 89f, 89t
systemic model of change, working with, 90–91, 90f, 91t
systemic patterns, 88
setting goals after, 109t
therapeutic approach, 108–109, 108t
treatment contract, 108–109, 108t
Family-focused therapy (FFT), 242
Family-focused treatment for bipolar adolescents (FFT-A), 345
Family function
illness impacts on, 304
impacts on illness, 303–304
adherence to treatment, 304
factors, 303
gender matters, 303–304
health beliefs, 304
Family genogram, 97f–98f, 101
The Family Guide to Mental Health Care, 109
Family identity, 66
Family intervention
in medical illnesses, 345–346
strategies of, 137–149
emotional experience, techniques for expanding, 139–140
family reality, techniques for construction of, 149
family structure, techniques for reorganizing, 143–146, 143f
insight and conflict resolution, techniques for increasing, 147–148
interpersonal skills, techniques for developing, 140–143
psychoeducational approach, 138–139
Family life cycle, 42–50, 48f, 89t
and adult development, 43t
child-focused years of, 43t
children and shifts in function, 48–49
companionship and, 47
couples/marital, 44
family structure and, 49–50
individual life cycle, 42, 44
intimacy and, 47
marital coalition, 46–47
phase of relationship and tasks, 45–46
courtship and early marriage, 45
marriage in mid-adulthood, 45
marriage in older adulthood, 45–46
sex and, 47

Family members, 5
conflicting interests of, 360–361
controlling, 274
in family evaluation, 86
family therapist and, 164–165
symptomatic, 360
Family myths, 73–75
Family of origin model, 123–124
approach, 18
issues, 333–334
Family participants, 176–178
caregivers, 178
extended family, 177–178
significant others, 177–178
Family problem, 97–98, 97f–98f
Family Process, 372
Family psychoeducation, 7
Family Psychologist, 371
Family reality, 149
Family resilience, 53
Family secrets, 172–173
Family structure
family life cycle and, 49–50
identifying, 90
techniques for reorganizing, 143–146, 143f
Family Systems–Illness Model, 304
Family tasks, 50–53
age-appropriate childrearing techniques, use of, 51
basic needs, provision of, 51
generational boundaries, maintenance of, 51
offspring, enculturation of, 53–54
parental coalition, maintenance of, 51
sexuality, 51–52
sibling coalition, support of, 52
Family therapist, 360–363
Family therapy, 7
for acute treatment, 293–294
adolescent as identified patient, 333
adolescents in, 178–180
for adult disorders, 343
focused family therapy for bipolar disorder, 343
major mental illness, 343
schizophrenia, 343
brief, 326
for child and adolescent disorders, 344–345
anorexia nervosa, 345
bipolar disorder, 345
delinquent adolescents and, 344
externalizing disorders, 344
multisystemic therapy for youth at risk, 345
substance abuse, 344–345
child as identified patient, 332–333
children in, 178–180
clinical experiences in, 370–371
clinical practice implications, 18, 186–187, 327, 336, 352, 373
collaborative, 176
in combination with other psychosocial therapies, 184–186
contraindications, 185
diagnosis, 185
effective family intervention, 186
formats and strategies, comparison of, 186, 187t
goals, 185
practical guidelines, 185–186
sequencing, 186
untoward effects, 185
competencies in, 368
concurrent, 176
conjoint, 176
conjoint couples therapy, 176
in context of other special problems, 264–282
child abuse, 278–279
family violence, 265–267
intrafamilial child sexual abuse, 275–278
suicidal patient and family, 279–282
contract, 108–109
contraindications, 334–335
cultural/religious prejudices are present, 335
family as whole denies having family problems, 335
family/therapist thinks risks of therapy outweigh the advantages, 334–335
psychopathology in one family member makes family therapy ineffective, 334
couples and, 9–10
data from outcome studies, clinical implications of, 351–352
definition of, 9–10
differential use of basic strategies, 149–150
disconnection in, 167–173
duration and intensity of, 325–327
effectiveness of combining medication and, 346
ethical issues inherent in, 360–364
conflicting interests of family members, 360–361
gender, gender roles, and sexuality, 363–364
HIPAA violations, 361–362
managed care policies, 364
secrets and confidentiality, 362–363
family crisis therapy *versus* hospitalization, 325, 326t
family of origin issues and, 333–334
family participants and, 176–178
fees, 182–183
field, development of, 6–9
financial issues with, 365
formats and strategies, comparison of, 186, 187t
inability to engage and premature termination of, 350–351
indications for, 319, 322–325
in individual psychiatric disorders, 231–260
anxiety disorders, 248–250
borderline personality disorder, 246–248
cognitive disorders, 251–253
eating disorders, 253–254
major depressive disorder, 243–246
mood disorders, 239–242
obsessive-compulsive disorder, 250
persistent depressive disorder, 243–246
posttraumatic stress disorder, 250–251
schizophrenia, 233–239
substance-related disorders, 254–256

versus individual therapy, 322, 322t–323t, 324
informed consent in, 364–365
limitations of, 346–347
long, 326–327
managed care and, 324–325
models of, 122t
negative effects of, 347–350, 348t–349t
versus other psychotherapies, 16–18, 17t
packages, 149
professional issues with, 365–367
in psychiatric disorders of childhood, 256–260
ADHD, 257–258
anxiety disorders, 259
autism spectrum disorder, 256–257
CD, 259
intellectual disability, 256
mood disorders, 259
obesity, 260
ODD, 259
psychotherapy relationship to, 137
record of treatment, 183
resistance in, 167–173
scheduling, 182–183
setting, 182
sex therapy for sexual problems, 325, 325t
studies result, 340–341
team for, 181–182
therapists uncomfortable with family groups, 335–336
time, 182–183
time-limited therapies, 157–161
training issues in, 368–370
Family therapy fellowships, 372–373
Family therapy schools
clinical practice implications, 127
cognitive–behavioral model, 125–126
experiential therapy, 126
family of origin model, 123–124
goals, 128–135
clinical practice implications, 134–135
final, 130
individualizing, 130–132
mediating, 129–130, 133
and related strategies, 133–134
relation to process and content issues, 132–133
insight-awareness model, 123
narrative approach, 126
psychoeducational model, 126–127
structural model, 124–125
systemic-strategic model, 124
Family violence, 265–275
and alcohol/drug abuse, relationship between, 269
assessment of individual and family systems issues, 269–271
causes of, 269
cognitive-behavioral models of, 273
COVID-19 pandemic and, 274
cycle of, 269
definition of, 265–267
degree of danger, 271
physical and psychological consequences of, 271
power imbalance and, 274
shame, 267
therapists, clinical issues for, 274–275
trauma bonding, 268–269
trauma repetition, 268–269
treatment, 271–274
approaches, 273
family dynamics, exploring of, 273–274
mandatory reporting laws, 271–274
safety, 272–273
time-out procedure, 273
Family warmth, 286
Father–daughter incest, 275–276
Father-headed single-parent families, 61
Father–son incest, 276
Feedback, 13
Feedback loops, 13, 68
Feelings, 217
FFT. *See* Family-focused therapy
FFT-A. *See* Family-focused treatment for bipolar adolescents
Final goals of family therapy schools, 130
Financial issues with family therapy, 365
Focusing, 145
Frames of reference, 96
Framo, J. L., 124
Freud's psychoanalytic approach, 68
Functional families, 41–42, 41t
belief systems, 53
clinical practice implications, 53
couples and family life cycle, 42–50
cultures, 42
family as system, 40–42
individual life cycle, 42, 44
processes, 41t
resilience, 53
tasks, 50–53
Functional single-parent family, 26, 60–61

G

GAP diagnostic scheme, 107
Gay/bisexual individuals, marital issues in, 212
Gender, 7, 303–304, 363–364
differences, 46, 196
roles, 363–364
General systems theory, 10–11
Generational boundaries, maintenance of, 51
Genograms, 89, 89f, 91, 97f–98f, 101, 124
Global Assessment of Relational Functioning (GARF) Scale, 107
Global Assessment of Relational Functioning Scale, 41
Goals of family therapy schools, 128–135
clinical practice implications, 134–135
determining strategies after, 130t
final, 130
individualizing, 130–132
mediating, 129–130, 133
and related strategies, 133–134
relation to process and content issues, 132–133

Grandparent-headed families, 63
Grandparents, 177
Group for the advancement of psychiatry (GAP)
 proposal for specific family systems
 competencies, 368, 369t
Group therapy, 7

H

Haley, Jay, 121, 124
Health beliefs, 304
Health care system, 9
Health Insurance Portability and Accountability Act
 (HIPAA), 361–362
Heroin, 213
Heteronormativity, 32
Hierarchy, 221
HIPAA. *See* Health Insurance Portability and
 Accountability Act
HIV, 213
Hoffman's time capsule, 15f
Homeostasis, 15–16, 30–31
Hospitalization *versus* family crisis therapy,
 325, 326t
Human open systems, 14
Human sexual behavior, 212

I

Identified patient
 adolescent as, 333
 child as, 332–333
Illness
 clinical practice implications, 311–312
 family coping and adaptation to,
 304–306
 learning to, 306
 therapeutic space, 306
 family function impacts on, 303–304
 adherence to treatment, 304
 factors, 303
 gender matters, 303–304
 health beliefs, 304
 family interventions and, 310–311
 family support, 310
 multifamily groups, 311
 psychoeducation, 310
 systemic interventions, 310–311
 family systems interview for families with,
 307–310
 affective involvement, 309
 affective responsiveness, 309
 behavior control, 309–310
 communication, 308
 problem solving, 307–308
 roles by gender, 308–309
 impacts on family function, 304
Immigration, 22
Incest, 275–277
 father–daughter, 275–276
 father–son, 276
 mother–child, 276
 sibling, 275–276
Individual life cycle, 42, 44
 early adulthood, 44
 mid-adulthood, 44
 older adulthood, 44
Individual psychiatric disorders, 231–260
 anxiety disorders, 248–250
 borderline personality disorder, 246–248
 cognitive disorders, 251–253
 eating disorders, 253–254
 major depressive disorder, 243–246
 mood disorders, 239–242
 obsessive-compulsive disorder, 250
 persistent depressive disorder, 243–246
 posttraumatic stress disorder, 250–251
 schizophrenia, 233–239
 substance-related disorders, 254–256
Individual therapy *versus* family therapy, 322,
 322t–323t, 324
Infidelity, 197–198
Information, 14
Informed consent in family therapy, 364–365
Insight and conflict resolution, 147–148
Insight-awareness model, 123
Insight-oriented marital therapy for marital distress,
 341
Integrative behavioral couple therapy, 125
 for marital distress, 341
Integrative interpersonal model, 16
Intellectual disability, 256
Interpersonal distress, 6
Interpersonal skills, 140–143
Interpretation, 147
Interracial families, 65–66
Interview for family evaluation, 87
Intimacy, 46–47
Intimate partner violence, 266
Intrafamilial child sexual abuse, 275–278
 assessment, 277
 family issues, 276
 individual issues, 276
 larger system issues, 276–277
 overview, 275–276
 treatment, 277–278
Issue of commitment, 197–198

J

Jacobson, N., 125
Journal of Family Psychology, 371

K

Krasner, B., 124

L

LAT. *See* Living apart together
LCSW (licensed clinical social worker), 372
Lesbian, gay, and transgender families, 63–64
LGBTQ (lesbian, gay, bisexual, transgender, queer)
 couples, 27–28
Licensure, 373
LICSW (licensed independent clinical social worker),
 372

Lies My Father Told Me (1976), 177
Living apart together (LAT), 62
Living systems, 14
Long-term family therapy, 326–327

M

Major depressive disorder, 243–246
Major mental illness, 343
Male erection problems, 205
Managed care, 324–325
Managed care policies, 364
Marital coalition, 46–47
  on amount of shared activities and values, 46
  on closeness-distance (emotional intensity), 46
  on inclusion and exclusion, 46
  on intimacy, 46
  on marital commitment, 46
  on power, 46
Marital commitment, 46
Marital distress
  emotionally focused couples therapy for, 341–342
  insight-oriented marital therapy for, 341
  integrative behavioral couple therapy for, 341
Marital issues in gay/bisexual individuals, 212
Marital rape, 276
Marital separation, 57–58
Marital therapist, 216
Marital therapy, 7
  approach, 142
  conjoint, 330
  for depression, 342
  for marital distress, 341
Marriage and family therapy (MFT) programs, 371
Marriage counseling movement (1930s/1940s), 123
Marriages, 5, 7, 42, 56–57
  depression in, 243–244
  divorce and, 25–26
  in its historical context, 194
  in mid-adulthood, 45
  in older adulthood, 45–46
  secular view of, 24–25
  structures of, 25
  Westernized, 194
McFarlane, W., 126
McGoldrick, M., 124
McMaster model of family evaluation, 95–100
MDFT. *See* Multidimensional family therapy
Mediating goals of family therapy schools, 129–130, 133
  attempted solutions, clarification of, 129
  communication skills, improvement in, 129
  increased family knowledge about serious psychiatric illness, 130
  individual desires/needs, clarification/specification of, 129
  individual expectations/needs, modification of, 129
  insight regarding historical factors, 130
  mutual contribution to problem(s), recognition of, 129
  redefinition of problem(s), 129
  shift in disturbed, inflexible roles and coalitions, 129
  specification of problem(s), 129
  strategies, 133t
  working alliance, establishment of, 129
Mediation in separation, 219
Medicaid, 8–9
Medical Family Therapy (MedFT), 311
Medical model, 165
MEI. *See* Multifamily educational intervention
Mental illness, 6
  of family member, family responses to, 287
Microenvironments for siblings, 52
Mid-adulthood, 44
Miklowitz, D., 126
Milieu therapy, 7
Minuchin, Salvador, 121, 124–125
Mood disorders, 239–242
  in children, 259
  rationale, 259
  treatment, 259
Mother–child incest, 276
Mother-headed single-parent families, 61
MPF. *See* Multiple-partner fertility families
Multidimensional family therapy (MDFT), 344–345
Multifamily educational intervention (MEI), 344
Multifamily group (MFG) psychoeducation, 310–311
Multifamily Group Therapy, 127
Multiple-family groups (MFG) therapy, 343
Multiple-partner fertility families (MPF), 65
Multisystemic therapy for youth at risk, 345

N

NAMI. *See* National Alliance on Mental Illness
Narcotics, 213
Narrative model, 126
National Alliance on Mental Illness (NAMI), 236, 289, 297
National Consensus Statement on Mental Health Recovery, 9
Neuropeptides, 5
New Freedom Commission on Mental Health, 9
New mothering, 66
Nonshared environment, 52
Nonverbal communication, 96

O

Obesity in children, 260
Objective burden of family, psychotic illness, 287–288
Obsessive-compulsive disorder (OCD), 250
  family intervention in, 250
  treatment, 250
OCD. *See* Obsessive-compulsive disorder
ODD. *See* Oppositional defiant disorder
Offspring, enculturation of, 53–54
Older adulthood, 44
Operative family beliefs and stories, 105
Oppositional defiant disorder (ODD), 259
Overt control, 266
Overt power, 274
Oxytocin, 5

P

Painful intercourse/female orgasmic disorder, 210–211
Panic disorder, 249–250
Paradoxical techniques, 146
Parental coalition, maintenance of, 51
Parental quarreling, 219
Parents/parenting, 29–30
  depression in, 244
  with a gender nonconforming child, 65
  trends in, 66
Pedophilia, 276
Perpetrators of violence, 275
Persistent depressive disorder, 243–246
  depression in adolescents and young adults, 243
  depression in parents, 244
  depression in partnered/married people, 243–244
  rationale, 243–244
  treatment considerations, 245–246
Physical violence, 266
Polyamory, 29
Pornography, 211–212
Postdivorce treatment, 220–221
Posttraumatic stress disorder (PTSD), 250–251, 342–343
  rationale, 250–251
  symptoms, 251
  treatment for, 251
Power, 46
Power and Control Wheel, 266
Power imbalance in family, 274
Premature (early) ejaculation, 210
Privacy, 362
Problem-oriented school of brief therapy, 161
Problem-solving, 103, 141–142, 307–308
Process *versus* outcome research, 339–340
Professional issues with family therapy, 365–367
Psychiatric disorders of childhood, 256–260
  ADHD, 257–258
  anxiety disorders, 259
  autism spectrum disorder, 256–257
  CD, 259
  intellectual disability, 256
  mood disorders, 259
  obesity, 260
  ODD, 259
Psychoanalytic thinking, 178
Psychodynamic/psychoanalytic school. *See* Insight-awareness model
Psychoeducation, 186, 219, 310
Psychoeducational approach, 138–139
Psychoeducational model, 126–127
Psychologists, 371
Psychology, 8
Psychopathology, 18, 68
Psychopharmacologic treatment, 7
Psychosexual disorders, 210–211
Psychosis, 276
Psychotherapy
  elements of, 137
  outcome research, 338–340
    efficacy *versus* effectiveness, 339
    process *versus* outcome research, 339–340
    qualitative *versus* quantitative *versus* exploratory *versus* confirmatory research, 339
    specificity, 339
  relationship to family therapy, 137
Psychotic illness, family burden in, 287–288
PTSD. *See* Posttraumatic stress disorder
Public Health Service Act, Title III, Section 303(d), 7

Q

Qualitative research, 339
Quantitative research, 339
Quid pro quo agreements, 125

R

Race
  definition, 22
  versus ethnicity, examples, 23
Rape, 212–213
Rebellious/inappropriate behavior, 139
Record of treatment, 183
Recovery, 9
Reframing, 145
Relational diagnoses, 105
Relational ethics, 360
Remarried biologic parents, 224
Remarried couple, 62
Resilient families, 305
Resistance in family therapy, 167–173
  clinical practice implications, 174
  definition, 167
  family, emanating from, 167–168
  family secrets, 172–173
  in ongoing treatment, 171–172
  stages of treatment, 169–171
  techniques to deal with, 173–174
    assume nothing, 173
    collaboration, 173–174
    emphasizing family responsibility, 174
    focus on present, 174
  at termination phase of therapy, 172
  from therapist–family system, 168–169
    common systems to be considered, 168–169
    disagreement as to treatment goals, 168
    mismatch between therapist and family, 168
  therapists, emanating from, 168
Resistances in learning skills, 166

S

Sandwich generation, 31–32
Satir, Virginia, 121, 126
Schizophrenia, 7, 233–239, 343
  development of, 233–234, 234f
  family's role in etiology of, 233
  living with/supported by families of origin, 237–238
  married, with/without children, 238–239
  rationale, 233–234
  treatment considerations, 235–237, 235f, 235t, 237t

Secrecy, 362
Secrets, 362–363
Sederer, Lloyd, 109
Selective serotonin reuptake inhibitor (SSRI) medications, 210
Self-harm (cutting and self-mutilation), 247
Separation, 215–220
  communicating issue of divorce to children, 218
  family conflict and, 219
  immediate issues, 218–219
  individual therapy in, 216
  leading to divorce, 217–218
  marital therapist and, 216
  mediation in, 219
  overview, 215–217
  therapy for families facing divorce, 219–220
  trial, 216
Serial relationships, 226
Sex, 47
Sex addiction, 211–212
Sex therapy for sexual problems, 325, 325t
Sexual abuse, 212–213, 266
Sexual contact between siblings, 275–276
Sexual desire, lack of, 209
Sexual dysfunction/dissatisfaction, 205–206
  after medical illness, 213
  assessment of, 206–209
  clinical practice implications, 214
  couple discord co-occurs with, 206
  in elderly, 213
  secondary couple discord, produces/contributes to, 206
  secondary to couple discord, 206
  treatment of, 209–212
    erectile disorder, 209
    lack of desire, 209
    painful intercourse/female orgasmic disorder, 210–211
    premature (early) ejaculation, 210
    psychosexual disorders, 210–211
    sex addiction and pornography, 211–212
  without couple discord, 206
Sexual function, 205–206
Sexual identity, 212
Sexual issues, couples therapy for, 331
Sexuality, 51–52, 363–364
Sexual life, 204
Sexual orientation, 212
Sexual performance, 205–206
Sexual problems, sex therapy for, 325, 325t
Shame, 267
Sibling abuse, 276
Sibling coalition, support of, 52
Sibling incest, 275–276
Sibling perpetrators, 276
Significant others, 177–178
Single-parent families, 26, 60–61, 221
SMT. *See* Systemic-motivational therapy
Social classes, 31
Social learning theory, 142
Social system, 75
Social work, 8
Social workers, 372
Solution-as-the-problem approach, 72–73
Solving Your Problems Together: Family Therapy for the Whole Family, 110
Spectrum of sexuality, 212–213
Splitting, 247
Stepfamilies (blended families), 26–27, 62–63, 222–225
  emotional climate in, 225
  evaluation, 223–225
  goals for therapists working with, 222
  versus nuclear families, therapeutic implications, 223t
  treatment, 223–225
Strategic systems model, 166–167
Structural model, 124–125
Subjective burden of family, psychotic illness, 287–288
Substance abuse, multidimensional family therapy for adolescent, 344–345
Substance-related disorders (SUDs), 254–256
  assessment and treatment guidelines, 255–256
  children of alcoholic parents, 256
  family-focused interventions in, 255
  rationale, 254–255
  screening instruments for, 255
Substance use disorders, 344
SUDs. *See* Substance-related disorders
Suicidal patient, 279–282
  acute management, 280
  discharging hospitalized, 282
  epidemiology of, 280
  family evaluation, 280
  family treatment, 281
  involving family in treatment, 281
  overview, 279
Systemic model of change, 90–91, 90f, 91t
Systemic-motivational therapy (SMT), 255
Systemic reality, 145
Systemic-strategic model, 124
Systems approach to problems and dysfunction, 69–73
  current perspectives, 70–71
  family resilience key processes, 71
  historical perspectives, 69–70
  solution-as-the-problem approach, 72–73
  structural and organizational problems, 71–72
Systems theory, 5, 10–15
  continuum of natural systems, 12f
  control over and adaptation to environment, 13–14
  energy, 14
  general, 10–11
  hierarchy of natural systems, 11f
  Hoffman's time capsule, 15f
  and homeostasis over time, 15–16
  Minuchin's description of boundaries of, 13, 13f
  organization, 12–13

T

TBCT. *See* Traditional behavioral couple therapy
Team for treatment, 181–182
Temporary triads, 144
Termination phase, 156
Therapeutic alliance, 164–165
  coaching model and, 166
  conflict model and, 166
  family therapist and, 164–165
  functions of, 164
  medical model and, 165
  strategic systems model and, 166–167
Therapeutic approach, 108–109, 108t
Therapist combinations, 181–182
  co-therapy, 181
  working as team, 181–182
Therapy for families facing divorce, 219–220
Time-limited family therapies, 157–161
  behavioral and emotional rehearsal, 160
  brief family/couples intervention, indications for, 157
  course of, 158
  crisis intervention, 161
  family reconceptualization, reinforcement of, 159–160
  family strengths, reinforcement of, 159–160
  homework and family tasks, 160–161
  problem-oriented school of, 161
  setting limited goals and definite end point, 158–159
  techniques, 158
Time-out procedure, 273
Toxic secrets, 78
Traditional behavioral couple therapy (TBCT), 341
Training, 373
Training issues in family therapy, 368–370
Training programs in family psychiatry, 371
Transference, 123
Trauma bonding, 268–269
Trauma repetition, 268–269
Treatment contract, 108–109
Treatment packages, 149
Trial separation, 216
Triangles, 72
Triangulation, 72

U

Unbalancing techniques, 145
Unmarried couples, couples therapy for, 332
Unresolved grief, 78

V

Vasopressin, 5
Verbal abuse, 266
Veterans Health Administration, 9
Videotape playback, 156
Violence in family, 265–275, 342
  and alcohol/drug abuse, relationship between, 269
  assessment of individual and family systems issues, 269–271
  causes of, 269
  cognitive-behavioral models of, 273
  COVID-19 pandemic and, 274
  cycle of, 269
  definition of, 265–267
  degree of danger, 271
  physical and psychological consequences of, 271
  power imbalance and, 274
  shame, 267
  therapists, clinical issues for, 274–275
  trauma bonding, 268–269
  trauma repetition, 268–269
  treatment, 271–274
    approaches, 273
    family dynamics, exploring of, 273–274
    mandatory reporting laws, 271–274
    safety, 272–273
    time-out procedure, 273

W

Westernized marriages, 194
Whitaker, Carl, 121, 126
Williamson, D., 124
Women, 66

QUADM1024